Sandplay: the Image Speaks for Itself

by the same author

Foundation and Form in Jungian Sandplay
Lenore Steinhardt
ISBN 978 1 85302 841 0
Large print ISBN 978 1 84985 280 7
eISBN 978 0 85700 147 4

On Becoming a Jungian Sandplay Therapist
The Healing Spirit of Sandplay in Nature and in Therapy
Lenore F. Steinhardt
ISBN 978 1 84905 338 9
eISBN 978 0 85700 686 8

SANDPLAY
THE IMAGE SPEAKS FOR ITSELF

Signposts, Symbols and Themes on the Path of the Sandplay Journey

Lenore F. Steinhardt

Jessica Kingsley Publishers
London and Philadelphia

First published in Great Britain in 2026 by Jessica Kingsley Publishers
An imprint of John Murray Press

1

Content Warning: This book mentions physical abuse, child abuse, death, kidnapping, trauma, war and violence.

A CIP catalogue record for this title is available from the British Library and the Library of Congress

ISBN 978 1 80501 428 7
eISBN 978 1 80501 429 4

Printed and bound by CPI Group (UK) Ltd, Croydon, CR0 4YY

Jessica Kingsley Publishers' policy is to use papers that are natural, renewable and recyclable products and made from wood grown in sustainable forests. The logging and manufacturing processes are expected to conform to the environmental regulations of the country of origin.

Jessica Kingsley Publishers
Carmelite House
50 Victoria Embankment
London EC4Y 0DZ

www.jkp.com

John Murray Press
Part of Hodder & Stoughton Limited
An Hachette UK Company

The authorised representative in the EEA is Hachette Ireland,
8 Castlecourt Centre, Dublin 15, D15 XTP3, Ireland (email: info@hbgi.ie)

Dedicated to my children, Gabriel, Yael and Michael,
my grandchildren, Maytal, Dana, Michal, Shachar, Gal,
Yahli, Ari and Rene, and my future great-grandchildren
who give me much joy as they form their individual paths,
with creativity, exploration, depth and relationship

Contents

Part 4: Sandplay and Mythology

Figures

Plates

Acknowledgments

As a sandplay therapist, I value the art of the creative psyche and the visual sandplay language of the unconscious. I am enthralled by images and their transformations in a sequence of sandplays. They form paths whose stages are linked together by symbols, with personal and universal relevance that can only be understood at the end of the journey. A sandplayer's unconscious history and more conscious relationships to personal stages of growth, to body, family, emotion and development are embedded in these images. I thank the many clients whose sandplay journeys have paved the path of this book, for their trust in me and for permission to reproduce photographs of their sandplays and excerpts of their insights. The children in my family played freely in my studio whenever they wished, creating art and sandplays. I am quite sure that their early creative interaction with sand, objects and materials has contributed to their creativity and achievements today as adults. I thank Carol Proudfoot Edgar for her spoken story of Jumping Mouse, in the preface of this book, whose journey and transformation resonates with the sandplay journey. Special thanks to Joyce Camuyrano Cunningham, editor of the *Journal of Sandplay Therapy*, for her permission to cite excerpts from two of my articles that were originally published in the *Journal of Sandplay Therapy* (all rights reserved, permission granted to reprint):

Steinhardt, L. (2020) "Jasmin, thirteen sandplays: From divination to archetype." *Journal of Sandplay Therapy 29*, 1.

Steinhardt, L. (2016) "Casting an invisible net into an invisible unconscious ocean, catching a reflection of the psyche on an invisible map." *Journal of Sandplay Therapy 25*, 2, 179–189.

Preface

I have been very fortunate to work primarily as a sandplay therapist, teacher, supervisor and writer about sandplay for more than 30 years. I have enjoyed learning from my colleagues about integration of sandplay with bodymind disciplines and about research on human brain functioning that has led to the formation of specialized trauma techniques that help understand and treat trauma in general and in specific situations. My own understanding of creative work was initially formed as a child during World War II, playing on a quiet sea beach and in open fields, and later studying art in New York City. I began writing this book with a focus on themes that pertain to observation and unconscious apperception of the visual, non-verbal environment that constitutes a sandplay setting and small details that impact on the formation of images, symbols and their journeys. I also wrote about some unusual sandplay settings, organized in response to unusual clients or to natural or man-made traumatic events.

I did not know that a horrific mass trauma would take place closer to home, on a quiet Saturday morning in October 2023, or that improvised sandplay settings as a therapeutic intervention would be offered to large groups of civilians who had experienced collective devastation and loss, evacuated to hotels with no home to return to. On October 7th, several thousand heavily armed terrorists invaded Israel's southern border, pillaged and destroyed villages, slaughtered over 1000 civilians and took hostage several hundred people. The evacuees were placed in hotels, where schooling for the children and immediate therapeutic care were provided. Improvised sandplay rooms in several hotels, equipped with donated sandtrays and miniature objects, were staffed by volunteer sandplay therapists and others specializing in treatment of trauma. In Chapter 3, I have included a brief account of these unusual group sandplay settings that were spontaneously formed as a therapeutic response to the shock of this mass trauma.

The title of this book—*Sandplay: the Image Speaks for Itself—Signposts, Symbols and Themes on the Path of the Sandplay Journey*—suggests that the range of representations in sandplay images can be studied using several approaches to observing an image. As the sandplay journey unfolds, the meanings in each image become more clearly defined. The goal or quest of a sandplay journey is at first diffuse, but an actual path may take form in the sand in an early sandplay. Like a map through the maze of conscious and unconscious personal memory, archetypal aid and expanded potential, this path predicts a possible route with stages arranged by a collective unconscious universality. The theme of the "site-specific" environment of sandplay and the "site-specific" sandplay in a sandtray as an "art form" was introduced in my two previous books, *Foundation and Form in Jungian Sandplay: An Art Therapy Approach* (2000) and *On Becoming a Jungian Sandplay Therapist: The Healing Spirit of Sandplay in Nature and in Therapy* (2013). The theoretical lenses that support a sandplay process are Jung's writings on the structure of the psyche, Neumann's developmental theory, and the work of theoreticians that help understand trauma, the brain and the healing process.

In this book, detailed observation of the sandplay setting and of the image that is formed has been given a larger scope, so that visual aspects of the image itself will become a consciously noticed language. Symbolic reality is written in sand form and in the relationships of objects, color, number, materials and placement within the limitations of the sandtray, producing symbols whose range of meanings extends well beyond what logic first perceives. The choices of the therapist who creates the sandplay environment and arranges its physical components influence the formation of images in the sandtray. The style of a therapeutic relationship and co-transference permeate each image as it opens a door to a new image, in segments like a crystal developing from an invisible inner pattern into its pure form. The therapist reflects on many images over time. The image reflects upon itself, and when it is time, a new image begins its incubation. A higher perspective on all the sandplays at the end of a process reveals the order, sequence of connections between images, their stages, transitions and goals that tell the story of the sandplay journey. Case examples of adults and of children illustrate the merger of psychic content with an innate sensory awareness, perhaps inherited from our ancestors whose survival relied on precise observation of their environments. The figures from this book can be viewed and downloaded from https://digitalhub.jkp.com/redeem using the code HKBCCCS.

Journeys

In the 1990s, I attended several Bear Medicine Workshops at a ranch in Montana, a land of natural forests, rock formations and caves, where artifacts and structures made by the Native Americans who once lived there could still be found. The workshop leader, Carol Proudfoot Edgar, taught forms of traditional healing to the women who had traveled here from distant places, and also spoke oral versions of Native American stories. Carol gifted me with her versions of two stories, "Turtle Island" and "The Covenant between River, Salmon and Bear" as the prefaces of my first two books on sandplay (Steinhardt, 2000, 2013). In September 2019, after the ISST Berlin Sandplay Conference, I visited the German countryside with some artist friends. As I sat painting under a wide sky in a wild field, "Jumping Mouse" fell from above and leaped into my consciousness, together with a realization that I would write a third book, as if he knew that his transformative journey complemented the sandplay journey. I had heard Carol speak the story of "Jumping Mouse" and his "call" to discover the source of a roaring sound that no other mouse could hear. He left his sheltered mouseland on a long and dangerous journey that led to River, Magic Mountain and "powerful medicine." He met great wounded powers, Buffalo and Wolf, and helpers such as Raccoon, Frog and Bear, experienced fear and pain, and voluntarily gave his eyes to heal others' wounds, becoming a blind wounded healer, until his final transformation to Eagle.

Jumping Mouse offers a call to leave worn-out points of view, to receive guidance from wise powers, to attain new vision and final transformation. In a sandplay process, puzzling images sprout up along the path, but when viewed from the higher comprehensive perspective of Eagle at the therapeutic journey's end, we see that the road map to individuation is universal, and has been guided by helping entities. The call to adventure comes on the wind and blows an invitation into our consciousness, and if answered, the journey begins. Once more, I thank Carol Proudfoot Edgar for gifting me with permission to include "The Story of Jumping Mouse and His Friends" in the preface to this book. The spoken story was transcribed by Cally Davis and Cheryl Ban from old recordings. I apologize that it has been slightly edited to fit the limitations of text in this book.

NOTES FROM THE ROAD

The Story of Jumping Mouse and His Friends

CAROL PROUDFOOT EDGAR

Once there was a little mouse who lived in a very special Mouseland where all the mice had just about everything they could want. In this village there lived a few very wise old mice, and some who weren't so wise but had some learning, and lots of new mice coming in. But one little mouse kept getting a really serious headache. He said to his brother and sister, "I hear a roaring in my head." And they would say, "There is no roaring. Leave us alone." And Mouse would feel unhappy for a while because nobody understood. Then the roaring would come back, and he'd say to a brother or sister, "My head hurts; there's a roaring in my head. Please help me." And the brother or sister once again would say, "Quit bothering us. There is no such thing as a roaring anyway." And Mouse grew lonely and decided to find out where this roaring came from. He began walking towards the edge of Mouseland. But every mouse knows that the one way to stay safe is to stay home, so nothing will eat you.

At the edge of Mouseland, he heard a voice say, "Mouse, what are you doing out here? You're going to get into trouble." And Mouse said, "Who's that?" And the voice said, "I'm Raccoon. I'm your brother." And Mouse said, "I've never heard of a raccoon. I'm here because I have a big roaring in my head, and no one believes me." And Raccoon said, "Oh, that's the river you hear." And Mouse said, "What's a river?" And Raccoon said, "Come, I'll take you down. I'll show you where that roaring's coming from." But Mouse said, "No, I can't go unless you protect me all the way." And Raccoon said, "Look, here's a path, it's not far. The roaring's very close and that's why you have such a bad headache." So Mouse followed Raccoon down a path through the woods, and then the roaring got louder and they came to this huge, great thing that Mouse had never seen before. And Raccoon said, "This is River." Mouse looked at River, and said, "It's awesome!" And Raccoon said, "Yes, River's great. Now I've got to leave you, but you can talk with my friend out there."

Mouse looked way out, and there in the river was a green thing with a white belly, sitting on a green leaf. And Mouse said, "What are you?" And the green thing said, "I'm a frog." And Mouse said, "Frog? Aren't you afraid way out there all by yourself in this big river?" And Frog said, "Oh no, I live here, I love it here. Most of the time I live under this great being, but right now you can see me above, where the world is green." Mouse pondered this and asked, "How can you live in both worlds? And Frog said, "Mouse, you have an awful lot of questions. Why did you come here anyway?" And Mouse said, "I heard a roaring in my head, and I met Raccoon who brought me here, and I saw you way out there." And then Frog asked, "Mouse, would you like some Medicine Power?" "Me? Medicine Power? A mouse?" And Frog said, "Yes." And Mouse said, "Oh yes!" And Frog said, "Okay, crouch as low as you can crouch, and jump as high as you can jump, and tell me what you see." So Mouse crouched as low as he could crouch, and he jumped as high as he could jump, and then he saw all the way to the Sacred Mountains. And then he fell into the water. He got up and said, "You tricked me, Frog; you got me all wet!" And Frog said, "Settle down; don't let your anger blind you. What did you see?" And Mouse said, "I saw the Sacred Mountains." And Frog said, "Yes, and that's where you need to go; that is where the Medicine Power is. And now your name is Jumping Mouse! Don't forget it." But Mouse replied, "I'm going home to tell my brothers and sisters that there is a roaring and it's called River, and that there are Sacred Mountains. They'll be delighted and I can take them with me."

So Mouse scooted back through the grass to Mouseland and gathered all the mice together. "Come, come, I've got great news. That roaring that was in my head is real and it's called River. And in the River is a green thing with a white belly sitting on a green leaf, that's called Frog, and he told me to crouch as low as I can crouch, and jump as high as I can jump. And I saw the Sacred Mountains where the Medicine Power is! Come with me! Let's go!" And there was absolute quiet. Mouse saw that his brothers and sisters were turning their heads, saying, "Oh, there's no such thing, and everybody knows a wet mouse is so foul-tasting that nothing wants to eat it." Mouse really felt bad and went to dry off. He thought that maybe his brothers and sisters were right: he had made this all up; he just needed to have a drink. Time passed, and he got busy collecting wonderful things in the woods, but his head started aching again, and his brothers and sisters could not help. Then Mouse remembered what Frog said. "Frog told me to turn my back on Mouseland and go straight ahead and I would find the Sacred Mountains."

So Mouse packed his little bag, put it on his back and went to the edge of Mouseland. He was really quite afraid. He had no idea what was out there or what would happen to him. The most he had ever seen was a raccoon and a frog and a river. But he began to walk and pretty soon he came to a wonderful stand of sage, and mice love the fragrance of sage. "Mmm," he thought, "I could take some of this sage back to my brothers and sisters, and maybe they'd follow the smell and go with me to the Sacred Mountains." And then a voice said, "Hello, Mouse, what are you doing here?" And Mouse saw an old mouse in a rocking chair, and said, "I didn't know any mouse lived this far out." And the old mouse said, "Oh, I'm so wise and I know so much I had to leave the village. There was no more I could teach, and no more they could learn. So I'm out here to just observe." And Mouse said, "Well, do you know what I found out? There is a roaring thing called River, and there are Sacred Mountains with Medicine Power in the distance. Do you want to go there with me"? The old mouse said, "There's no such thing as Sacred Mountains, and there's no such thing as Medicine Power. Now, there is a river, I grant you. I heard that once before." And Mouse looked at this wise old mouse and thought, "Maybe I'm wrong." And then he crossed to the other side of the shelter and looked at the old mouse and thought, "That mouse looks like it's almost glued to a rocking chair. I don't want to spend all my days in a rocking chair." And he said, "I'm really sorry but I've got to leave." And the old mouse said, "Oh, please spend the night with me, or a few days, or at least a month or a year with me." And Mouse says, "Oh no, I've got to go."

Mouse took off and he was really afraid, for the seasons had changed. He was so small and the grasslands seemed to him like a huge forest. Now he was out where those things he heard about, called eagles, fly. And every mouse knows that the one thing that will eat them for sure, once it spots them, is an eagle. He looked up to the skies, and hid in the grasses and tried to make his way keeping Mouseland at his back. He was afraid that at any moment one of the spots above would come down and eat him. And as he walked and worried how to cross these grasslands, he heard a loud snorting in the grass. Mouse looked up and walked around a great being, and said, "What are you, Great Being?" "I'm a buffalo," the great being said, snorting and gasping. And Mouse said, "What is wrong with you?" And Buffalo said, "I'm dying. And I've been told...that the only thing...that can save me...is the eye of a mouse. But there's no such thing as a mouse." And Mouse jumped back and said, "The eye of a mouse? He wants my eye." He started to run away and hide. Then he stopped and said, "How can I let such a great being die? I have two eyes." So he went close up to this big head there in the grass, and said, "Buffalo, I can't let you die. I have two eyes, and you can have one of mine." And as soon as Mouse said that, an eye flew out of his head right into Buffalo's head, and Buffalo got up and he was cured. He looked down from his massive high place at this tiny weak creature in the grass and said, "I know about your journey to the Sacred Mountains, to the place where there's Medicine Power. I will help take you there. I know you fear the eagles in the air, and they are everywhere. You can walk beneath my belly, and we will cross the prairie together. The eagles cannot see you, and I'm too big for them to attack." And Mouse said, "Good," and he got under Buffalo's belly and they started to cross. The whole earth shook with Buffalo's hoofs clopping heavy and slow, and Mouse was scared out of his wits. Finally, Buffalo stopped. But now Mouse's paws were sore and soaked in blood, because the prairie was dry and full of burrs. Burrs stuck to his belly too, and it was sore with blood. And Buffalo said, "I'm sorry for all your bleeding, but this is the way we had to go. We're not there yet. Through the forest you have to go, and I'm too big to get through the trees. But in there, you will find a friend of mine. And you will know, by the sound she makes, that she's a friend of everyone who through the forest comes." And Mouse said, "Will this friend help take me to the Medicine Power?" And Buffalo said, "Oh yes. Oh yes"

Mouse was now really excited, and he gathered up his courage and tried to make it fast through the forest, with his tail in the air, and his little whiskers going, and the blood dripping, because he was just so sore, and then he heard a loud screeching and yelling and hid under a bush. He peeked out and whispered, "What is that?" Then a loud screech trailed off into a sobbing moan and then a deep breath. And Mouse said, "I am a mouse. Who are you? And what is wrong with you?" And this big thing said, "I am Bear. I have lost my cub and my heart is breaking. I have no one for which to care, and no one to share the fall and winter with." And then Bear crumpled to the ground. And Mouse leaned over and said, "Oh, Bear, please don't die, such a great being you are." And Bear said, "Well, I think I will get well if you will stay with me." And Mouse said, "Oh no, I've got to go to the Sacred Mountains and get my Medicine Power." So Bear said, "Well, at least I can show you how to get to the foot of the Sacred Mountains." And as they went down the trail through the forest, Bear saw the wounds on Mouse's feet. And she very gently lifted up Mouse in her paw and said, "Mouse, can you see how wounded you are? You cannot go like this; you will not make it through the winter, and will not reach the mountains. Let me clean you up and heal your wounds, and then you can sleep the winter with me. When you wake, you'll be well." And Bear took Mouse down to the river where she went to fish and wash, and very gently she put Mouse into the river and cleaned his fur, his belly and his little paws, and washed his wounds. And Mouse softly, gently fell asleep.

Bear took Mouse to her cave and held him close, and so they slept the winter long. And while they slept, Mouse dreamt about Mouseland, Frog and a thing called River. And he even dreamt that Frog told him to crouch low and jump high, and that he saw the Sacred Mountains, and that Frog told him he was Jumping Mouse, and he should remember his name. And then he slowly came awake, stirring against this thick, nice fur, and he looked up into the face of the most beautiful animal he had ever seen. He had soaked in her fur and in her love and warmth the winter long, and now he was healed. But Bear was sleeping for it was not time for her to wake. So Mouse very gently whispered in her ear, "I love you, Bear," and he kissed Bear on the cheek. He gathered his courage and left Bear's cave, for the love he had now gave him courage.

As he reached the edge of the wood, he watched for the eagles. And from there, but maybe not too far, he saw the foot of the Sacred Mountains. He crouched low and jumped high, and yes, indeed, they were the Sacred Mountains. So he said, "I'll gather my courage, stiffen my tail, turn my whiskers right, keep the one good eye open and head out." And he got across, and then at the base of the Sacred Mountains, he saw this being sitting there, saying, "Kwahf, kwah, waf!" And Mouse said, "Who are you?" and got a little closer, and said, "I think he's lost his memory." So he said, "Do you know who you are?" And the creature said, "Kwah, waf...I think I know...well, I don't know, I just don't know." Mouse looked up again at this very beautiful creature and said, "All right, I know what could cure you. You can have my eye." And his one good eye flew out of his head and into Wolf's eye, and Wolf was suddenly well.

But now Mouse was totally blind, and he could not see the path or the eagles, and could not even see Wolf, whose health he restored, or see Bear again. And then he heard Wolf howl with joy, "All is well, all is well." And Wolf leaned down very close to Mouse and said, "You have come to the Sacred Mountains to get some Medicine Power, haven't you?" And Mouse said, "Yes, but I can't see anything, and I can't find my way up there. I'm so tiny, and I'm sure the eagles will get me." And Wolf said, "Yes, they will get you, but I am the pathfinder; I will take you up there. I sit down here at the base of the mountain so I can take people up to get their Medicine Power. That's been my job all these years, but I lost my mind, and I couldn't remember. Now I remember because you gave me your eye. So I will take you up and you will hang on tight to the end of my tail with your two little paws and not let go. I'll go very slow and warn you when there's a big stone or a puddle." Mouse hung on to the end of Wolf's tail, and Wolf was so gentle that Mouse had no trouble just using his two little hind legs to go up the mountain hanging on the tail. They climbed higher and higher, and Mouse, because he was blind, could really hear the sound of feathers in the air. And he sensed the shadows on his body and felt the shadows on his back and felt all around him the very thing he feared. And the higher they went, where eagles nest and dwell in the mountains, the more he heard these beings in the air. But he held tight to Wolf's tail, and they went way up to the very top. And Wolf said, "Mouse, I've got to leave you here. I must go down to the base of the mountain and wait for another to appear. That's my job in life. But thank you for restoring my health to me, and my memory, for I wished to remember why I was sent here." And Mouse said, "Ooh, you're welcome," but didn't dare tell him how really scared he was, because he could not see and Wolf was leaving. So he crouched really low, and even though he could not see, tears of fear in his eyes dropped and dropped.

And suddenly he heard the sound of flapping everywhere and shadows all around, and his little body started to shake and quake. And he tried to get as low as he could, to disappear into the earth where no eagle could grab him. And just as he thought that he almost made himself disappear... PEEEUUMWMPFFF!!!...then slowly Mouse began to stir and move his head...and look down...and he thought that way, way, down...he saw his reflection in the lake on the mountain top...and everything so far away looked so clear to him. And then a voice behind him said, "Do you want some power?" And he said, "Oh yes, oh yes!" And the voice said, "Trust the wind. Trust the wind." And Mouse felt the wind blow below him, under his belly and his arms. And suddenly the wind lifted him, and now he was flying over the land, over the lake, and he looked down and saw Wolf, and Wolf looked up and said, "Hello, Eaglemouse!" And he flew further and saw Bear, and cried out from high in the air, "I love you, Bear!" And then he saw Buffalo and dipped his wing in honor of Buffalo who protected him at the start. And then he crossed over the old mouse alone in his little sage hut, nodded his head to him and just kept flying along. And then he was near Mouseland and saw Raccoon, and finally he came to the roaring river, from which all this began. And he swooped down, and Frog looked up. And Frog said, "See, now you know. When you hear a roaring in your head, and every time there is something that you fear, crouch as low as you can, jump as high as you can, and what you see, you go there, and everything will change. And every time you will come back with a name you have never, ever heard before."

Introduction

Playing with sand and water on my childhood beach, I considered the sand as mine alone. I was oblivious to the possibility that every sand form that I sculpted or drew had already existed somewhere, for someone else, on every beach at every time in human history. Perhaps the sand itself held memories of several thousand years of children playing on it, memories that remained in the sand and permeated the forms that I made. I wonder now about the first humans, our remote ancestors, who played as we do during their short lives. Children played while fathers fished far into the sea and mothers gathered shellfish in estuaries and mud flats. Or perhaps adults ritually cast a gift or object of penance into the sea, encountered sea shells suitable for adornment or grave goods, or placed them on mud constructions to attract the blessings of nature spirits. Perhaps their presence still dwells in the sand we bring into our sandtrays.

Our ancestors lived within a respectful relationship to nature powers in accordance with the inherent possibilities of their environments. Their spiritual beliefs supported their biological existence and became myths, enacted through story, movement, music and ceremonial costume. Archetypes of play, creativity and spirituality formed in their psyche, integral to their survival. My childhood beach sandplay was an unplanned creative form of emotional and spiritual survival that flowed into making art, teaching art and becoming an art therapist. Later, chance or destiny contrived together, in 1987, in an expressive therapy colloquium, to guide me towards a workshop entitled "Sandplay." The experience activated my love of sand and confirmed the path of becoming a sandplay therapist. My first meeting with clinical sandplay aroused a familiar sense of timelessness and space, inner and outer, that I had known in childhood. I formed the sand as usual, added objects and adjusted their placement. My hands were now framed by a very small rectangular sandtray, my gaze was selective; the sense of unrest and creative urgency continued until the image was right (Steinhardt, 2018).

The evolving sandplay environment—from Lowenfeld to Kalff, to today's sandplay therapist

Dora Kalff studied music, Eastern philosophy and then Jungian studies. Jung recognized her natural understanding of children and, in 1955, suggested that she study sandplay with pioneer child psychiatrist Margaret Lowenfeld in London. Thirty years earlier, Lowenfeld had founded a children's clinic, influenced by a little book entitled *Floor Games* by H.G. Wells (1911/2016), who played with his children in a room filled with various materials for constructing different worlds. Lowenfeld allocated separate rooms in her clinic for art, drama and construction, and another for play equipped with 200–300 figurines and two random-sized trays with sand or water, made of plastic, metal or wood. The children added objects to the trays and called their scenes "worlds." Lowenfeld termed this phenomenon the "World Technique" and later lectured widely with slides of the children's worlds, as well as on her other innovative methods (Lowenfeld, 1993). Kalff studied for a year with Lowenfeld, returned to Zurich and integrated the basic setting of Lowenfeld's sandtray method with her own knowledge of Eastern philosophy and a Jungian understanding of healing through the collective and personal unconscious. Accordingly, she displayed unlimited types and numbers of figurines on her sandplay shelves and offered two wooden sandtrays of specific geometric proportions, painted light blue inside, one filled with wet sand for molding and its opposite with dry sand that cannot hold form. She called her approach "Sandplay," emphasized "delayed interpretation," provided a "free and protected space" for spontaneous play with sand, water and objects, and established a warm, supportive relationship with her patients. In the 1960s, she began to teach her method to Jungian analysts, and also taught in other countries. The International Society of Sandplay Therapy (ISST) was founded in 1985, and sandplay literally traveled around the world. Other mental health practitioners began to train in sandplay, and today sandplay therapists from many orientations and cultures adapt Kalff's guidelines to their local social, generational and therapeutic conditions. International congresses and workshops continue to bring Kalff's sandplay method into a technological world and restore the emphasis on a therapy where natural instinct and non-verbal communication heal and enrich therapists and their clients.

The sandplay experience of the sandplay therapist

Not all sandplay therapists have played in childhood in the sand of a sea or ocean, and not all sandplay clients have played freely on a beach or have experienced joy after creating something from themselves. Clients in therapy can choose whether or not to work in the sandtray. But the sandplay therapist must complete a personal sandplay process with a certified sandplay therapist before studying Kalffian Sandplay. Undergoing a personal sandplay process reveals its power, mystery and depth, but it is required rather than personally initiated therapy and can be met with resistance. When the therapeutic relationship goes well, when a perception or emotional or spiritual insight emanates unexpectedly from an unseen world and resolves into a visual expression in the sandtray, resistance can turn into appreciation. But given the limited availability of certified sandplay therapists, finding one can involve travel, time and expense. Some sandplay candidates choose to experience their personal process with a sandplay therapist in another country or culture. They may make several trips, stay for several days each time, make one or two sandplays per day and complete the recommended 25 sandplays. After certification, sandplay is not required. But in the psyche, another sandplay is always waiting. The author and a group of sandplay colleagues meet yearly for one day each summer to experience together creative unconscious expression in sandplay (Steinhardt, 2013, pp.179–199).

Sandplay is a creative, non-intrusive method of therapy. Non-intrusion is intrinsic to the role of the therapist-witness, who has experienced a personal process, is comfortable with silence and is prepared for difficult themes that intrude into consciousness in spontaneous sandplay. Within a positive co-transference, themes of healing increase as therapy continues (Bradway, 1991/2022). The self-healing knowledge of the therapist activates the self-healing potential of the client. It then becomes possible for a client to accept painful and hidden shadow aspects. One experienced sandplay therapist writing up a final case for certification realized that a powerful turning point in her client's sandplay process contained the same symbols that she had once used in a turning point in her own personal sandplay process.

Sandplay literature and writing

In each session, a sandplay therapist takes notes and photographs sandplays. Records of entire processes of children and adults of different ages and diagnostic characteristics are filed away for years. Sometimes, the therapist opens this store of data when a theme seems to need clarification and sifts out notes on symbols, patterns of non-verbal behaviors or verbal communication, or styles of constructing an image, and begins to write.

The first sandplay book in English was the translation from the German of Kalff's book *Sandplay* (1980/2020). Following were books written by Jungian analysts and other certified members of the International Society of Sandplay Therapy (Bradway *et al.*, 1981; Weinrib, 1983; Ammann, 1991; Ryce-Menuhin, 1992; Mitchell and Friedman, 1994; Bradway and McCoard, 1997). In the 1980s, psychiatrists, psychologists and social workers entered the sandplay world, and not long after, expressive arts therapists discovered sandplay. Research was published on the use of sand and stages of children's play with sand (Lowenfeld, 1979; Jones, 1986 in Mitchell and Friedman, 1994). The psyche's relationship to spatial-visual phenomena was researched by Ryce-Menuhin (1992) who diagrammed specific placement of material from three levels of the psyche—the collective unconscious, the personal unconscious and consciousness. Ammann (1991) discussed placement in quadrants, relating the far and near areas of the sandtray to the masculine and feminine, and the left and right sides to the past or unconscious, the present and future, with the ego in center. Mitchell and Friedman's second book, *Supervision of Sandplay Therapy* (2007), gave voice to the many therapeutic orientations and cultures that sandplay therapists come from, and to different approaches to sandplay supervision and the varied populations with whom they work (Steinhardt, 2007). *The Journal of Sandplay Therapy* was founded in 1991 by the STA (Sandplay Therapists of America) and continues to publish important articles on sandplay twice yearly in English, written by American and international sandplay therapists.

In my first book, *Foundation and Form in Jungian Sandplay* (Steinhardt, 2000), I focused on the symbolic meanings of universal sand forms built in play on the beaches of the world and in the sandtray, the physiological and psychological impact of blue as the color of the inner surface of the sandtray and the client's intuitive choice between art or sandplay. Ten years later, the process of becoming a sandplay therapist and appreciation of the healing potential of sandplay inspired a second book, *On Becoming a Jungian Sandplay Therapist: The Healing Spirit of Sandplay in Nature and in Therapy* (Steinhardt, 2013). Now, after another ten years, my writing quest focuses on detailed observation of the sandplay environment and the image itself, its sources and the unfolding sequence of images in the sandplay journey. Jumping Mouse, whose story is in the preface of this book, began his journey when he left home. Our sandplay "home," the sandplay environment, is the starting point in each session for that day's journey. In the small, receptive space of the sandtray, each image is a step in an invisible path, whose threads weave together the known and unknown content of one's life and the inherited knowledge within our psyche. As James Hillman has said, we are in psyche rather than psyche being in us (Hillman, 1990).

The chapters

This book is divided into four parts and 11 chapters. The first three chapters (Part One) focus on environments from nature to clinic, the physical and symbolic qualities that make each setting unique, the choices of the therapist who constructs it and variations on its use. In Chapter 1, the differentiation of similar natural environments by geologic, seasonal and atmospheric conditions is compared to differentiation of similar sandplay environments whose ambience results from each therapist's preference, age, culture and previous therapeutic profession. The unique atmosphere, boundaries and content of a sandplay setting, and the therapist as part of it, separate it from the outside world. The sandtray's boundaries separate it from other content in the room. A client, seeing natural sand inside a tray, a multitude of objects, creating a sandplay, being witnessed, not having to explain or clean up in a "free and protected space" can have a "first-time" experience of surprise and awe. Sandplay recalls the human need to create within an environment, like the marks etched by our ancestors on natural surfaces, which in time transitioned to skill in painting, sculpting and stone construction. A child's efforts to build a pyramid in the sandtray may echo the aspirations of past civilizations to construct monuments as a way of serving invisible powers that determine our physical, emotional and spiritual wellbeing. In our time, in the years after World War II, creative artists of all kinds left their "site-specific" studios and used their artistic skill to form a new profession—creative arts therapy, therapeutic work with groups in psychiatric hospitals and schools. Jung's analytic concepts and work with the unconscious attracted many creative arts therapists, and around the 1980s, some discovered sandplay. Other artists had begun in the 1960s to work in natural environments with on-site materials, creating Land Art, or "site-specific" art. Their works were photographed and left to disintegrate, similar to photographing a sandplay and then dismantling it. Creativity, therapy and environment join together in the "site-specific" sandplay setting, whose materials fill a small but symbolically immense sandtray with images. And the presence of light, embodying spirit and numinosity in the sandplay setting, is discussed in the work of certain artists, and exemplified by the light that enters Dora Kalff's sandplay room through a wall of windows (Kalff, 2020).

Chapter 2 is a review of the physical components of the sandplay setting and their symbolism. Each therapist makes choices that fill the enclosed space of the room. The client's "net of imagination" opens and scoops up in each session a limited group of themes that are transposed into symbols in the sandtray, embodied in form, form as the habitat of life (Bachelard, 1994). Several "invisible maps" that guide a sandplay into existence are discussed—the inner psychic maps of a session and of a journey, the imagined map of the space inside the rectangular sandtray, and the co-transference. The influence of the sandtray's rectangular form on its content is compared to the influence of a circle-, square-, hexagon- or octagon-shaped tray. The opposites in the setting, two trays and dry or wet sand, are linked to cyclical aspects of nature. The author's small sandplay studio is referenced as a symbolic center of the four directions. The origins of sand, living with the miniature collection, controversial objects, materials that objects are made of and the energies present in the setting complete this chapter.

Chapter 3 surveys some variations in sandplay settings when budgets are limited, when work with unusual clients or disabled or very young children necessitate inventiveness, when sandplay is integrated into a clinic for verbal or arts therapy and the boundaries of either method must be preserved. Dumped sand or breaking objects and coping with water and flooding or fire and burning are illustrated with case examples. Sandplay therapists also respond to emergencies caused by natural and man-made disasters. Several examples of improvised sandplay settings are described, with a brief report on the months-long temporary sandplay rooms for thousands of homeless evacuees living in hotels, whose villages on the southern border of Israel were destroyed in a horrific terrorist attack. Sandplay enabled silent expression of acute trauma.

In Part Two, in Chapters 4, 5 and 6, human experiences with nature, creativity and quests for transformation in a wider world are connected to their activation in the sandplay environment. Chapter 4, "Nature and Its Teachers, Observation and Differentiation," links human adaptation to an environment to observation and differentiation between animals and plants and acquired knowledge that may be stored in our own collective unconscious. Our animal and plant miniatures represent instinctive knowledge and can activate a response to the wonder and beauty of nature, still preserved in the unconscious and in dreams (Hillman, 1990). Our opportunities to observe animals and plants in their natural setting are few, but beyond labeling their miniature representatives as symbols, the therapist may have knowledge of biological and botanical aspects represented by our objects which resonates in the co-transference with a client. Differentiating between the symbolism of realistic animal miniatures and the imaginary cartoon creatures on our sandplay shelves corresponds with Psyche's first task, sorting out a pile of different grains with the help of ants (Neumann, 1971). A sandplayer first observes, then intuitively sorts out choices that gain access to the collective unconscious (Shamdasani, 2015). In sandplay, plants are less represented than animals, but the sandtray itself is a symbolic "soul-garden" (Ammann, 1994). The therapist as "master gardener" understands plants, seasons, cycles, healing and growth, and fosters this knowledge in the apprentice gardener, the client.

Chapter 5 links creative urgency to an inner drive to form visual images on various natural surfaces, as long as 500,000 years ago in a geometric zigzag scratched on a shell in Indonesia. This altered shell records the creative impulse of one man, who chose an object from the sea for his image, perhaps a talisman calling for spiritual nurturance combined with physical nurturance. Humans gradually invested time and aesthetic intent in making art, drawing visual images of edible animals on cave walls, handprints in high caves, carving totems or building monuments in which to worship divine powers. Themes of food and nurture were depicted on ancient Egyptian grave walls, in Renaissance paintings of luxurious foods and in contemporary pop-art depicting street food. But in sandplay, the act of filling the sandtray with various objects can represent self-nurture, nurturance from the therapist and from therapy. Creative urgency channels the need for love, and emotional and spiritual nurture into a sandplay. In Chapter 6, pilgrimages to "power spots" in nature and quests towards general goals in reality are compared to the "sandplay quest" as a path to transformation. It has been postulated that beautiful natural places, and shrines and temples built there, are situated on "ley lines," part of an energetic global network. Pilgrimages are made to chosen destinations by travelers who wish to communicate with divine powers that are said to visit these spots. Sandplay is more of a wandering quest whose initial destination changes as responsive energies coagulate towards a truer goal. Perception of the sandplay setting changes from a playroom to a "power spot" and each image crystallizes its place in the journey The process of change can be explained to a client with a simple drawing task based on the "hero's journey" (Lahad, 1997). But resistance often accompanies change (Montecchi, 2004). Blocks and wounding can be expressed as images in the sandtray or through transference to the therapist until healing energies appear in the sand.

In Part Three, the range of non-verbal symbolic language in sandplay images is considered, through different theories and case examples, from a single image to the interactions between images in the unfolding journey. Chapter 7, "The Sandplay Image Speaks for Itself," contains research done by Ryce-Menuhin (1992) and Ammann (1991) on the universal meanings of placement on the sandtray map, and a comparison of the effects of rounded or angular forms, colors, number and materials on content, before considering the identities of objects. Symbols of transference in sandplays can be represented by objects pointing towards the therapist or when two objects are placed together. Conscious and unconscious co-transference in the levels of client–therapist interaction activate the therapist's role of "healer" in the client and the client's wounding in the therapist. The case of Helena, a 50-year-old woman, illustrates the slow transition over 16 years of her defensive isolation, symbolized in central solitary mounds in the sandtray center, to central mounds that portray relationships and healing.

In Chapter 8, paths constructed in the sandtray in early stages are seen as maps of potential stages and ensuing transition of themes from wounding to healing. Paths incised on the sand, cut through to the blue bottom, pieced together with different materials, tracks and paths of mourning, blocked paths, or sandplays with no path that show early neglect are illustrated with sandplay examples. A spiritual sandplay process of Tara, a 50-year-old woman, illustrates paths that begin and end in the sandtray center, place of origin and return.

Chapter 9, the 13 sandplays of Jasmin, a 32-year-old woman, convey the power of sculpted sand as symbol and invite archetypal amplifications, with almost no objects. Jasmin constructed her images from all sides of the sandtray and observed them to read her fortune, like the Turkish coffee-mud fortune-telling practiced in her original family. She had broken contact with her unstable mother, but the gentle touch of her hands created sand mounds and mud balls that echoed a pre-conscious memory of a loving mother (Winnicott, 1971). Her love of sand and rejection of objects may have been a preference, or a sign of early trauma.

In Chapter 10, Neumann's stages of ego development of children (1973/1988) confirm the stages of spontaneous developmental sandplay of two boys and a girl playing alone in the author's sandplay studio from early to middle childhood. Photographs of their sandplays and their stories were saved and dated, and reviewed many years later. Their sandplays conform to Neumann's developmental stages and their relationships to family and siblings, and to themselves. Personal and universal core themes and some differences between boys and girls are identified. Stages of the use of sand according to age and sex (Jones, 1986) clarify the inner developmental map of Oron, from two years ten months old to five years eight months old. Campbell's (1949/1973) stages in the journey of Theseus, an orphan who became a hero, support Ben's journey in sandplay from age two and a half to seven years old, leaving the matriarchate and transitioning to the patriarchate. Maya's sandplay process from age two years ten months to 11 years six months reveals her unspoken reactions to the births of her sisters and later to her parents' divorce. Her own needs remained in shadow until she accepted their separation and could focus on herself.

In Part Four, Chapter 11, eight Greek myths are summarized with commentary on the history of these myths in ancient Greece and Rome, and amplification of symbols and patterns of coping with obstacles in each myth that resonate today in our unconscious psyche. The telling of each myth was part of the curriculum of a sandplay training program followed by experiential individual sandplay, bridging collective unconscious themes and the personal in the sandtray. The myths are: Demeter and Persephone; Amor and Psyche; Theseus, the Minotaur and Ariadne; Ariadne and Dionysus; Asclepius God of Healing; Orpheus and Eurydice; the Journey of Odysseus; and Hecate, Triple Goddess of Night, Crossroads, the Household and Magic. A workshop at a sandplay conference designed around Hecate's healing presence is described.

The conclusion of this book, "Listening to the Unconscious," summarizes the personal and professional process of expanding a vision of sandplay by opening the scope of relevant realities, resources from inherited knowledge, personal unconscious and conscious knowledge, and new ingredients from the contemporary abundance of theories and methods that can amplify not just a symbol but the creation of a sandplay and of the sandplay journey. A brief case example of a six-year-old boy, traumatized before birth, concludes this chapter.

PART ONE

THE SANDPLAY ENVIRONMENT

Place, Presence

1

The Sandplay Environment

The word environment is defined as "a surrounding or associated matters that influence or modify a course of development." It is synonymous with the words ambience, atmosphere, climate, medium, milieu, mise-en-scene and surroundings. It is relevant to words such as habitat, backdrop, background, context, setting, situation and status. It also infers a boundary that encloses something within it, separating the inner area from things beyond its fringe (*Webster's Collegiate Thesaurus*, 1976, p.291).

Environments, from nature to clinic

The sandplay environment replicates some of the natural elements that make up a beach environment, such as its sand, water, blue color and various objects. The natural unstructured approach to play at the beach is encouraged in clinical sandplay. In both environments, linear time is forgotten. At the beach, the diffuse space of air, sky and light above touches two imprecise boundaries, a horizon that separates sky and water and its opposite boundary, the shoreline, between water and sand. Children build their imprecise and impermanent mud structures here and embellish them with stones, shells, sand forms and debris. The moods of this environment shift from calm and clear to turbulent and dark, in response to the seasons, sunlight and the phases of moonlight at night. All beach environments are similar, yet each has a unique local quality defined by light, the colors of sky, sand and water, local rocks and plant and animal life forms specific to its location.

When sandplay therapists visit each other's sandplay clinics, they tend to notice the miniatures and their arrangement on the shelves, then the light and space of the room, the type of sand and the height and boundaries of the sandtrays, and compare these with their own sandplay clinic. Like natural environments, the site-specific content of each sandplay setting creates its own ambience. Closer attention to the sandtrays, miniatures and whatever populates the space reveals the therapist's interpretation of the sandplay guidelines. As architect of this environment, the therapist is almost a part of it, having sensed the shape, proportions, color and location of the entire content of the room, as separate from the outside world. The therapist has crafted an environment, either a private clinic or public facility, that offers a large symbolic vocabulary of sand, water and objects. The room and the supportive therapeutic relationship contain the creative expression that will be experienced freely and safely by the client's body and psyche. The sandtray contains the image, framed by the sandtray's boundaries and separated from the contents of the room surrounding the sandtray.

Entering the sandplay environment for the first time

First-time experiences alert the senses. Entering a sandplay environment for the first time can be a completely new experience for a child or for an adult. In that first moment, the richness of the setting may be unconsciously absorbed, but each client has an individual pace of exploration and discovery, for several or many sessions or even years. Each session is also a "first time" of exploration, attunement, discovery of objects on the shelves. Creative possibilities and new configurations and stories can emerge into a more conscious reality, visually, verbally and symbolically. Being witnessed, receiving silent support, submitting to guidance from the unconscious, or gazing at a finished sandplay and not speaking, with a non-intrusive therapist can be a strong "first-time" experience. After observing a sandplay together, some children begin to "tidy up" at the end of the work and put objects back in place, when the therapist suggests that they leave the outer image untouched, while a complete internalized image will be taken with them in memory. A less trusting client might enjoy making a sandplay, but reject support from a therapist, object to the therapist writing notes during the work, as if it were a diagnostic test, and even destroy the final sandplay so that its "secrets" cannot be photographed and revealed. For the mistrustful client, the setting itself becomes "the therapist." The therapist learns to maintain the right distance for this client. After a client has gone, photographing the sandplay is a therapist's opportunity to focus on its components and then dismantle it in an order that may convey some of the emotions felt by the client. The sandplay setting, like a natural environment, returns to its original state after each session, and everything begins anew with the next client.

Art forms within environments and their connection to sandplay

Our ancestors were skilled observers, perceiving tracks and minute signs left on the environment by passing animals or humans. They also incised petroglyphs, stenciled hands in high caverns and aspired to perfect their drawings of animals and hunting scenes in caves around the world. The human creative urge in our genes was integral for thousands of years for the first artists who invested time and effort in creating ceremonial symbols to honor higher powers. Monuments constructed of quarried stone still stand, in the Maltese Ggantija temple (3600 BC), Stonehenge in England (3000 BC), the Egyptian pyramids (2630 BC), the Mounds of Native American civilizations (from 500 BC), and the Mayan Chichen Itza in Mexico (250–900 AD). Other extraordinary pyramids and stone complexes continue to be excavated or reclaimed from deserts, jungles or cities sunken under the sea. A child's impulse to construct a pyramid in sand at the beach or in the sandtray and decorate it with shells and pebbles is perhaps the legacy of our ancestor's desire to achieve artistic, architectural and technical excellence. An art movement that began in the 1960s, known as "Environmental Art" or "Land Art," attracted artists to restore their personal connection to nature and use wood, stone, leaves, feathers, water, sand, snow and light to create "on-site art." Natural materials disintegrate over time, so these works are preserved in photographs (Goldsworthy, 1990). Some colossal Land Art projects do remain in nature, such as the Spiral Jetty in Utah (Smithson, 1972) and the Roden Crater project in Arizona (1970–2024) in which natural light is a creative material in concordance with phases of the sun and moon, as in ancient great temples (Turrell, 2023).

Environments do not immediately reveal their details. The trees in a forest may look the same at first, but each tree knows its place among others, and every bird knows the branch it prefers to sit on (Wagoner, 1972). Although a sandplay environment has immense content, each client will focus on what is intuitively needed for making an image. The client inhabits this setting each session, for a short but immense time, selecting and arranging materials that transform inner urges and ideas into a site-specific completed sandplay for a therapeutic purpose. The finished work may feel larger than its physical size. Bachelard's philosophical category of "intimate immensity" inspires contemplation and transports the "day dreamer" outside the immediate world to another infinite world. Bachelard writes, "Immensity is within ourselves. It is attached to a sort of expansion of being that life curbs and caution arrests, but which starts again when we are alone" (1994, p.184).

Creative environments, creative therapeutic studios and sandplay settings

Creative people tend to choose and arrange the objects in their work spaces so that they feel surrounded by themselves. I once visited an exhibition of life-size photographs of the work spaces of several well-known writers, their names printed on a label on the museum wall. The writers were not present in the photographs. The order or disorder of each intimate writing space, its light, shadow, color and objects such as a desk, typewriter, chair, note papers, pencils, books and pictures defined the character of the unseen writer who created this environment. The room became a portal to a world of invisible words. In comparison, artists' studios have large windows and light-filled open space. Paintings are stacked against smudged white walls pinned with notes and drawings. A bare floor stained with colors is littered with scraps of materials whose smell is part of the space. A chair could be anywhere; a canvas might be on the floor, on the wall or on an easel. Tables with paints and brushes, with buckets beneath, drawers and shelves holding tools are near an easel ready for work or for viewing finished work. Sculptors are surrounded by blocks of stone or wood, clay, plaster, metal, with tools for cutting, molding, welding, gluing, polishing and shaping materials. The physicality of an artist's studio may seem chaotic, but for the artist, it is an alchemic womb for the process of coagulating an idea into a finished image.

In the late 1940s after World War II, and in the 1950s, the writer's study, the artist's studio and ateliers for acting, dancing and music were the precedent for the first creative therapeutic spaces established in psychiatric hospitals and therapeutic boarding schools. Artists provided creative therapy for children or adults in groups, so that more patients per hour could benefit than in individual therapy (Junge, 2010). Verbal therapy was usually provided by psychologists. By the 1980s, the therapeutic power inherent in the expressive arts therapies was recognized, and formal training programs for creative arts therapists were established, primarily in the United States and in Great Britain. Jobs opened in schools, clinics and psychiatric hospitals. Creative therapies activate communication with the unconscious psyche, and Jung's concepts of the structure of the psyche became a relevant theoretical base for these practitioners. From there, the path led many to Kalffian Sandplay.

My first ISST sandplay conference in San Rafael, California, in 1992, was attended by over 200 analysts, psychologists and social workers and eight art therapists. Sandplay therapists who had studied with Kalff presented cases with photographs of their sandplay settings, sandtrays, shelves, figurines and accessories. As an art therapist, I valued these examples of coordination of a setting as a form of visual guidance that helps to begin the work. In 2003, I began to teach sandplay, with an initial focus on the ambience of the sandplay setting and its connection with the therapist who created it. A setting should feel comfortable for therapist and patient, with a selection of objects and natural materials wide enough to support an entire range of emotional expression, from pain and wounding to healing and individuation. Sandplay students who have yet to construct their own setting often have experienced only one sandplay setting—that of the therapist with whom they did a personal process. Although most settings conform to the basic guidelines for a "good enough" sandplay environment, each setting is inevitably personal. In 2011, I created a presentation about sandplay settings with photographs of the sandplay clinics sent by several sandplay colleagues from different countries. At an ISST-sponsored International Sandplay Workshop in Poland, some of the therapists who had sent me photographs participated in the presentation and discussed various details of practice. For example, the therapist may remain stationary during verbal therapy but change seating during sandplay. Some therapists sit opposite the client and do not take notes. Others take notes as the client works, and sit somewhere behind the client, on the left or right, or unseen.

Light, windows, spirit and numinosity

In a filmed interview, Dora Kalff sits outdoors in her garden and describes the concept of free and protected space in sandplay and the relationship between ego development and the Self. She then continues inside her sandplay room with its magical atmosphere, the sandtrays, the shelves filled with unique miniatures, chairs and surfaces for art making (Ammann, 1972). Part of the enchantment that pervades Kalff's sandplay setting comes from illumination of the room by natural light that enters from a wall of windows looking out onto the dark green garden. Light bridges outer and inner, nature and the room, the visible and what is intuited. The presence of natural light in a room can improve mood and productivity. Light carries color and penetrates transparent materials such as glass, water, plastic and air. Architects often plan windows for maximum natural light or install electric light that mimics natural daylight. A sandplay therapist's clinic may not be near a garden or have large windows, but good lighting, whether natural or electric, complements the inner light of spirit that is sometimes encountered as a numinous presence emanating from certain sandplays.

Artists seek light that resonates with their artistic goals. Strong direct sunlight produces intense color, which brought Van Gogh to Arles, Gauguin to Tahiti, and Matisse to Morocco. Matisse stated that a painting can light up a room, and that "Color helps to express *light*, not the physical phenomenon, but the only *light* that really exists, that in the artist's brain" (Cowart and Schneider, 1992). The entire north wall of Paul Cezanne's studio in Aix-en-Provence (1839–1906) is constructed of windows. Diffuse skylight illuminates the interior with subtle transitions between light and shadow that reveal the form and color that is essential to Cezanne's painting (Aix-en-Provence, ville de Cezanne, n.d.). Vermeer (1632–1675) repeatedly painted clear diffuse Dutch light breaking through a window into a room's interior, suggesting a divine presence that illuminates people and objects in soft lush color (Schutz, 2012). The recurrent theme of Edward Hopper (1882–1967), tinged with an unfathomable longing, was the oblique rectangular shape of sunlight entering a window, falling on a room's slightly darker wall (Berman and Hopper, 2005). In paintings by Caravaggio (1571–1610) and Rembrandt (1606–1669), a mysterious and spiritual light emerges from darkness, and dramatically illuminates people's faces and hands, defining three-dimensional form and revealing underlying human emotions (Schutze, 2021; Bockemuhl, 2000). Outdoors, light creates rainbows and reflection, and, when magnified, creates fire. Our eyes and skin absorb light from its source, the sun, which nurtures everything on earth. Ancient monuments attuned to the equinoxes and solstices commemorate these points in the sun's celestial journey and the numinous moments of its daily rebirth in the east and its "death" at sunset in the west. Artist James Turrell constructs small empty structures called "sky-spaces" into which light enters through an aperture in the ceiling open to the sky. Time and the trajectory of the moving sun in the sky become visible as the shape of light on the floor moves from place to place in an almost tactile presence of light, a spiritual experience of wordless thought and the sense of presence of space as an entity (Turrell, 2023).

2

The Physical and Symbolic Sandplay Setting

Qualities of sandplay settings

When planning a sandplay setting, in a public facility or in a private clinic, the practical variables are the actual space available and the budget allotted for content. Then the therapist refers to the sandplay guidelines and makes the many decisions that go into creating a "good enough" setting. Decisions are inevitably influenced by the therapist's age, sex, culture, country and previous therapeutic profession. The relationships between components in the available space will project an essence beyond the physical and convey something of the therapist's personality. Sandplay settings will all have similar details but will be unique as complete frameworks.

Space and imagination

Our imagination lives in a kind of unlimited space, like the infinite space in the sky above us. When the sun or a cloud during the day, or the moon, stars and galaxies of the night become focal points in the sky, they give presence to the space surrounding them. The open space of imagination contrasts with the physical and mental boundaries and social rules of behavior that guide our daily life. In the closed space of the sandplay room, the sandtray's small boundaries provide a limited but safe arena to contain inner themes, as they become focal points within which sand forms and symbolic objects merge. They take their places within the sandtray space, guided by invisible territorial and developmental maps unconsciously sensed by a sandplayer.

The ambience of a room, the shape of space, the form of content

The walls of a sandplay room, its windows, doors and inner content (furniture and shelves, sandtrays) vaguely define a protected space for the sandplay setting, a temenos. Within this room, a sandplayer engages in unconscious access to the invisible formless expanse of imagination, with no preconceived intention and with no mind to receive a specific image. The net of our imagination will scoop up in each session a relatively small, manageable catch of images. The specifically proportioned rectangular sandtray becomes a receptive container enclosing a protected space with low walls, open and accessible from above. With our bodies safely ensconced in the room, our imagination wanders in invisible unconscious space, and our eyes survey the visible room space and the inner sandtray space. In imagination, innumerable images drift. An invisible psychic net is cast into this unconscious "ocean" to catch themes (yearning, abandonment, anger, confusion, fear, anguish, or peace, protection, wholeness and balance), themes that mirror archetypal and personal unconscious and conscious aspects of one's inner world. What is caught in the net is at that moment differentiated from the endless "ocean" substance and merged with a sand form or miniature, creating a symbol. This symbol is then installed within the sandtray, in a specific area. No two directions, no two spaces are the same. The location chosen then also becomes a symbolic space that confers on the symbol additional meaning connecting it in time to past, present or future, or to feminine and masculine principles (Ammann, 1991, p.47; Ryce-Menuhin, 1992, pp.91–97).

What has not been framed, formed and accommodated in the sandtray space continues its enormous dark drift, somewhere, elsewhere, indefinitely. The act of visible creation began with the casting of the psychic net into that pre-existing dark drift, to retrieve a theme and invest it in physical matter. The sandplayer's psyche, eyes and hands collaborate and work with no consciously declared intention to turn passive objects into meaningful symbolic imagery. The sandtray itself may have no mind to become that unintentional mirror of a theme that casts its reflection transposed into symbolic form, arranged on the tracks of that day's journey, on the invisible map of the sandtray terrain. Theme, when embodied in form, becomes accessible to ourselves and others. "Form could not possibly exist without content, form is the visible shape of content" (Shahn, 1957/1972, pp.60–61). French philosopher Bachelard writes that nature endows itself with form, that life originates forms, and that "form is the habitat of life" (1994, p.114).

In sandplay, we can choose an already formed object to embody a theme that is not yet completely known. Or we can impact our hands on the sand and create a new form, moving like wind or water that encounters a natural substance and changes its form. In sandplay, forms are early messengers of the story that will eventually be told. Without any conscious predetermined order, sand form, objects and location transpose into a specific content, both physical and psycho-spiritual (Steinhardt, 2016).

Sandplay's invisible maps

The Oxford Dictionary of Current English defines a map as "a flat representation of the earth's surface, or part of it; diagram of a route; similar representation of the stars, sky, moon, etc.; diagram showing the arrangement or components of a thing" (1992, p.541).

In sandplay, there are invisible maps—for example, the sandplayer's inner psychic map of this day's journey; another map of the stages of the unfolding, individual but universal sandplay process (Weinrib, 1983, p.98; Jackson, 2008, pp.53–64); and the invisible map of the inner rectangular space of the sandtray: its corners, imaginary diagonals and center, its left and right sides, near and far levels (Ammann, 1991, p.41). And in relation to where the sandplayer stands, the sandtray becomes a horizontal or vertical rectangle, each direction with its own purpose: the horizontal parallels the earth (feminine) and sky (masculine); the vertical emphasizes ascent from earth to sky, from body to spirit. Each object and each form that populates the sand terrain will move or be moved, loyal to these invisible maps until it marks its spot and direction. Placement is a natural language that in sandplay can be felt as if nature speaks to us through our primitive tracking instinct.

Blue as a map into distance

The color blue is suitable for the inner sandtray surface, leading the psyche into ascent or descent, always receding from the eye, detaching from the concrete and distancing us from the themes of our dramas (Steinhardt, 2000, 2023). Color enters the body through the eyes and affects the human nervous system psychologically and physiologically. Blue has a calming effect on human behavior and thinking. Blue colors in water or sky change according to atmospheric conditions, time of day, season and depth or height. Blue pigments, such as ultramarine, cobalt, cerulean, manganese, and Prussian blue, each have a specific aura and as a painted surface in the sandtray cannot really approximate the blues of sky or water. Cobalt could be considered the bluest blue. Other blue pigments may tend towards green, violet or black. Any blue mixed with white becomes lighter and may be pleasant, but diffuse. A dark blue that tends towards black draws the emotions towards depression or disconnection from ordinary reality. I prefer cerulean blue for the dry sandtray as it is clear and powerful with less depth. Cobalt blue has depth that corresponds to the symbolic depth of water in the wet sandtray (Steinhardt, 1997, 2023). When the entire inner bottom and inner sandtray edges are colored blue up to the top inner edge, leaving the rim and outside of the tray white or the color of wood, there is a clear visual separation between "inside the tray" and "outside the tray."

Sand: an overview

The sand's color reverberates with the particular shade of blue chosen, and, as in nature, mirrors the dialogue between the elements of sand, water and sky (Steinhardt, 1997). Sand provides witness to the history of time, geology and evolution of life. The grains of sand scattered on this planet have been compared to the innumerable clusters of stars in an infinite blue space, which are said to outnumber our sand grains (Willis, 2013). Sand itself is a mirror of the world evolving and devolving on a vast scale. The *arenophile*, a sand collector, classifies a sand's identity for texture, color, mineral base and location. The sandtray boundaries are a partition that separates the mundane aspects of the space around the tray and the extraordinary events that emerge within the tray. Natural boundaries created by nature—membranes, shell, skin, bark, hide—are protective partitions that enclose the inner content of all living things within an outer environment. The skin envelope is our personal boundary, with body apertures for the entrance and exit of substances. But our imagination lives in unlimited space. When our imagination meets the sandtray, we begin to sense the metaphoric dimensions of inner space. "One must go beyond logic in order to experience what is large in what is small" (Bachelard, 1994, p.150).

Natural sand is an ever-present base in the sandtray. It holds the memory of substances that were present on earth before life forms existed. Sand encourages forming and objects evoke choosing. Clients combine them differently to illustrate the unconscious themes of their psyche. Some clients ask, "Where did you buy this figurine?" But others ask, "Where did you get this sand" or "What beach did this sand come from?" All sand is composed primarily of beige quartz and feldspar from rocks that are fragmented by wind and water over thousands of years and flow in rivers that reach oceans. My sand has a light beige color and fine texture, and is perceptibly darker when wet. Its prehistoric origins began eons ago in the mountains of Central Africa as rock, fragmented into smaller pebbles that reached the Nile River and were pulverized into sand and carried by the river to the Egyptian Delta, and into the Mediterranean Sea. Currents moved the sand eastward until 1970, when the new Aswan High Dam blocked the Nile's annual flood of water and sand into the sea. With less sand pouring in, beaches and estuaries receded. Today, barriers protect the remaining sand. Many beaches of the world are presently endangered because sand is quarried extensively for building construction and industry. This erodes rivers and seacoasts and causes sea levels to rise. In many countries, it is illegal to remove sand, pebbles, shells, sea glass and driftwood from a beach, punishable by fines or prosecution. It may be awkward for a sandplay therapist to obtain natural sand for the sandtray. Some therapists buy ground quartz used in play therapies, or kinetic sand for the sandtray. These products have their own potential but are not from a natural source and cannot replace the ancient presence, depth and history of real sand and all that it contributes to Jungian sandplay.

Sand and color

Sand takes the color of the mineral content of local mountains and of pulverized coral and shell. The sands of the Atlantic or Pacific Oceans are usually white-beige. In the Bahamas, pink sand comes from coral and pink marine shells. In Hawaii, black lava rock which sometimes contains the mineral olivine is naturally pulverized into black or olive-green sand, and on Kaihalulu Beach on Maui, iron in cliff formations gives the sand a red color. For the sandtray, pale white-beige sand with a fine texture may be best, but any local natural sand can become a physical and symbolic base that represents evolution, time, journey and transformation. Dry sand is light in color, is enlivened when light falls on it and moves loosely. Wet sand is darker and has sculptural potential. Light falling on dark wet sand enlivens it, but where light does not fall, shadows add depth and three-dimensionality to its structure.

Sand, light or dark, analogous to white or black

In the sandtray, the sand's color is a background for the colors of objects placed on it and will influence an object's appearance. Dry and wet sands are usually visual opposites of light and dark, similar to the opposites of two non-colors, white and black. Kandinsky (1914/1977, p.39) described white as symbolizing a world without color far above us, whose silence is like an impenetrable wall that "shrouds its life from our understanding. White therefore, has this harmony of silence...not a dead silence, but one pregnant with possibilities...the appeal of the nothingness that is before birth." The light beige dry sand, like beige or brown paper, may feel warm and supporting; its texture and quartz granules sparkle and fill the surface so that it does not seem "empty." It is comparatively close to white and may have some of the "harmony of silence" that Kandinsky describes. Kandinsky considers black, the darkest non-color, as "a totally dead silence...with no possibilities...burned out, like the ashes of a funeral pyre...motionless like a corpse. The silence of black is the silence of death." Black is lifeless in itself, then, but it gives life to all other colors placed on it. The darker wet sand in the sandtray, while not black, does have a dark primal quality that encourages creation of forms whose themes might be deeper than what would emerge in dry sand or with objects. Von Franz (1997, p.48) points out that white is associated with joy and purity but also with snow and coldness. Mourning clothes and burial shrouds can be either white or black. As the colors of death, they are interchangeable, although ghosts are usually draped in white, and demons covered in black. The clothes of priests, preachers, imams and rabbis are often black, sometimes with white collars or shawls. Hindi religious leaders wear white, the color of purity.

Physical and symbolic darkness

Darkness is embodied in the surface color of wet sand and in shadowed crevices where light does not reach. The ecology of the psyche needs the light of consciousness as well as the dark personal shadow, and the dark and light of archetypal images. On the sandplay shelves, we position black witches, demons, Cerberus, bats and Batman, as well as black-clothed religious figurines, intuitively placing "dark" and "light" objects near or far from each other. Dark meaning can be connected to figurines of sorcerers, monsters, snakes, worms, ants and beetles that digest dead matter. The lotus, beautiful Buddhist symbol of perfection, is tied with long roots to deep, dark muddy water soaking up from below the nutrients it needs. Some sandplay therapists might feel revulsion for a snake or cockroach and would prefer not to display them in their own object collection. But the personal psyche needs to project its opposites onto objects as symbols, and to experience fear or repulsion until the source of these emotions is understood.

A sandplay example: the great good mother, destruction and darkness in a boy's sandplay

In his ninth sandplay, an intelligent nine-year old boy from a well-to-do family experienced one regressive creative moment. He constructed two sand mounds like big breasts with nipples on them, singing and patting down the sand as he inserted an English flag into one nipple, saying that this was a nude woman in the bath. He loved touching the nipples and repaired them when they fell apart, saying, "Poor thing." He pushed the breasts into the far-left area, giggled, turned them into mountains and opened a round shape in front of them that resembled a vagina. He then flattened everything and went to the bathroom. On his return, he placed a series of "containers"—houses, a sarcophagus, pyramid, a closed treasure chest, a Buddha and a castle—in the front-right corner with a large bell hanging out of the sandtray. Two bridges placed left of center were separated by a small mound with a black hour glass on it. He printed my name stamp on his hand several times. At the onset of therapy, he had no friends, was afraid of thieves and closed the window shades of his family's sixth-floor apartment so no one could spy on them. His sandplays were constructed from many points of view. Disastrous fires, hopeless wars, earthquakes and volcanoes always destroyed mounds and houses connected by bridges, leaving many graves. The sand breasts and nipples seemed to access a brief comforting unconscious memory of a Great Mother figure (Neumann, 1983). Two weeks later, his scenes of destruction actualized. His father was arrested for embezzlement, and therapy was suddenly terminated. His fears that time was up were confirmed, symbolized by the hour glass and a warning bell.

Kalff's rectangular sandtray

The Kalffian sandtray is a rectangle with specific measurements (approximately 49.5 x 72.5 x 7 centimeters). Its size comfortably receives a person's whole field of vision. Kalff used the measurement of the sandtray's short axis to draw a square, and a diagonal from the front-left corner to the far-right corner that, when dropped down, becomes the length of the longer edge (Jackson-Bashinsky, 1994). Kalff's sandtray sides have an inner height of 7 centimeters which may be impractical when working with children who tend to throw sand around. An inner height of 8 or 9 centimeters is more containing and will not obstruct photography. The rim and walls of the sandtray, their color, width and depth frame the inside space of the sandtray and guide the sandplayer's eyes to focus on the contents within.

The rim's width of at least one centimeter and not more than two (3/8 to 3/4 of an inch) will feel solid and stable but not draw attention to itself. Rims are also horizons beyond which lies an unknown amorphous space.

The sandtray is a rectangle. Its parallel opposite sides are equal, but one pair is longer than the other. When viewed facing the longer side, a horizontal rectangle parallels the supporting earth (the feminine, close to the body). Young children's picture books or landscape paintings and still-lives primarily use horizontal rectangles. A vertical rectangle has a narrow base and emphasizes height as if ascending from earth to heaven (the masculine, distant from the body) which is suitable for newspapers, textbook formats and for portraits or photographs of a single person, directing the eye upwards to the subject's face. Whether horizontal or vertical, the left side of the sandtray usually contains unconscious content, while on the right side more conscious material such as relationships in the home and in the outside world is represented. These tendencies of placement have been researched and diagrammed by Ryce-Menuhin (1992) and by Ammann (1991) and are discussed in Chapter 7. The sandtray rectangle is large enough to move the hands freely, and watch them move, apart and together, far and near, from the less conscious left side to the more conscious right side. Invisible diagonals extend from corner to opposite corner and are the longest distances in the sandtray. Objects placed spontaneously in opposite corners often represent opposites in the personality. Where the two diagonals cross, they mark the center. As the sandplay process progresses, the opposites may meet in the center, the place of ego, and the Self–Ego axis. The arrival at the Self–Ego axis can take a mandala form. Thus, the rectangle is the most dynamic shape for a sandtray and for finding the center alone.

Other geometric shapes

Sandplay students question if a square, circle or hexagon shape is suitable for a sandtray. Artists are aware that different outer shapes influence inner content to arrange itself differently. They choose contours to suit the content that is aimed for. A square's equal sides infer a center and create tension with less depth. A square "flat" format was preferred by abstract artists Piet Mondrian (1872–1944) and Joseph Albers (1888–1976), and by painter Neil Welliver (1929–2005) for his large, dramatic landscapes (Seuphor, 1956; Albers, 1975; Welliver, 1999). A circle is always balanced and calls attention to its center, which is equidistant from any point on its circumference. The Tondo, a circular painting or carved relief, was popular during the Italian Renaissance for depicting the primal relationship of Madonna and Child.

The six-sided hexagon and the eight-sided octagon have straight sides of equal measurement, and, like the square and circle, have an already present center, equidistant from each side. These four shapes—square, circle, hexagon and octagon—project a sense of harmony and balance and easily offer a center. As shapes for a sandtray, the goal might be related to symmetry, center or to the number of sides.

My first sandtray was constructed according to the measurements printed in Dora Kalff's book on sandplay in English (1980). Kalff's original centimeters were incorrectly converted into inches. The vertical sides are several inches longer than Kalff's so there is less difference between the lengths of both sides. This sandtray has a laminated white surface with a cobalt blue waterproof Perspex box fitted into the interior space. I like its proportions and the work done in it has been very powerful. The proportions of my wooden dry sandtray conform to Kalff's measurements. Inside, it is painted cerulean blue.

Two sandtrays: concrete and symbolic opposites

Jung understood the goal of therapy as enabling the opposites in the personality to approach each other, and begin to work together, to complement rather than remain in conflict (Jung, 2014, para. 705). We usually use two sandtrays with identical measurements, filled to half with either dry, flowing sand or with wet sand that can be molded. These two sandtrays are a pair of opposites, implying an unconscious mirror of opposites in the psyche. The sands are opposites of wet and dry, like opposites of sand and sea. Clients in countries with a seacoast will associate sand with the beach and may be surprised to see something as familiar as sea sand in trays in a closed setting. A client living far from a sea may react to sand in trays inside a room as magical and unfamiliar.

I collected the sand in my sandtrays long ago from the beach I usually visit. I have never changed it. I do wash it periodically. I sense its ancient memory in nature and its more current history of being touched and formed for many years in my sandtrays. In nature and in our sandtrays, sand fluctuates between being wet and dry, between being dark and light-colored. Both wet and dry sands are porous and three-dimensional, with a visible surface and unseen depth, but they move differently. Dry sand shifts easily when touched or blown upon; its impermanent form echoes involuntary change. Physical effort of the arms and hands is needed to mold wet sand. Its dark color and texture hints at deeper, darker emotions. These opposite states of sand reflect natural transitions such as rhythms of night and day, or seasonal change, and cycles of sea tides that turn dry sand into mud and recede, leaving the sun's heat to dry the sand again. Some clients resist work with sand, wet or dry. Its passivity, depth, texture and small particles that lodge like filth under the fingernails may evoke disgust, fear of penetration or touch, but also resistance to movement that brings change and transitions. Two sandtrays are sometimes used in the same session by a child or adult. The objects and scenes in each tray are usually opposites in the psyche that need separate representation at this stage. Internal conflicting states, such as aggressive or gentle feelings, inner masculine and feminine opposites, or a boy's transition from the matriarchal to a patriarchal stage, can be expressed by using two trays. Outer situations expressed in two trays may be parental divorce, leaving one location for another, or being adopted and living in a concrete present life, but having an unknown imaginary life elsewhere. Some clients use the distance between the sandtrays as a symbol, move them apart or together, sometimes bridging them with an object.

Sandtrays and wood

My sandplay studio is in my garden near many trees and plants whose leaves and branches are sometimes used in a sandplay. Wood, the gift of trees, has always been a primary resource for humans to build houses, boats, furniture such as a bed, chair or table, a coffin, or to sculpt masks, totems and religious figures such as a Madonna, a Buddha or Kwan Yin (Cooper, 1978). Scientific research reveals the botanical processes of plants and trees during night and day, their healing or poisonous properties, their fruits, underground root networks and their fungi companions. Carpenters or sculptors choose hard or soft woods for furniture or for carving. A diagnostic drawing test of a tree correlates human relationships to the way a tree's foliage, trunk and connection to earth are drawn. Consciousness and ego are projected into the structure of the trunk, to our primary caretakers in the roots and connection to earth, and to contact with the environment in branches, leaves, flowers or fruit. Trees are venerated in some cultures and in others they are seen as commercial timber. Tree lore may be forgotten, but sometimes we may feel the spirits that dwell in a favorite tree and unconsciously respond to a tree as a symbol of our human inner nature. Wood, then, is a suitable material for constructing a sandtray. A block of natural wood can also be a useful, even mysterious, symbolic natural object inside the tray.

My sandplay room

Sandplay rooms are usually rectangular, with continuous walls, a door and window. In a large room, movable sandtrays can stand in the center of the room, accessed from all sides. The shelves and miniatures, and tables for other creative work may be comfortably distant. In smaller spaces, two sandtrays are often placed side by side on a table near a wall. When a client stands to work in the sandtray, breathing and body movement are freer, and the arms can reach the entire inner space of the tray, activating movement in the psyche. While sitting, the client's small wrist movements touch less sand and access less of the space.

My small studio is shaped like an irregular rectangle. On the side facing west towards the garden, a large central window and two smaller diagonal windows on either side allow a maximum of light to enter. Under the windows of this almost "rounded" wall is a sofa for the client. The opposite wall towards the east is continuous, with no windows, so that the wet sandtray, shelves for miniatures, a small wooden stool and my wooden chair can be placed along it. Although it can't be seen, the sandplayer faces east, the birthplace of the sun each morning, when working in this tray. Sandner (1979/1991, pp.206–208) describes traditional Navajo healing chant ways that honor all directions and their properties. Sand paintings for healing are designed so a patient sits on the center facing east. The color of east is usually white. Its wider symbolism includes new beginnings, spiritual purity and the blessings that the sun may give each morning as it rises. This sandtray is used more often than the dry sandtray. With children, I tend to sit fairly close as they may ask me to participate, to hold objects or to search under the sand in the tray for something that the child hides there. When adults work in this tray, I distance my chair towards the door, take notes and sketch the image from there. At the close of work, I move my chair closer. The client faces the tray sitting on the wooden stool, and we observe together. Under a small diagonal window to the north is the dry sandtray, and above it two shelves with containers of animal figurines. The space around the sandtrays and shelves is open and accessible. On a small wall facing north-east, a chest of drawers with shelves is filled with odd objects and accessory materials. During verbal interaction, my chair remains in its place opposite the client on the sofa, facing west and the garden. Near the door on the south wall is a table for art, and a chair for the client (Figure 2.1)

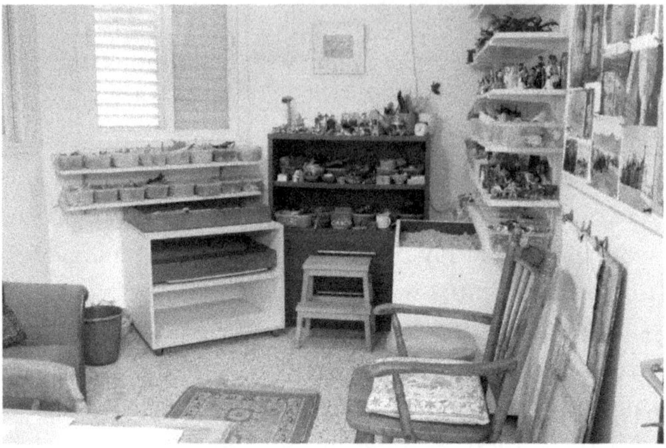

Figure 2.1 *The author's sandplay studio*

Living with the miniature collection

Miniatures can be purchased or come from the places we visit in the world, from flea markets, received as gifts or made by the therapist. They represent every culture and era throughout history and amplify our understanding of the magnitude of human outer and inner worlds. Even when our shelves are fairly full, and we have an ongoing personal relationship to objects already there, each new figurine is a source of pleasure. Today, therapists on opposite sides of the globe order figurines online from the same sources and display identical figurines on their shelves. When objects are ordered online, it may be practical to check their actual size or if they are breakable before buying. Miniatures are usually between 3 and 10 centimeters high and made of resin, plastic or sometimes metal. Glass and ceramic objects can be breakable.

As the collection grows, objects communicate with each other on the shelves and form unpredictable combinations in the sandtray. The therapist decides what to buy and where to place an object on the shelves, and notices how it is used, by whom and how its symbolic meaning varies for different clients. An object that is used by different clients in the same day or week seems to absorb multi-layered meanings and energies that pass from client to client. I have received gifts of very large objects that I would not have thought to buy—a large winged horse, huge snakes, centipedes, gorillas and goblins. I have been surprised when these large, frightening creatures become symbolically useful when children place them near tiny Smurfs, Mickey Mouse and Donald Duck. An enormous spiraling red-and-yellow centipede was placed over the center of the sandtray by two adult women in therapy at different times. The centipede may have been the only symbol that could convey the looming catastrophe and hopelessness felt by their parents as Holocaust survivors, that was silently present and absorbed during their childhoods.

My shelves

My shelves are white, which emphasizes the identity, form and colors of miniatures. They are 20 centimeters wide, which for me feels supportive and allows many figurines to share a small space. My instinct decides if I place an object free-standing or in a container, on the left or right side of a shelf, in categories or at random, on a low or high shelf. Above the wet sandtray on the lowest shelf are eight plastic boxes for various figurines of people arranged from left to right: Native Americans, women, men, babies, farm workers, dwarfs, elves and clowns, sportsmen and superheroes. The shelf above holds containers with food, furniture and small houses on the left, followed by free-standing objects of buildings, country women and men. The third shelf holds boxes for trees, flowers, vehicles, boats, airplanes, Playmobil® doctors and hospital equipment, small monsters and angels. The fourth shelf is visibly higher, filled with free-standing goddesses, musicians and fairy-tale and film characters. On the fifth shelf, figurines connected to firepower are lined up—costumed soldiers, cannons, totem poles, witches, dragons, mythological beings, but also a lone fisherman. Buddhas, Kachinas and other deities stand on the sixth and highest shelf. I may shift a container, move a figurine to another place or remove objects from a crowded shelf to a box. But unique objects always stand alone and remain at their original height. Because of the room's shape, the dry sandtray stands near a small north-facing wall with two shelves above it, holding containers of wild and domestic animals arranged from left to right in evolutionary order. Skeletons, bones, dinosaurs, amphibians, snakes, bats and rats, insects, small wild animals and farm animals inhabit the lower shelf. Above are the elephants, rhinos and hippos, bears and monkeys, tigers and lions, deer and giraffes, fish, larger sea creatures, birds and horses. On the north-east wall on a chest of drawers with shelves between the dry and wet sandtrays are accessories in containers: tiles, feathers, fabrics, wooden sticks, pebbles, mirrors, metal objects, marbles, stone eggs, crystals, corks, toothpicks and tiny musical instruments. Natural materials such as sea glass, stones, shards, shells, dried plants and fruits are arranged in baskets on the floor (Figure 2.2).

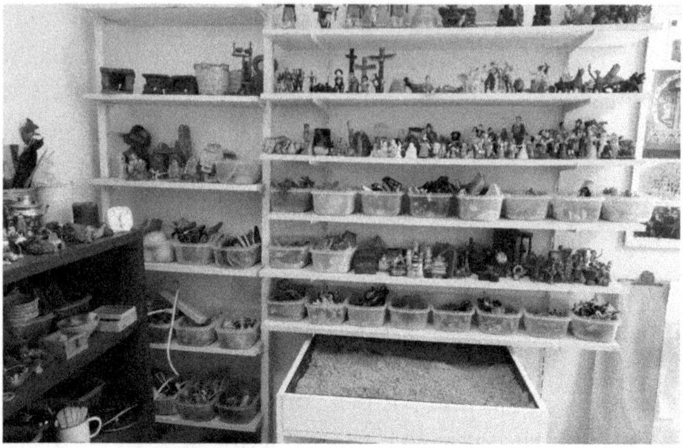

Figure 2.2 *The author's shelves*

Controversial objects

Frightening, repulsive, realistic or imaginary animals, demonic gods, monsters, snakes, bats, rats and insects need representation in a miniature collection. Their presence may upset some clients, and sometimes the therapist as well. Perhaps a smaller devil or a cartoon cockroach representing an unacknowledged shadow element in the psyche might be acceptable. Frightening objects provide the option of relating in some way to the many sides of a symbol and eventually to a clearer perception of its personal meaning. A therapist who dislikes an object can work through resistance in the personal sandplay process, in supervision or in art. But some clients might feel so threatened at the sight of a figurine of a naked woman giving birth, an unclothed goddess, a black witch, a Batman or an ethnic mask, for religious or personally traumatic reasons, that they leave the room or even stop therapy. The threatening object may have to be removed when that client is present. For me, a "Hitler" miniature is far too offensive to include on my shelves. Other figurines can represent evil, madness and cruelty. Another type of replica that might have landed on a sandplay therapist's shelf are figurines of grandiose equestrian statues placed in public places to glorify conquest, exploitation or denigration of others because of race or gender. Some of these offensive monuments are being demolished and replaced by sculptures of leaders for civil rights, women's rights, gay rights or environmental protection. Miniatures of popular monuments such as the Eiffel Tower, the Empire State Building, the Statue of Liberty, the Little Mermaid, a church, synagogue, mosque or Buddhist temple have their own historical or religious connotations. The therapist can choose what is relevant but not offensive for a client group.

Acceptance or rejection of objects, or of sand and water

It is often a pleasure to hear children express enjoyment at the option of free play with the many objects, sand and water in the sandplay setting, just for them. Some objects become emotionally attractive. A child may want to take a figurine home, trade it for one of their own toys, or just put it in a pocket. Sadly, I say that the objects belong to the room and can't leave it, but anything they draw or sculpt can be taken home at the end of their process, together with photographs of all their sandplays. Years later, in some public space, a smiling adult may approach me and tell me that they have kept all their art and sandplay photos from their childhood therapy process.

Adults seeing a sandplay setting for the first time may smile at the many figurines, gaze at the shelves, examine exotic and beautiful objects, and before sitting down, ask if this is for adults. Some casually draw their fingers through the sand in a sandtray before sitting. But a few seem to ignore the presence of the sandtrays and objects, as if they were not there. An unspoken painful aspect of childhood, dislike of touch, unpleasant memories of sand, play or objects can continue throughout therapy. If this person is occasionally attracted to a figurine to express a personal issue, it will be placed from above without the person touching the sand, which can be marked or moved with a stick or rake if necessary. Both wet sand and brown clay are materials that can provoke disgust or revulsion in some adults (and children), connected to dirt, burial, penetration of the body or uncontrolled body excretions.

On the other hand, some adults sculpt and move with the sand and rarely choose objects. Renouncing objects may be an expression of disturbing memories of lost, broken or stolen objects, objects that belonged to others, connected to longing, guilt, pain, shame and jealousy. An endless search for an object that is not there, criticism of what is there, letting something fall and break "accidentally" may be a form of deep loss, or resentment that the sandplay room is used by others. An adult who consistently chooses beautiful crystals and natural objects may be avoiding ugly or frightening objects in order to "make a good first impression" on the therapist. Later, expression of difficult material may eventually break through. But avoidance of almost all objects might reflect pain connected to objects. Absent parents may buy their children objects as a substitute for love. Toys may be left behind when a family moves, is separated or in war. Physicians distract children with toys before performing painful medical procedures, linking toys to trauma and betrayal. An adult who as a child had no toys, and learned to "do without," can fill the absence by creating everything alone in sand, forming a world just from moving the hands and sand, re-experiencing loss, with the therapist as witness (see Chapter 9).

One sandplay student began her personal sandplay process with a lecturer in her training program a few months before the teaching began. She enjoyed sandplay and was pleased that she did not have to speak. In class, her therapist presented slides of past sandplay cases, where she saw the same shelves and objects that she had used in her sandplays. She suddenly realized that the objects she chose were not hers alone, and became angry that she had to share them with others. In childhood, she had shared space, objects and her mother with her siblings. She made one final sandplay, refused to work through these shadow elements and left the sandplay training program.

Objects made by the therapist

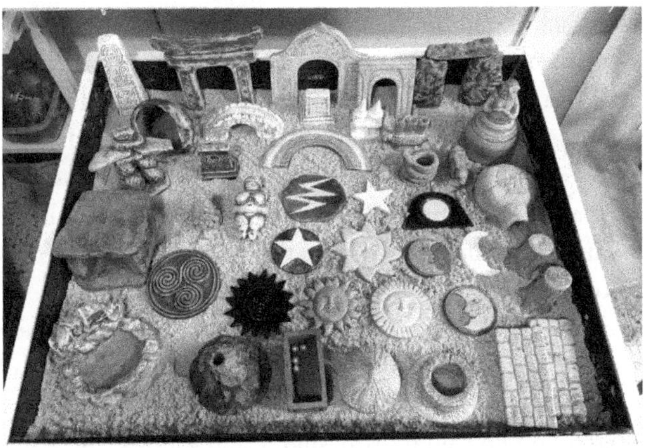

Figure 2.3 *Self-made ceramic objects*

Interesting and unique objects that I notice in case presentations or other sources are often powerful handmade symbols that can't be bought. When I sculpt with clay, I save leftover bits to make small objects for the sandtray, and glaze and fire them. Archetypal symbols such as lightning clouds, suns with differently shaped rays and different colors, phases of the moon, stars, a rainbow, portals, dolmens, stone walls, tombstones, wells, bridges, caves, tree stumps, volcanoes and campfires have an intensified presence when made of fired clay. I have made yellow, blue and black suns with rays that are straight, curved or pointed, in different widths. Each sun elicits a different emotional response. A sun is often a symbol for a parent. Warm yellow shades with wide curved rays convey warmth and love. A reddish orange can project anger. Straight rays in cool yellow seem authoritative and distant. A black sun projects a sense of trauma, hopelessness and disappointment. A blue sun can represent divine sun power. Some sandplay therapists make their own essential objects such as a house, tower, tent, well, bridge or volcano from cardboard, fabric, mosaic, wooden sticks and natural objects. Handmade objects may appear less slick than a manufactured object, but choosing them for a sandplay may reflect a comfortable transference to the therapist (Figure 2.3).

Materials that objects are made of and their origins

Much of our sandplay work honors unconscious, instinctive knowledge, archetypes, and the invisible origins of whatever exists in our current outer and inner world. The inanimate figurines on our shelves have obvious identifiable forms, but a client may select them for the material they are made of, holding and silently feeling them before placement in a sandplay. The material substance of an object and its identity co-exist, and both are part of their sandplay history. Years ago, handmade objects were formed from metal, wood, clay and glass—materials that added their character to the object's identity. Our mass-produced plastic miniatures are chosen for their identity, but not for their material. When frequently used objects such as houses, cars, certain animals, plants and mythological or film characters are made of wood, ceramic, glass or metal, these materials add to an object's symbolic range.

Sometimes, all the different objects in a sandplay are made of one material substance such as metal. The material itself then becomes a symbol. Metals have accompanied the history of human cultural development and ingenuity since the discovery that metals mined from the earth could be melted in fire and molded into permanent shapes, as coins, jewelry, tools, utensils, sculpture, weapons and toys. Metal as a symbol in sandplay can represent permanence, weight, value or even a certain god. Clay, a material made of quartz and feldspar from fine earth, can be molded, fired and transformed into hard ceramic ware, sculpture and toys. Sand is melted by fire into glass. And the sand in the sandtray has also undergone its own transformation from its original rock, coral or shell origins, pulverized into tiny grains in rivers or on the ocean's floor. But plastic, the most versatile of all materials, is produced from fossil fuel, with origins in the plants of the vast primeval forests of 500 million years ago, that decomposed under heat and pressure beneath the earth's crust. In 1907, Belgian-American chemist

Leo Baekeland manufactured Bakelite, the first plastic, from oil. His success led to mass production of useful objects made of Bakelite that could be molded and colored, and to the invention of all the forms of plastic in use today. Identical figurines are produced in quantity and are purchased by all sandplay therapists to fit any role our clients imagine for them. Their sandplay history co-exists with the hidden primeval origins of oil.

The horses of sandplay

Horse figurines are popular as sandplay symbols. Horses combine intelligence and emotion, physical strength, grace and beauty of movement. Horse miniatures range from medieval to military, from farm to race horses, from simple differently colored plastic horses with different positions to Chinese blue ceramic horses and purple or pink cartoon horses with long manes that children like to brush. Mythological centaurs, such as Chiron, the wounded healer, white unicorns, and the winged white horse Pegasus elevate horse symbolism to relationships between body and spirit.

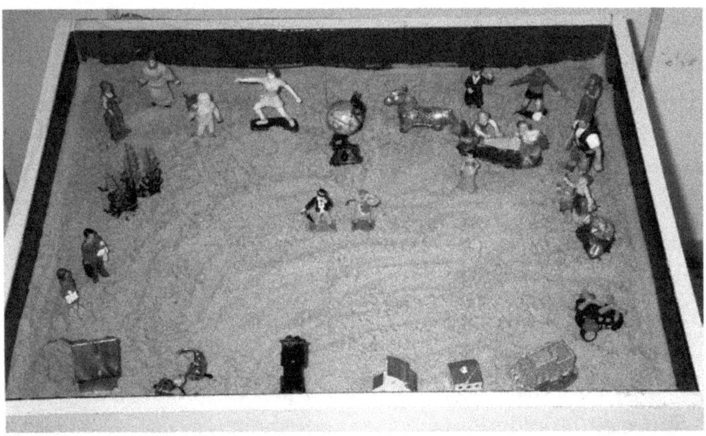

Figure 2.4 *Dina: Final sandplay, mandala with archaic horse*

A middle-aged woman mourning a son who had been killed in war, wore dark clothes and almost never went out to visit her relatives. When social services offered her sandplay, she agreed. In each session, she slowly and silently formed a large circle of human figurines on the sand without touching it. In her fifteenth sandplay, she lined up three vertical rows of 14 plastic horses and placed the fifteenth, an elegant white horse with a brown mane, slightly apart from the others. In another sandplay, she lined up a group of soccer players, with one soccer player falling down. I felt that the white horse and the falling soccer player represented her son. Later, towards the end of her Sandplay process, she constructed a large family circle and placed figurines representing herself and her husband in the center. Just above them, without comment, she placed an archaic silver metal horse that for me resembled a monument honoring her deceased son (Figure 2.4). (Steinhardt, 2000, p.160).

Constancy and hidden energies that remain in the physical sandplay environment

Over the years, the same sand may remain in the sandtrays, and many familiar miniatures remain in their places on the shelves, like a secure anchor that balances the changes in a client's inner and outer worlds. Small changes, such as adding new miniatures, may be spotted immediately by some clients, while others will notice something that has been on the shelf for years and ask if it was always there. And sometimes an object unused for years is chosen by two people in the same day or week, or the same sand forms or combinations of miniatures appear in different clients' sandplays. A client might exchange one object for another during a sandplay, repeated by the next client with almost the same objects as if the energy was somehow transferred. Meanwhile, the expanding content of the therapist's unconscious becomes a multi-layered reservoir of knowledge, memories and energies that blend together sandplay images and meanings from past and present. The life in the object, in the sand, in the therapist's unconscious and in other entities that may be present seems to be absorbed into the unconscious activity of a present client. Hegeman (1992, p.103) quotes Alexander Von Berghes who describes the atmosphere of the sandplay room and the miniature collection as a balance between several inner and outer worlds that connect the inner and outer worlds of therapist and patient. At the end of a session, Von Berghes returns the figurines to their places and, in Native American tradition, thanks them for the work they have done. He also thanks the spirits of place and whatever entities dwell there.

3

Variations in the Sandplay Setting

Therapists who study sandplay have already attained professional therapeutic status in verbal or arts-based therapy. They may wish to add the sandplay setting to their existing work space as a practical option. When combining two fundamentally different therapies with different settings in a single environment, clear boundaries are needed to protect the integrity of each discipline. In a verbal therapist's clinic, lighting may be indirect; a comfortable chair for the client is placed opposite the therapist near a table with a few interesting objects on it, bookshelves filled with professional literature on a wall behind. The proximity of a sandplay area to the client's chair might divert a client's contemplative thought towards active play. If the client is working in the sandtray, the chair's presence might be a cue to verbalization rather than a focus on silent hand movement and sensory creativity. A screen divider, a wall or doors can separate the analytic area and the creative sandplay area.

Sandplay and creative arts therapy are both are non-verbal therapies that use materials for creative symbolization, but their methods and goals are different. Clear spatial boundaries and separate areas are essential when sandplay is included in the creative art therapy setting. Creative arts studios are well lit for art activity with materials in view, a sink for water and clean-up and tables, easels, walls and floors for making art. Art therapists encourage directive exploration of feelings and emotional blocks with materials. This helps to lessen anxiety and develop self-awareness, social skills and self-esteem. Releasing aggression through materials is permitted, such as pouring paint within boundaries, tearing paper or throwing clay at targets. Sandplay therapists are silent and often indirect. Silent witnessing and delayed interpretation with no obvious intervention, is central to sandplay and allows the senses and the unconscious to lead, through choice, touch and hand movement. When a sandtray is close by and accessible, this may be construed as permission to spill paint or throw clay into the sand, remove sand to mix with glue or paint on paper or on clay, or paint miniatures with gouache as part of a construction. This contaminates sandplay materials and compromises the symbolic potential of a sandplay process. In a shared setting, the "free and protected" space intertwines with a co-transference between therapist and client on the conscious and unconscious levels. Some sort of separation would protect against the fusion of two non-verbal methods. A therapist might be aware of differences between his or her non-verbal participation in healing and any verbal or creative expressive exploration of wounding.

Setting up a sandplay clinic, sandtrays, miniatures and other objects in various contexts

Kalff's clinic with two sandtrays and hundreds of miniatures standing on shelves has become the guideline for sandplay therapists. Beyond that, chairs, tables, rugs, pillows and other accessories are added by each therapist. In cold climates, some therapists install heaters under their sandtrays so the client's hands touch warm sand. In the past, sandtrays, stands and shelves made of wood were ordered from carpenters. The particular blue hue painted on the inner surface of the tray could be waterproofed or made of Perspex. Today, when purchasing a sandtray online it is practical to check the measurements, the inner blue hue and waterproofing of sandtrays. The width of a sandtray rim, when 1.5 centimeters or ¾ inch allows the rims to function as boundaries that protect inner content, or become a symbolic horizon for amorphous space beyond the tray.

Miniatures are easily purchased in quantity on the internet and shipped directly to one's home. An entire collection arrives all at once and quickly fills the shelves. The therapist's relationship to large groups of new objects may be less personal than to those objects that were collected slowly. Unique, beautiful and interesting objects impress clients who may enjoy "possessing" them for a moment in the sandtray, but they can be seductive. "Beautiful" sand pictures might conceal creative uncertainty, resistance to expression of pain, unwillingness to allow a therapist to witness shadow imagery or allow the Self to lead. "Beautiful" objects may disappear. I once noticed that a large diamond, a green jade Kwan Yin and an ostrich egg were no longer in their usual places. They were never found. Other objects are sometimes taken without permission not for their beauty but because of a strong emotional attachment to them (Talamini, 2010).

Sandplay therapists who work in schools, hospitals and public facilities may face a range of populations, limited budgets and space shared with other therapists. Plastic sandtrays or other containers will be accompanied by inexpensive miniatures, natural objects, contributions of toys or objects made by the therapist. They may have to work with small groups of children and provide separate sandtrays. External noise, the view from a window or the path that leads to the sandplay room are out of the therapist's control. One sandplay therapist working with inner-city adolescents in a neighborhood clinic kept a box of broken part-objects and body parts for these children who expressed their lives in the sandtray more with damaged rather than perfect miniatures. In the closed adolescent ward of a psychiatric hospital, an art and sandplay therapist secured a small room and gave lectures to various donors so she could purchase good-quality sandtrays and miniatures. During art therapy sessions, she covered the sandtrays and hid the miniatures with a curtain that was moved aside for those who were able to work in sandplay (Abramovich, 2015).

In facilities for developmentally delayed children and others with special needs, children may be referred before the age of two. One therapist saw very young children climb into a sandtray on a low table and sit inside, with no interest in the sand. She left two sandtrays with sand on tables and placed a third empty tray on the floor. The children sat in the empty tray and brought miniatures with them to play inside. A few sessions later, they began to stand and place the miniatures in a sandtray on a table. An art and sandplay therapist noticed that small children were afraid to draw on large paper (50 x 70 cm) about the same size as the sandtray. She offered three different sizes of paper, and many children chose the smallest size. She then added two sandtrays, each smaller than the other, in the same rectangular proportions for the children to choose from, from small to the largest standard sandtray. In a school for children with serious physical disabilities who used wheelchairs, or who were unable to communicate verbally, the sandplay therapist placed a stand for a sandtray on the children's wheelchairs, close to a child's vision. The children could touch the sand and indicate where to put the miniatures they chose. A few children were able to undergo a sandplay process with some symbolization.

Unexpected situations can arise in ordinary sandplay settings, such as a child's sudden urge to throw sand or scatter miniatures around the room. This may not be dangerous but it does challenge the therapist to preserve the setting, maintain a positive attitude and identify the emotion behind the act. Large plastic sheets on the floor can be placed under the sandtrays to collect the fallen sand so it can be returned to the tray. Dumping miniatures may surprise the therapist who has told the child, "You can use these objects in any way you want." For a child, this might be an authentic expression of an undifferentiated primal state, although a child (or adult) may dump deliberately, unconcerned that the therapist must return everything to its place later.

The fire and water of nature may need to find a place in the sandtray

Extreme imbalance when using either fire or water in the sandtray can be dangerous. Both elements challenge the therapist to find safe expressive solutions and identify the emotional origins of uncontrolled expression through them. In ancient Greece, fire was kept alive by vestal virgins in temples devoted to Hestia, Goddess of the Hearth, and in the Athenian household by the women of the family. If the fire died out, it could bode ill for the city. Men were the carriers and keepers of fire in a similar tradition in indigenous Native American communities (Kimmerer, 2013, p.364). In Chinese medicine, the body's life depends on the warmth, light and energy of the fire element, connected to the heart and the small intestine, delegating warmth to its flows and excretions (Connelly, 1994). In nature, fire appears as the sun, stars, lightning, volcanoes or spontaneous combustion. Fire cooks and transforms food, burns dead flora to clear land, burns bridges in war, releases fragrances from burnt plants for incense and purification, releases spirit from the body in cremation after death, although heretics and witches were punished by fire while alive. A circle of people around a bonfire energizes a sense of community. Candles, a safer form of fire, are lit on birthdays or as commemoration for someone departed. Their smoke rises and reveals the movement of air as it disappears.

A depressed young boy entered therapy four years after his mother awoke from a year-long coma after an operation. She returned home, suddenly reborn and alive but with limited functioning (Steinhardt, 2013, p.167). He would stack objects one on top of the other in the sandtray and hang things in the air above them. In his eleventh session, he hung five butterflies, a spider and a bird's nest over the dry tray. Suddenly, the electricity went off. I lit several candles, and soon he moved them underneath the butterflies until the session ended. In the next session, he lit candles, melted wax with the fire, then hung birds and a nest in the air over them. He sat a fisherman on the front-right corner edge, fishing in a well on the sand and said, "Everything is high except the well." In his thirteenth session, he placed 13 objects in the tray that were symbolically connected to fire—six kachinas, four witches and three small dragons—and lit several candles with matches. The rising smoke became for him a magical genie. He asked the genie to grant his wish for a happy life and to become a good soccer player.

A married woman expressed anger and pain with fire in the sandtray. She had fallen in love with a co-worker, a married gay man. She drew symbols of her feelings on pieces of paper, inserted them between mounds in the sandtray and burned them with many matches until only black ash remained. The sand had to be washed later to clear the ash and the burnt smell.

In Chinese philosophy, all forms of water are believed to be controlled by dragons that are usually symbols of luck and success. Water is usually in constant movement and change, from vapor to flow or to ice when thawing, as well as flooding. Stagnant water becomes putrid. Two-thirds of the human body consists of water. Water is the womb of all life. Human emotions are expressed by release of liquids, tears, saliva, sweat, vomit, urine and diarrhea from different body organs. Even a small amount of water in the wet sandtray can accelerate a need to express endless tears and sorrow by flooding. Excess water can demolish sand constructions in the sandtray, but water can safely overflow when a small plastic tub is placed within a larger tub that can contain the excess water. Water is sometimes used ceremonially in the sandtray to purify and clean. A six-year-old boy orphaned of his father needed deep water. He filled a tub for many sessions, then floated boats or drowned masculine figurines, until he was able to work again with solid forms in the sandtray. A hyperactive seven-year-old boy suddenly flooded his first carefully built sandplay, and watched as the rocks and sand collapsed. After the session, he opened the water hoses in my garden and released a flood. Unfortunately, his parents ended therapy without notice. His flooded collapsed sand may have mirrored something that he unconsciously knew: that his attempts to express something of value in himself would be terminated too soon.

Catastrophic disasters and war, and improvised sandplay settings to treat large group trauma

The sudden shock from earthquakes, tsunamis, erupting volcanoes, train or airplane collisions and war create havoc and trauma for hundreds of people simultaneously. Immediate action on personal and community levels is needed to treat confusion, the sense of helplessness, pain, loss and despair. Therapeutic first aid after exposure to catastrophic trauma can prevent the danger of post-traumatic stress disorder (PTSD). Short-term sandplay interventions that reached as many trauma victims as possible were organized for children in New York City schools immediately following the terrorist attack on the World Trade Center on 9/11. A form of sandplay known as "symbol formation" was introduced, carried out by teachers and others who were given on-the-spot training for work with large groups of people in response to the attack (Winter, 2002). In 2018 in Hawaii, when Mount Kilauea erupted, mobile sandplay therapy units were organized to respond to individual and group disorientation in improvised therapy centers (Freedle *et al.*, 2021).

On February 24th, 2022, Russia invaded Ukraine, forcing thousands of Ukrainians to flee their country. Some found refuge in Israel, where they were housed in hotels and received food, clothing, schooling for the children and therapeutic support from Ukrainian-speaking therapists. Art and sandplay therapy were offered in improvised creative studios. Those who decided to remain in Israel found themselves facing another war, that began at 6 a.m. on October 7th, 2023, with an unprecedented terrorist attack on civilian communities on the southern border of Israel. Villages were blown up, homes pillaged, and civilians of all ages kidnapped. Thousands of traumatized survivors hidden in bomb shelters were exposed to sounds of unimaginable brutality, mutilation and killing. Later evacuated to hotels, they were provided with emergency medical care, food, clothing and therapeutic services by government agencies and volunteers. Schooling and activities for the children were immediately organized, to allow parents time to grieve, receive support and re-orient themselves. Members of the Israeli Sandplay Therapists Association (ISTA) set up open sandplay rooms in many hotels, equipped with individual tables with donated small plastic sandtrays and tables with boxes filled with miniature objects. Several sandplay therapists were present in each room, as individuals or groups might wander in at any time. As a child approached a sandtray, chose miniatures and silently created a scene in the sand, other children might do the same or play on the floor while a mother sat silently on the side. After several weeks, scheduled sessions enabled therapists to give personal attention to children who might want to tell a story of their scenes. Recurring symbols such as Israeli flags, small and large soldiers, superhero figurines, tanks, missiles, ambulances, rows of cars, fences, shelters, watch towers and umbrellas were prevalent in many initial sandtrays. In some, heavy greenery hid upheaval and destruction depicted on the sand below. In later sandplays, greenery, ordinary people, household and marketplace scenes and symbolic water returned, like a glimmer of resilience, emotional strength and sense of control. Group supervision helped the therapists understand their own feelings, consciously and unconsciously, and recurring symbols in the traumatic images of shock and fear or denial that they had repeatedly witnessed and absorbed.

PART TWO

NATURAL FORCES IN A WIDER WORLD

4

Nature and Its Teachers, Observation and Differentiation

Appreciation, reverence and gratitude for nature's gifts

James Hillman points to the illusion of human superiority over nature and the human reverence for consciousness that would free us from nature and the unconscious. This misunderstanding has resulted in denial of dependency on the fundamental gifts of nature—air, water, earth, plants and animals. Lack of appreciation of the beauty of our earth has furthered the slow destruction of its natural resources (Hillman, 1990, pp.69, 253, 293). But nature and animals remain in our unconscious and in our dreams, and might be accompanied by a sense of loss. For Hillman, psyche, the anima mundi, the world soul is in all things. Everything is alive and in psyche; we are in psyche rather than psyche being in us. All animals, with their "miraculous shapes and behaviors" (Hillman, 1990, p.70) have something to teach, before we label them as symbols or place them in a sandplay as a miniature object. Living with reverence for the power and beauty of animals is the purpose of much of the ancient art of Central and South America, or the half-animal, half-human gods of ancient Egyptian art. In sandplay, psyche reconnects us to the natural world and to unconscious memory. A simple plastic replica of an animal might activate a longing for a dream interaction with animals who speak, a hunger for a guardian totem animal and spirit guide, or a plan to adopt an unusual animal as a pet and remember one's relationship to nature.

Animal teachers

Natural environments are shared by humans and other more-than-human entities, earth, water, rock, plants and animals. All living creatures have their own forms of consciousness and subjective experience of themselves which develop through interactions with their surroundings. Although we can never really understand what the interior world of an animal is like, a child, for example, may choose a shark or whale miniature for a sandplay, accompanied by sound and movement as if enacting the experience of being a whale or shark. Indigenous peoples comprehended all their co-inhabitants as being animate, listened to their languages and observed their lifestyles and changes through the seasons of the year (Kimmerer, 2013). Animals developed life-survival patterns, defended their territories, built habitats, played, mated, raised and protected their young, and established a niche for themselves in their surroundings. The vegetarians among them differentiated between edible plants and those that were poisonous, hallucinatory or medicinal. Their composite knowledge and behaviors guided human understanding of the reciprocal relationships between all species, plant and animal. Humans transposed this knowledge into stories, myths, superstitions and predictions. An owl's hoot might be warning of imminent death, but its hunting accuracy in the dark and wide range of vision made it Athena's symbol of wisdom. The eagle, symbol of her father Zeus, soars higher than any other bird in circles towards the sun, in a symbolic connection with the Great Spirit. It is also a precise, aggressive hunter, monogamous for life and tender when feeding its chicks (Ronnberg and Martin, 2010). Fair or stormy weather could be predicted according to the height of a certain bird's flight, or a frog's evening song that welcomed a pleasant new day. The coming winter might be hard if ant hills were built high in July, if spiders spun larger webs than usual, if squirrels cached nuts in many hiding places before hibernation. The architectural craft wisdom of mollusks, birds, insects and small mammals, taught humans about materials, and about safe and aesthetic habitats and form as function. Animal clan guardians were honored in tribal dance, in portable carved amulet sculptures and on carved cedar wood totem poles that protected a clan and also accessed their guardian's potency. On the north-west coast of North America and Canada, totem poles in one clan portray eagle, hawk, raven, whale, bear, beaver or frog with large and staring eyes, while in another clan, piercing slanted eyes are emphasized. Eagle's high gaze encompasses a wide perspective, bear looks forward, beaver observes small details. Our animal figurines unobtrusively represent the wisdom acquired by each species for survival. They gift our sandplay images for our benefit and psychic survival in our own environment (The Canadian Encyclopedia, 2017).

Sandplay trainees research two symbol papers for certification and at first may be attracted to power animals such as owl, eagle, lion, snake, dolphin or whale. Animals are amplified through symbol dictionaries, biology, myth, the arts, Jungian theory and sandplay literature. Observation or experience of the singularity of an animal in nature is less common, but when possible, endows understanding. Similar species such as dog, wolf, fox, jackal and coyote all retain the general characteristics of their common ancestor. But their individual natures have diverged in response to specific environments and as a symbol are not interchangeable. Whales, dolphins, seals and walruses are mammals that returned to the sea at some point in their evolution. In symbol papers, they are sometimes mistakenly labeled as "fish," misunderstanding their evolution, lifestyles, intelligence, group loyalty and ability to navigate entire oceans. Post-menopausal grandmother whales help young whale mothers to care for their young for years. Their great size makes them symbols of the womb and rebirth. In cultures dependent on the sea, they are worshipped as gods and celebrated in totems and temples. In sandplay, whales and dolphins can symbolize instinctual ability to navigate the unconscious.

Various animal objects are chosen by different clients, but those that are alive in the therapist's psyche may resonate more strongly in the client's unconscious. A bear and a grasshopper have been part of my inner and outer reality for many years. I first envisioned bear as a guide to fishing and healing with plant medicines, and later was healed by him in Bear Medicine Workshops. Later, two grasshoppers jumped into my sandtray in a workshop, facing each other and sharing information about the events on each side of the sandtray. Then, in a shamanic workshop, a huge silent grasshopper presented himself as my teacher, and a few years later, a large grasshopper attached himself to my window for a few hours. Recently, while sitting on a shady bench at the beach, three ravens perched on the bench near me, turned in unison towards the eastern sun, opened their mouths wide and remained in this position for a long time, even when I photographed them. When they left, their gait was clumsy, but their transition to flight was smooth and powerful. I understood these happenings as invitations to sculpt these animals in clay. When a sandplay client chooses a bear, grasshopper or raven, I sense a deep co-transference of unconscious communication, an unspoken "resonance" (Ammann, 1994), or connection through the "underground river" that flows between one unconscious and another (Oda, 1997).

I also recall how a woman transferred her interaction with an animal miniature to an idealization of a dog in her childhood reality. During art and sandplay therapy, she realized that when at a young age she had been sent to live in a foster home, it was because of her parents' inability to raise her and not through any fault of her own. She then recalled her love for a small dog and found a similar dog, ill and neglected, at an animal shelter. She proudly nursed him back to health but decided not to have him trained, as she loved his free instinctual nature. When he barked at people and other dogs on outdoor walks, she proclaimed, "Nobody messes with him." He began to bite and had to be muzzled, and at home she began to feel threatened by him. By now, he was too old to train out of his regressive instinctual behavior and she had to place him in a "foster home," a boarding home for dogs, where she visited him regularly from behind a fence

Differentiation between nature's creations and imaginary cartoon creatures

Since the birth of Mickey Mouse in 1928 at the Walt Disney Studios in California, children have grown up with cartoons of animals, superheroes and aliens from other planets, and participate in their battles between good and evil. The superheroes of my childhood—Superman, Batman, Spiderman, Captain Marvel, and Wonder Woman—live again today alongside the New Mutants, Power Rangers and Guardians of the Galaxy. They still conceal their secret identity and protect civilization from unimaginable disaster. Superheroes and cartoon animals now speak many languages and enter our lives in films, comics and books, as toys, mechanical pets and as figurines in sandplay. Real animals can be seen at a zoo or farm, or in films about animals that can be compassionate but often grimly violent. On our sandplay shelves, cartoon animal figurines may outnumber biologically accurate representations of animals that still exist in wild nature. Lion, tiger, horse, bear, eagle, raven, bat, wolf, fox, snake, frog, mouse, whale, crocodile, in authentic miniature representations, may become "endangered species" on the sandplay shelves, outnumbered by cartoon creatures.

Plant teachers, the therapist-gardener, differentiation and the sandtray soul-garden

The enormous biodiversity of plant species in nature is the foundation of strong and balanced ecosystems. In our sandplay collection, plant miniatures are more limited, represented by several general categories of trees, bushes and grasses, and various flowers. Some of my clients have preferred live plants from my garden for a sandplay. Gardeners observe seasonal plants as they grow, flower and die in unison, returning nutrients stored in their bodies and roots to the earth. Deciduous trees annually release their leaves to the earth to decay and feed new growth, and the gardener who collects them into a compost heap becomes aware of the time it takes for natural rot until decaying leaves become fertilizer.

Fungi form another vast natural category of life which is neither animal nor plant, whose representatives can be microscopic or huge in size, who produce poisons, hallucinogens and healing medicines, and are silently active in affecting plant and animal forms of life. In natural environments such as forests, fungi form huge underground networks along the root systems of plants, and transform matter into nutrients that feed new plant life (Sheldrake, 2020). Growing interest in mushroom species as food and scientific research into the helpful or destructive presence of fungi in all life processes have provided more precise information on this life form. Mushroom miniatures in sandplay are often limited to cute conical spotted, red-topped types, which in actual nature may be poisonous or hallucinatory. Perhaps sandplay therapists could add other mushroom forms and colors to their shelves. In natural environments, plant species engage among themselves in reciprocal communication, much of it underground. The life process of each plant balances that of other plants in a territory and contributes its special chemistry to the environment. Plant lovers differentiate between plant personalities, their botanic intelligence and interconnectedness in the wild (Kimmerer, 2013; Calvo and Lawrence, 2022). And gardeners know each plant's life cycle, and its season for sowing or planting, in wait for a seedling to ready itself for its day of birth and ascend above earth to fulfill its destined life cycle.

Ammann (1994) transposes the gardener's knowledge into the symbolic language of the psyche in sandplay. She views the garden as a space that bridges nature and culture, and calls the sandtray a soul-garden, bridging the client's unconscious and consciousness, as a meeting place for the conscious and unconscious energies of the therapist and the client. The therapist–master gardener can relate to psychic growth in therapy as a natural cyclical process. In a therapeutic process, there will be at some point an unavoidable stage of metaphorical death, although at the same time an unnoticed seed containing a new life force can form and then transition to rebirth. The sandplay client is an apprentice gardener in the sandtray soul-garden, and unconsciously resonates with a therapist's understanding of healing and growth. Cycles of arid sand, watering, and preparation for growth appear in the sandtray before images of greening, grass, trees, branching out, flowers and fruit appear. Greening marks the return of life purpose, to grow and heal the soul in the sandtray. These stages parallel the physical and psychological processes and patterns we share with nature.

First tasks: becoming observant, differentiating, sorting

The first task of Psyche, the beautiful mortal heroine in the Greek myth of Eros and Psyche, was to sort a huge mound of different grains and seeds into separate piles by the end of the day. Aphrodite, Goddess of Love, was jealous of this young girl who was worshipped as more beautiful than she and instructed her son Eros to cause Psyche to fall in love with a monster. But Eros had Zephyr, the West Wind, abduct Psyche to his palace, and visited her each night, leaving before daylight (see Chapter 11). Psyche's sisters claimed that Eros was a monster, and encouraged her to see him at night while he slept. Psyche lit an oil lamp and gazed upon beautiful Eros, her hand trembling in awe. A drop of hot oil fell on his shoulder, waking and wounding him. In anger, he flew off to his mother, who decreed that if Psyche (who was pregnant with her grandchild) could complete four impossible tasks, the couple could reunite. A troop of ants helped Psyche to sort a mound of different seeds in her first task. Sorting can be done visually, noticing size, shape and color. But ants have a strong olfactory sense that may have helped them to differentiate between the seeds. Psyche became aware of differentiation, separated herself from her sisters and embarked on a path of individuation (Neumann, 1971).

The sandplayer's first task: passive observation and differentiation

A sandplayer gazes, moves the eyes over the figurines on the sandplay shelves and observes. Then an object differentiates itself from others, becomes unique, returns one's gaze and chooses you. Shamdasani (2015) describes Jung's emphasis on passive but careful observation in his practice of active imagination, contemplating the spontaneous changes of the image itself and allowing things to happen. A shaman's journey begins with a gaze, to identify a cave or hole somewhere through which one descends to the underground realm of the collective unconscious or ascends to the sky realm. There, one waits, gazes and accepts whatever entity presents itself. A spirit animal may give something, or wait for other animals to appear and communicate by their actions (Harner, 1990; Ingerman, 2008; Gallegos, 1987). The entire sandplay setting is both a physical and "other world" environment. Gazing at an object differentiates it from others, and can empower it to confer its gifts silently as an intermediary in the interchange between the sandplayer's consciousness and the collective unconscious.

5

Creative Urgency, a Human Legacy

Creative urgency in art and in sandplay: emptiness and fullness

Where will the image come from? The sandtray space is indeterminate and empty. A line drawn by a finger on the sand may imply a direction. Perhaps conscious choice of an object will lower one's trepidation and yield to an intention known to the unconscious. The process of connection to an image can be erratic, generate unrest and a sense of urgency to grasp an indescribable feeling and give it substance, as an image that can rest in the sandtray space. Artists and sandplay therapists that have experienced the unconscious transition to a clear creative moment can hold on to the belief that there is an inner intangible, indestructible creative spark deep within that will be reignited and fill a void with an image.

A shell unearthed in Indonesia dated at 600,000 years ago was scratched with a geometric zigzag design attributed to *Homo erectus*, a species that emerged in Africa about two million years ago, reached the island of Java, and became extinct around 140,000 years ago. At that time, a single individual experienced a confluence of conscious awareness and a creative urge to incise a movement on a hard durable surface, a sea shell. Once accomplished, this act may have inspired another creative act, with increased control and skill (Callaway, 2014). Archaeologists dig up utensils, tools, weapons and spiritual portable carvings. The incised or painted images that they discover on cave walls, stone, bone, ivory or wood confirm that on every continent except Antarctica, *Homo sapiens* invested time, effort and precision in making functional aesthetically crafted objects. In caves separated by continents, in Spain, France and South America, skillfully drawn images of animals from about 37,000 years ago may have served as hunting magic empowered by shamanic ritual. They confirm the great value attributed to craftsmanship and the efforts made to mine metal-based pigments from distant sources and process them through fire (Violatti, 2021; Bahn and Lorblanchet, 2017). American Northwest Coast indigenous artists carved wooden totem poles that gave presence to numinous totem animal ancestors, from the early 1800s. Early totem poles may have naturally decayed, but clan ancestors such as Whale, Eagle, Raven, Wolf and Bear continue to take their place on new totem poles and hold a group together today. These beneficent great nature spirits have eyes, beaks, hands, claws and wings that are carved to emphasize their power. Without the presence of these carved totem ancestors, life might be experienced as vulnerable, unprotected and incomplete. A spiritual center constellates around them when humans gather to speak their myths and enact their ritual in song and movement.

Sandplay, creative urgency, nurturance, love, food and fullness

Food is central to much of our activity in life. It is an absolute necessity that fills the body and sustains our physical world. It connects to land, agriculture and nature, or to supermarkets and restaurants. Its infinite variety is often a source of excitement that has elevated basic sustenance into a form of opulent pleasure. I live in Israel, where traditional and ethnic dishes are mainstays of holiday gatherings and family dinners, where mothers, fathers and grandparents invest days preparing their specialties for the extended family visit. Familiar aromas and olfactory memories connect food to love and family, but also evoke the shadowy underside of human relationships. Hunger imposed by difficult circumstances can be experienced as emptiness and suffering, both physical and symbolic, as if the world does not attend to one's needs. Food can also become a cultural obsession about the body and a method of control. When eating becomes repellent, it can symbolize an emotional reaction to undigestible emotional material, with no words that can describe it. Abstaining from food or regurgitating it after overeating can destroy the body and may replace expressing emotions outwardly or dull them.

But in art, food as nurturance and pleasure has always been immortalized, in ancient cave paintings of edible animals, carved images of grains, animals and kitchen scenes on the tomb walls of Egyptian Pharaohs, in opulent Roman mosaics, or in 16th-century Dutch paintings. Paul Cezanne in the late 19th century eternalized apples, Andy Warhol celebrated soup cans in the 1960s (Warhol and Figura, 2022) and Claes Oldenburg's voluptuous soft sculptures of pastries, fruit and hamburgers extol street food (Oldenburg and Oldenburg, 1992). Banquet tables are decorated with sculptures made of colorful fresh fruits and vegetables. Garbage, the end-product of commercial food packaging, has been transformed into art by sculptor Vik Muniz. He employed garbage pickers at a huge landfill in Brazil to collect thousands of food packaging waste products which he used to create enormous mosaics on the ground, of portraits of famous people and copies of paintings. He then photographed these from a high viewpoint (Muniz, 2010).

In the sandtray, a therapist might apply symbolic meaning to food items. Food is physical nurturance from the earth, from the archetypal Great Earth Mother, and in therapy is symbolic nurturance as love or the need for love from a primal caretaker. It can represent therapeutic nurturance and a growing ability for self-nurturance or self-love. Food miniatures are usually realistic small or large versions of fruits, vegetables, plates of cooked meals and dishes with sandwiches, cakes and desserts. The sandtray's inner space is a "bowl," a receptacle for any object that fills it. Food objects may be intended to be "just food" in a sandplay, perhaps food that is tasty, or that mother prepares, or does not allow, or as a desire or memory. Empty sand can be sensed as incomplete, mirroring a yearning to be filled with something missing, a physical, spiritual or emotional nurturance that any object can represent. Physically, an emotional void can be dulled temporarily by inserting real food into the body. But the emptiness of the sand in the sandtray rather than the body or the heart can be resolved symbolically by creatively filling the tray. Being able to fill an empty sandtray with a self-created image, including food objects, may bring joy and satisfaction. Inner emotional hunger is transformed and viewed as an external protected outer image. Time is invested in "preparing" the image, observing and ingesting it symbolically. A creative spark can be reignited with each sandplay, and can fill the empty hungry heart of the sand, with objects and forms that represent a theme of that day, bestowing symbolic nurturance on oneself in a visual image that began as a void.

6

A Wider World: Pilgrimages, Quests and Transformation

Earth energies and power spots

Earth environments can generate a sense of belonging and attachment in the unconscious of those who live in them, a reciprocal relationship with a local plot of land (Wheelwright and Schmidt, 1991). I experience this phenomenon each time I fly back to visit my New York birthplace. As the plane goes into landing mode above the Verrazano Bridge, I see below the small beach community at the tip of Brooklyn where I grew up. My body cells seem to compact themselves in recognition of this place that also recognizes me. In other countries, I experience a bodymind response to congenial or unsympathetic energies of place. I re-experience favorable sensations and memories of New York, San Francisco, Vancouver, Paris, Tibet or Montana as flashes of consciousness, as if a part of me is still in contact with those places.

Especially beautiful mountains, caves, waterfalls, springs and unusual rock formations are often considered "power spots." Shrines and temples are built there. Colossal temples in Yucatan, Asia Minor, India, Cambodia and Malta seem to have been constructed by colossal beings for humans. Researchers have posited that the sites of these temples were chosen because they sit on energy vortexes, points of intersection in a global energetic network of invisible "ley lines," powerful sources of earth energy (Newman, 2018). Their size emulates towering mountains whose axes are thought to hold the world together. Their structures are coordinated with points of transition of the sun and moon across the skies at certain times of the year. Each of these sites inspires pilgrimage for individuals or groups, a journey towards a chosen destination of spiritual significance, and an experience of transformation of the psyche (Devereux, 1990; Gray, 2007). The juncture of a river and a sea is also a power spot. Pure water descends from the sky as rain or snow, symbolizing a masculine penetrating spirit, and creates rivers, while feminine sea water contains minerals as in the human womb, and represents the unconscious. The meeting of these two waters integrates masculine and feminine, spirit and the unconscious. In the sandtray, "river" water joins sand from the sea, creating a symbolic "power spot."

Both quests and pilgrimages guide us towards a wider world. A quest, like a pilgrimage, begins with a journey. But unlike a pilgrimage, the destination of a quest can be unclear, not necessarily a place as a goal but a state of being within a place. The quests of the sandplay therapist and the sandplay client are intertwined, and for both, the material outer world and the illuminated inner world become wider, fuller and more fascinating as the journey continues. The history and energies of a sandplay environment itself and the energies absorbed in the therapist's psyche can permeate a client's sandplay quest, a journey through an inner landscape that leads towards clearer options. Two young women in my extended family, now adults after their army service, planned a year-long travel quest before going to university. Both had experienced sandplay therapy during a difficult period of latency. One chose the direction of the Far East, the other South America. Their choices were influenced by travel companions, friends' recommendations, family ties and cost, but underlying these was an attraction to the energy of a specific landscape, culture, language, type of food or music. On the road, they stayed longer in places where they felt more comfortable. One girl traveled through India, Nepal, Cambodia and South Korea where she felt "at home" and stayed on with local families. The second girl traveled through Argentina, Chile, Brazil, Bolivia and Peru. As an adolescent, she had learned some Spanish from watching an Argentinian television series called *Chiquititas*. She stayed on in Cuzco studying Spanish by day and dancing Salsa at night. A year of independent living in unfamiliar places reinforced both girls' trust in their intuition and authentic inner self. In retrospect, they recalled the flexible control and spontaneity of their sandplay experience as similar to their adjustment to unplanned events during their trips. After their return home, they both enrolled at a university far from home and continued their friendships with their travel companions.

Creating a power spot

The sandplay therapist's initial quest is to coordinate the content of the external sandplay environment, so that it conveys a balance of energies, with small adjustments as things are added. But as small as it may be, the setting is also immense, a landscape over which invisible entities hover as it continually recreates itself. The sandplay therapist repeats the acts of gazing and observing. This coagulates power and re-acquaints the therapist with minute relationships of the contents of the setting. For the client, gazing and observing is a mode of awareness that "precedes and underlies the literate intellect" and remains faithful to the sensuous world and to the other beings that surround us (Abram, 1996, p.264). Each sandplay client wanders through this territory, stopping here and there to observe something external that might become a bridge to their internal world. An initial uncertainty, an ability to cultivate and accept a lack of intention requires patience and the desire to stay with it until something shows itself. Landscape painter Neil Welliver, my teacher of color interaction at the Cooper Union in New York, stressed looking at something from all possible directions again and again. He himself practiced this daily in his walks through the old Maine woods near his home, his backpack filled with art materials. At first, no place seemed different from any other, full of non-descript corners, until something made him stop, move around and look, again and again until that particular spot became a place of power and the subject of his next painting. "If you give yourself to a place, you begin to feel its power" (Weber, 2013). In sandplay, meaning is never immediate, even after completion of the sandplay image and the closing observation together with the therapist. Musician John Cage wrote, "If something is boring after two minutes, try it for four. If still boring, then eight. Then sixteen. Then thirty-two. Eventually one discovers that it is not boring at all" (Cage, 1961).

The sandplay therapy quest, creativity and resistance

The sandplay setting is filled with attractive objects. The therapist is non-intrusive and non-directive, and sits silently without giving direction or interpreting the sandplay image. Parents of children in therapy and adult clients often ask how play and non-intervention can alleviate emotional pain and behavioral and trauma-related symptoms, and facilitate a positive rebalancing of the personality and a positive "return to the marketplace" of life. The path to the desired change through non-directive free play with sand and miniatures cannot be explained simply. The therapist understands the power of the environment, the conscious and unconscious levels of the co-transference, and the psyche itself that contribute to healing. An understandable explanation might be to describe sandplay as an emotional creative quest, a "hero's journey" with symbolic identifiable stages supported by the therapist in a "free and protected space." The six stages of a drawing assessment for children (Lahad, 1997) parallel the sequence of the process of therapy and explain the supportive role of the therapist. A small sheet of paper is folded into six numbered squares. A child is asked to draw a main character in the first square, his task or mission in the second square and the aid he receives to further his mission in the third square. These represent the client in therapy as the "hero," the desired goal and the therapist's help. The next three squares symbolize the therapeutic process. The obstacle to be overcome is drawn in the fourth square, the meeting between hero and obstacle in the fifth square and the outcome in the sixth square. Defenses and outer conditions that obstruct the journey are met by the "hero" with the therapist's help, and positive strengths are reinforced. The sandplay journey requires courage and external support, as difficult inner content is exposed. Children often let out the frightening inner imagery that they live with and build it in the sandtray, but adults may fortify their defenses and use modes of resistance in relation to the therapist or in relation to the sandtray. Montecchi (2004) describes "beautiful scenes" made to "please" the therapist, which actually conceal fear of inner content being exposed, or resistance, through refusal to touch the sand or use miniatures, or to refuse to do sandplay. A block can be authentically expressed with symbols of obstacles, blocked roads, cages or empty spaces in the sandtray. After building, observing and experiencing the obstacle is the next step in coping with it. Taking time to build self-acceptance, self-nurturance and preparation for an inner quest may then filter into outer reality.

A 32-year-old married father sought therapy because of the stress he felt each morning when he drove across the boundaries of his village into the next town. He refused to draw or work in the sand, but did choose miniatures to represent his extended family and himself. On a table, he placed a figurine representing himself and moved other figurines closer or farther away, to the left or right. One figurine represented a revered older brother who had died, now painfully absent from his life. Several times a year, the entire family visited the brother's grave together, but he had never gone there alone. He used miniatures to role-play a conversation with his deceased brother. His new goal was to cross the boundaries of the local cemetery alone and visit his brother's grave without his family. In this quest, he was able to feel his individual grief and express his love directly at his brother's grave.

PART THREE

THE LANGUAGE OF SANDPLAY

Images and Journeys

7

The Sandplay Image Speaks for Itself

Introduction

In the late 1950s, I was an art student at the Cooper Union in New York, deeply immersed in making art, talking about art and looking at every possible kind of art. All these aspects of creative expression merged together in a continuous process of seeing external visual reality, filtered through a personal sensibility to color and form. There were two different approaches to making art. A painting teacher would critique a painting with an intuitive approach of "what worked" or "didn't work." A more structured understanding of the elements of design and the relationships between line, form, color and format adhered to the principles developed at the Bauhaus in Weimar, Germany, from 1919 to 1933. With the rise of Nazism, the Bauhaus closed. Its founding theorists fled to the United States where their teaching influenced new concepts of architecture, design and the fine arts. Color theorist Joseph Albers taught at Black Mountain College, and at Yale University from 1950. His student, Neil Welliver (1929–2005) brought Albers's theories of two-dimensional design to the Cooper Union and confirmed that visual images conceived through formal concepts of color, line and plane had understandable relationships (Winton, 2016).

My transition from art to creative therapy and sandplay redirected my focus on images, from graphic aesthetics to expression of emotional themes that relied on spontaneity, containment, non-intervention and acceptance of an image within a therapeutic relationship. In sandplay especially, the client is encouraged to rely on an inner guiding sense of image-making, to allow movement and change as needed until the image feels right and "works." An aesthetic analysis of a sandplay image is not considered relevant in a therapeutic creative process. But the emotional truths that inspire the forms an image takes can sometimes radiate a vital, powerful presence of beauty and numinosity. The sandplay image is a three-dimensional form of "physical thinking" with height, depth and additional subtlety of detail in relation to its vertical and horizontal spatial directions (Gormley and Gayford, 2020). An image is the material form that an indistinct inner theme takes, and makes accessible its symbolic embodiment, as "form is the very shape of content" (Shahn, 1957/1972, p.53). The French philosopher Bachelard writes that nature endows itself with form, life originates forms, life is the cause of forms and "form is the habitat of life" (1994, p.114).

The non-verbal language of spatial-visual phenomena

Beyond the visible sandplay environment, several invisible factors influence the formation of sandplay images. The co-transference and its levels of energies resonate in a sandplay image and can manifest symbolically. The constant presence of an invisible map of spatial locations in the sandtray rectangle gives meaning to placement in each location. And as the process progresses, the psyche reveals its plan to arrive at the invisible Center, the source, place of return and of the Self–Ego axis. In this chapter, these invisible non-verbal language forms are discussed, closing with an example of the long sandplay process of Helena, a woman who began a sandplay process at age 45. Her evolving relationship to Center was first expressed as isolated central mounds, which gradually formed relationships to objects placed in corners and later became mounds of healing, growth and communication with the world.

Six channels of therapist–client co-transference: the relationship between wounding and healing

Figure 7.1 diagrams the six channels of conscious and unconscious communication in a verbal therapist–client interaction. Above and below, two parallel horizontal lines frame the therapist–client interaction on the higher conscious level and on a deep unconscious "hara" level, the "great underground river" that connects us (Oda, 1997). Two parallel vertical lines close the frame on the left and right sides and indicate the intrapersonal communication between the conscious and unconscious of either the therapist or the client. Two diagonal connections show the transfer of the conscious healing capacity of the therapist to the unconscious healing capacity of the client, activating it, and the conscious wounding of the client to the unconscious state of past wounds of the therapist, activating these. The therapist's acknowledgment of one's own wounding is a precaution to prevent harmful splitting and ego inflation in the therapist.

SIX CHANNELS OF COMMUNICATION BETWEEN THERAPIST AND CLIENT

1. Conscious level of communication between therapist and client
2. Unconscious level of communication between therapist and client
3. Communication between the therapist's conscious and unconscious levels
4. Communication between the client's conscious and unconscious levels
5. Communication between the therapist's conscious and the client's unconscious levels
6. Communication between the therapist's unconscious and the client's conscious levels

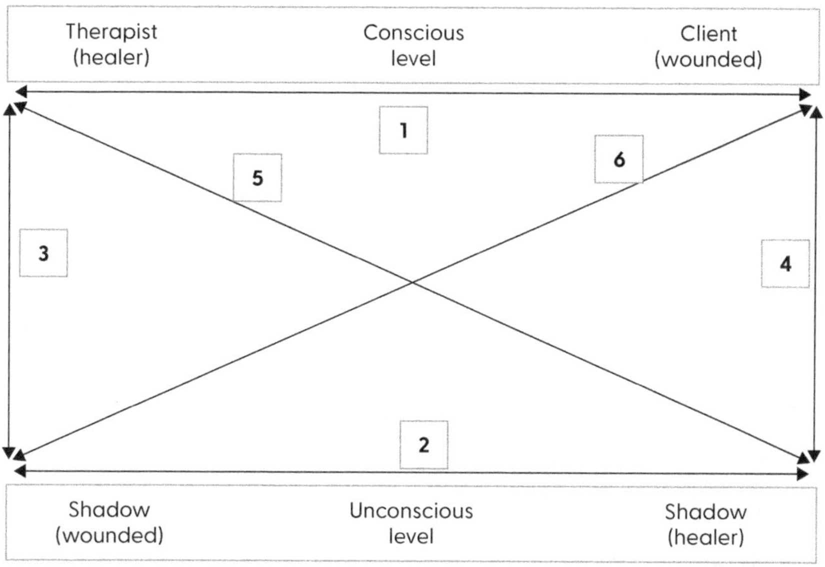

Figure 7.1 *Six channels of communication between therapist and client*

In a second diagram (Figure 7.2), the sandplay image is represented as a circle in the center where the diagonals of co-transference between therapist and client cross, a third entity holding a fusion of energies. Co-transference and symbolic representation of the therapist in a client's sandplay might appear as two empty chairs placed near each other as if observing the sandplay together. Beautiful crystals pointing to the therapist might represent a positive therapeutic relationship. A cannon, or witch, directed towards the therapist might express resentment or defense against intrusion. Whether the transference is positive or negative, the therapist's familiarity with unconscious guidance and authentic imagery can strengthen the client's trust in spontaneity.

SIX CHANNELS OF COMMUNICATION IN A SANDPLAY SESSION

1. Conscious level of communication between therapist and client
2. Unconscious level of communication between therapist and client
3. Communication between the therapist's conscious and unconscious levels
4. Communication between the client's conscious and unconscious levels
5. Communication between the therapist's conscious and the client's unconscious levels
6. Communication between the therapist's unconscious and the client's conscious levels

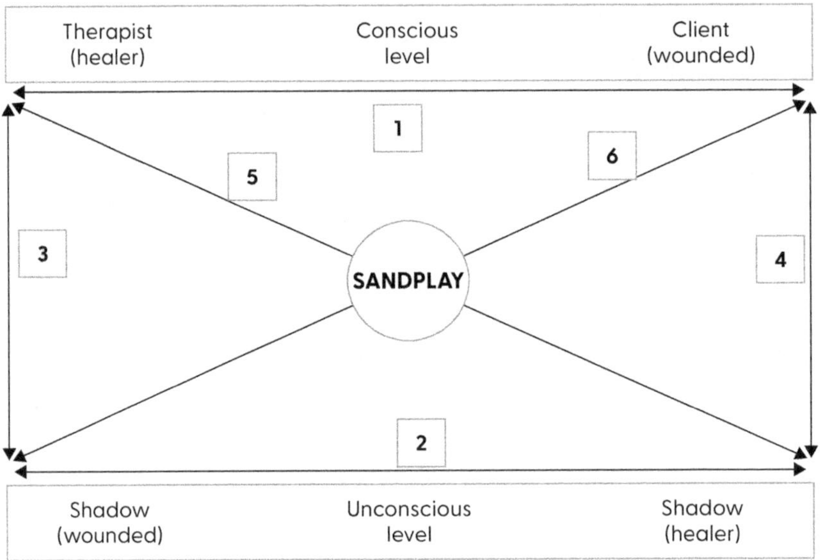

Figure 7.2 *Six channels of communication with central circle representing the sandtray*

The wounded healer

The title of "wounded healer," conferred on the therapist, is a term that originated in Greek myth. Chiron the Centaur became the first "wounded healer" after a poisoned arrow pierced his knee and caused him unending pain (see Chapter 11). He alleviated his suffering by applying herbs to his wound, and tutored Asclepius, who became a second wounded healer. Asclepius was cut from the womb of his dying mortal mother Coronis, by his father, the god Apollo. In Apollo's absence, Coronis betrayed him and was punished for this by death; Apollo saved their son by performing the first cesarean section. Asclepius acquired a healing power so great that, like the gods, he could bring the dead back to life. This threatened the boundary between humans and the divine. Zeus, God of Olympus, with the approval of Hades, God of the Underworld, killed Asclepius with a thunderbolt, but later relented and immortalized him as a constellation in the sky, as the God of Medicine. His temples of healing still stand in Epidaurus, Kos and other places (Graves, 1955/1960).

An invisible map in the sandtray

The sandtray is shaped as a rectangle with two parallel long sides and two parallel short sides, joined at four right-angled corners. The four sides frame a shallow inner space and separate it from space outside the sandtray. When standing opposite the longer axis, the rectangle seems horizontal, parallel to the earth, the feminine. This direction is usually chosen for sandplay. When standing opposite the shorter axis, the tray seems vertical, its short base and long sides imply ascent, aspiring towards achievement and intellectual growth, which are masculine attributes. Each direction, horizontal or vertical, impacts on forming the content of the inner space and its meaning. No matter which direction is chosen, there is always a center, left and right sides, horizontal and vertical axes, and far and near areas. A map of this territory would diagram the outer shape, direction of the short and long sides, and the external space. The inner space of the sandtray has invisible divisions that can be sensed as four equal quadrants with a center, with diagonal movements that connect opposite corners and also mark the center. The empty sand in the sandtray invites touch, the impulse to make a mark just as people centuries ago incised marks on shaped stones or arranged objects to intentionally form an image (Gormley and Gayford, 2020). In sandplay, the client's choice of an object, its color, size and direction, is experienced as personal. Placement is also experienced as personal but it is guided unconsciously by universal tendencies that perceive meanings for each inner location on the invisible spatial map created within the sandtray's boundaries. The final image and the specific locations that are occupied by objects in the sandtray space, must "feel right" to the client gazing on the image.

Research and definition of spatial phenomena in the sandtray

Joel Ryce-Menuhin (1992) and Ruth Ammann (1991) both correlate meanings to spatial locations in the sandtray, and both acknowledge that a therapist's personality and the atmosphere of the setting will also contribute to the content and organization of sand pictures.

Both interpret spatial phenomena in the sandtray using a consistent viewpoint from the front center of the sandtray. Ryce-Menuhin researched the designs of 1000 sandplays done by his adult patients and diagrammed eight universal sandplay patterns that he found to be most significant, which indicate "the tendency which the psyche takes in creating original and spontaneous sandplays" (Ryce-Menuhin,1992, pp.91–97). He correlated content from all three levels of psyche—the collective unconscious, personal unconscious and consciousness—with specific areas. Four of his patterns are organized around a central point—a mandala shape or central circle with content in four corners, an eight-pointed star shape—and the use of a central area to manifest the Self. Four other diagrams locate unconscious and archetypal material on the left or front areas, with more conscious and ego material located on the far and right areas. The three levels of psyche are projected into a sandplay in seven options. He found that in an adult patient's first sandplay, all three states (Level 7) are often present:

- Level 1: Conscious only
- Level 2: Personal unconscious only
- Level 3: Collective unconscious only
- Level 4: Conscious plus personal unconscious
- Level 5: conscious plus collective unconscious
- Level 6: Personal unconscious plus collective unconscious
- Level 7: Conscious plus both personal and collective unconscious levels.

In Ammann's diagram, the sandtray is divided into four equal quadrants created by a central horizontal line that crosses a central vertical line. I have added diagonals to Ammann's original diagram (Figure 7.3). The sand-player's hands move in this three-dimensional space from distant to close areas, and from left to right sides. In photographs, the left and right areas of a sandplay remain the same, but distant or close areas lose their spatial context and might wrongly be described as "top" and "bottom." Ammann sees her diagram as an aid, from which we rethink our understanding in light of each individual's personality and circumstances (1991, p.47).

In Ammann's sandtray map, the entire far half of the sandtray represents the patriarchal, air and spirit. The near area represents the matriarchal, related to earth, instincts and the body. The sandtray's vertical left side holds unconscious attributes and the inner world. The right side contains more conscious aspects such as family relationships and external social interaction. The four quadrants meet at the center of the sandtray, which represents the ego, immediate issues and the place of formation of the Self–Ego axis. Each quadrant combines the attributes of two locations, near-left, near-right, far-left, and far-right.

Content placed in the *near-left quadrant* may relate to the past, the body, early matriarchal stages and instinct. Unconscious attributes and new creative impulses emerge here from the "ocean of the unconscious." A leftward movement might indicate regression or a return of energies flowing back into the unconscious when no longer needed. A figurine in the front-left corner that faces left, or falls towards the amorphous space outside the tray, can point to fragility, a danger to life. Alternately, return to and collection of energies from the unconscious can be used to incubate a new goal, a new progression, an increase of energies from the body and the instinctual spheres.

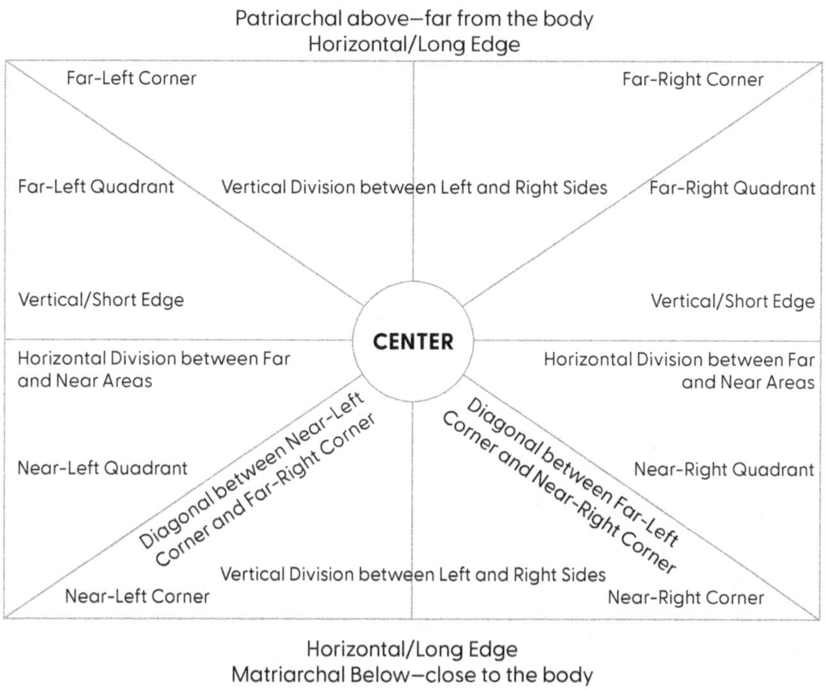

Figure 7.3 *Map of the sandtray with diagonals*

The *near-right quadrant* is close to the body and can represent conscious content such as the personal mother, primary others and the present family context. The *far-left quadrant* can hold powerful new spiritual, protective or frightening forces that enter or leave the sandtray through the far-left corner. The *far-right quadrant* may hold elements of the personal father, school, one's profession and goals. A diagonal of objects from the near-left corner moving towards the far-right corner can imply new energies and preparation to move out to the world.

Corners

A sandtray's 90-degree right-angled corners and their rim are visible stable structures. Ammann states: "Motifs which appear in the four corners of the sandtray provide a frame of reference for the unfolding of events. They represent the identifying individual strands, or components of the action" (1991, p.49). Corners are keepers of potent energies that either "wait" there, in preparation for a journey to the center, or, after a brief stay, will leave (Steinhardt, 2000, p.118). Diagonals from corner to opposite corner are the longest distance in the sandtray, analogous to the distance between opposites in the psyche. Two diagonals that cross mark the sandtray center. Objects with opposite qualities are often placed at either end of a diagonal. In opposite corners we might find a masculine aspect opposite a feminine one, a young and innocent aspect distant from an old and wise or dangerous aspect. These become the immediate central motif if they meet in the center.

Center, centering and off-center

Center is the meeting point between the quadrants, the diagonals and the location of the Self–Ego axis of the sandtray. Center symbolizes the place of origin and departure, and the point of return (Cooper, 1978, p.32). Centering is familiar to potters, who throw a lump of clay on the potter's wheel and coordinate the pressure of both hands on only one point of the revolving clay. They may breathe into the rotation of the wheel while their hands round the shape of the clay on the wheel, until it is a symmetrically balanced mound. The center of the clay is opened, an inner space is formed and "the center itself, in its initiating power, evolves in its form" (Richards, 1989, p.6). Centering clay relates inward to its own center of balance and is often a spiritual experience. The heart, the center of the body, circulates blood in two complementary movements, a movement away from center towards a journey into manifestation, returning to the heart center as a journey back to a spiritual center and to unity (Cooper, 1978). The center of the rectangular sandtray has to be discovered by the sandplayer, like a quest becoming clear during a wandering journey. Journeys are often off-center, not balanced or steady until the center manifests.

Ammann states: "I have found that mandalas are invariably located in the centers of sand pictures. They do, after all, represent the various aspects of the relationship of the ego to the Self and, moreover, symbolize the centering of the personality" (1991, p.49). Centering and constellation of the Self in sandplay is the fourth stage in Weinrib's eight-stage sequence of the sandplay process (Weinrib, 1983). It is preceded by a first stage of initial diagnosis and prognosis, a descent into the personal unconscious (shadow) revealing problems and healing potentialities more clearly, and then partial resolution of a major complex. Then, a central circular form manifests together with a form representing the number four. In the center is the constellation of the Self and the Self–Ego axis. The four corners can be anchored by objects that relate to whatever occupies the center.

HELENA, a sandplay example of center, from isolation to a place of relationship and healing

Helena, a 45-year-old woman, had suffered impingement, loss, violence, psychosis, neglect and rejection from early childhood. In almost 300 symmetrical sandplays done over 16 years, the center of the sandtray was her anchor and starting point. Her first isolated mounds in the sandtray center remained independent and unharmed, with nothing in the corners or in the sandtray space. Relationships were difficult and dangerous. She alone held herself together. But like wet sand that appears solid, its grains fall apart as it dries. Her first sand mounds were symmetrical, self-contained and made with enjoyment and a slow strengthening of the ego with the therapist as witness, perhaps as a symmetry between herself and the therapist. Jung (1953, para. 225) discusses the implications of the center and reflection in left and right symmetry: "Just as the 'right' denotes the world of consciousness and its principals, so by 'reflection' the picture of the world is to be turned round to the left, thus producing a corresponding world in reverse." Jung adds that "through reflection the right appears as the reverse of the left," giving both equal validity. Since the unconscious and its order are mostly unintelligible, "order becomes a symmetrical counterpart of the conscious mind and its contents, although it is still not clear which of them is reflected and which reflecting." In this relationship, the center is the point of intersection of "two worlds that correspond but are inverted by reflection."

Helena relived and shared her history through sandplay, replete with what she remembered and with what slowly reached consciousness. Her family came to Israel from Eastern Europe when Helena was 12 years old. Her psychotic father devoured her with love and may have abused her in early childhood, evidenced by lingering pains in her lower body. Rejected by her mother, she was raised by a "metallic" paternal grandmother who read her frightening fairy tales each day after school and forced her to write and eat with her right hand, as she was naturally left-handed. In Israel, she succeeded academically and, after her army service, married a quiet man with whom she had children. Her friendships were based on pleasing others. At times, her insecure, fearful inner world spilled over as inappropriate aggression, especially in groups. She instinctively left her technical profession and studied natural healing, art and sandplay. The sand mirrored her sensitivity to touch, movement and nature, but also accessed a repressed underground labyrinth where she faced a devouring, incestuous parental animus, an embittered cold mother and the terror of an evil grandmother witch. Her relationship to her husband deteriorated and they divorced. A memory of a childhood tree inspired her to spend time with old wise trees near her home. In a recurring dream, she fell into an abyss but always grabbed hold of something on the edge and pulled herself back to solid ground. In the first eight years of therapy, Helena made over 100 sandplays. In the next eight years, she came when she needed to understand a dream or a conflict with her family, co-workers or friends through work in the sand. In a final phase of therapy, powerful and previously unbearable themes found a place in the sandtray as well as images of healing and rebirth of her inner child.

Phase one, the first eight years

For eight years, a majority of Helena's sandplays featured symmetrical central mounds composed of all the sand in the tray with small variations on their forms. Most of the mounds were isolated in the middle of a blue surface with empty corners. Miniatures might be placed on or near a mound if a theme became conscious during the sculpting. A second type of symmetrical "butterfly" image appeared sporadically, with sculpted low sand forms defined by curved linear blue areas whose left and right sides accurately mirrored each other. After several symmetrical images, an unpredictable and unsymmetrical "realistic" scene might appear, with figurines involved in a story or quest. The first seven sandplays shown below represent eight years of work, moving Helena towards stabilization, ego growth and expanded meaning of her mounds.

In 13 sandplays chosen from the next eight years, central islands became receptive, the Self–Ego axis was formed and healing content appeared. Finally, she was able to express authentic central images that bridged her trauma and suffering with her innate sense of aesthetic beauty. The sandplays presented below were turning points in Helena's long journey towards a better relationship with herself and with others, and with internal and external renewal. Actual dates are listed on each sandplay to indicate the time in between sessions.

September 12, 2005: After father's death

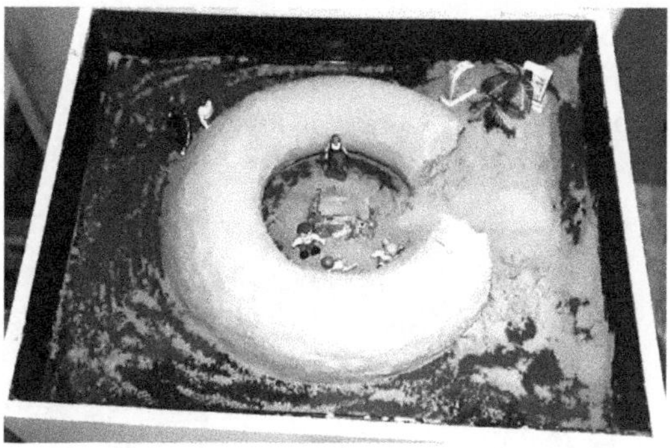

Figure 7.4 *Helena: After father's death*

Helena began therapy in 2003. Her mother had died some time ago, and she had not seen her father for years. She could not renew contact with him because of his irrational behavior. He was under psychiatric care and lived with his mother, the "metallic" grandmother, until she died. Helena made this sandplay in homage to both her deceased parents. The central sand ring is ruptured by a path to two graves in the far-right corner, under two palm trees (Figure 7.4).

August 6, 2007: An Eagle, a duck and her eggs

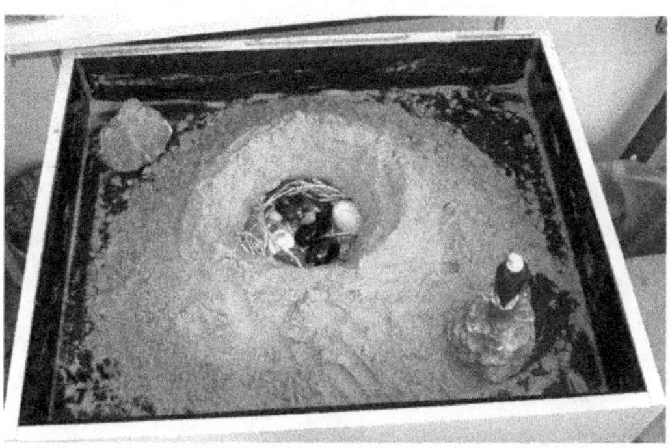

Figure 7.5 *Helena: Eagle, duck and eggs*

In the center of a symmetrical sand mound on a blue surface, a mother duck sits in her nest filled with beautiful eggs. Two large rocks in the far-left and front-right corners are diagonally opposite each other, outside the mound. An eagle standing on the rock in the front-right corner might be either protective or possibly dangerous. Helena thought that the eagle was a protective male presence, but he might also embody the ambivalent relationship with her father, confusing love and the danger of being devoured (Figure 7.5).

January 1, 2008: Girl wearing a red dress sitting on a whale

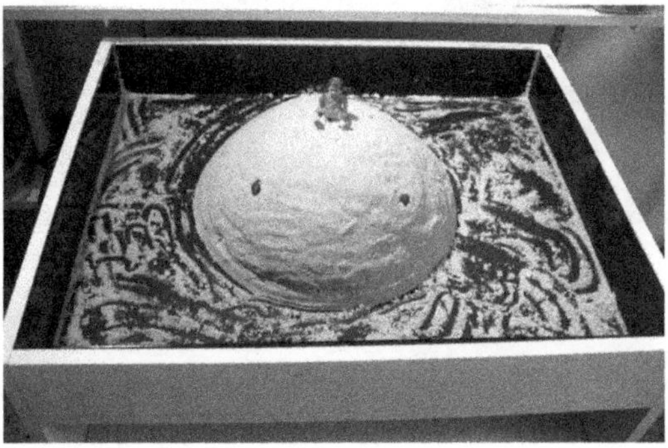

Figure 7.6 *Helena: Girl wearing a red dress sitting on a whale mound*

After ten sandplays with central mounds, and two unsymmetrical sandplays, this circular mound transformed into a supportive sand whale in an empty blue sea. A little girl in a red dress rides on its back. This is the first supportive relationship in the sandtray for the little girl, who will become the heroine of Helena's story (Figure 7.6). The whale is the largest creature that ever existed. Its brain possesses evolved cranial structures that link to compassion, self-awareness and linguistic expression (Ronnberg and Martin, 2010). Whale introduces womb, darkness, underworld, death and rebirth as Helena and the little girl begin their sandplay journey. This child will appear in nine sandplays in the next nine years. In 2017, she is joined in a sandplay by "Anastasia," an adult supportive companion. Their collaboration in six more sandplays enabled healing and closure of the sandplay process in 2019.

October 8, 2008: Kiva, babies, Poseidon and Mermaid, Turtle and Eagle

In the partly submerged center of the sandtray is a round structure that resembles a Kiva, a sacred, round ceremonial space used by the Pueblo peoples, usually the men, for spiritual gatherings. A bowl of many human babies in the center may be a transformation of the duck eggs in Figure 7.5, but the babies are alone. Two diagonal movements cross over the center. From a large construction in the far-left corner—a stone pillar, two crossed bridges, a fire and a large eagle—a strong diagonal moves through center towards the front-right area where a large turtle ascends a slope towards the babies. Eagle and Turtle, in opposite corners are powerful opposites; again, it is unclear if they are protective, or menacing, of each other or of the babies in the center. Eagle and Turtle might represent Helena's confusion between love and abuse in both masculine and feminine, in father and mother. Eagle represents solar power, wisdom, courage and strength.

Turtle is known as "Turtle Island" in Native American legend, her shell covered by mud brought up from a lake bottom which became the earth we live on. Turtle's outer shell is structured like a lunar calendar, with 13 central scutes representing 13 lunar cycles and a circumference of 28 plates, the number of days in a month. Three mythological creatures, Poseidon, Mermaid and Centaur, are joined by a man with a rifle. They stand opposite Turtle and seem protective. Poseidon, Greek God of the Sea, has human legs, while Mermaid with her fish tail and Centaur with a horse's lower body and legs are half human and half animal. Poseidon and Mermaid ascend from the depths of the unconscious as archetypal masculine and feminine powers. The Centaur may refer to Chiron, the first wounded healer who mentored Asclepius, God of Healing. A second diagonal moves quietly from a baby in a bucket in the front-left corner, through the center to a white swan in a small blue lake in the far-right corner. The baby and the swan face outwards, excluded from witnessing the events in the center, perhaps purification of the babies. As symbols, the baby and the swan symbolize a conjunction of masculine and feminine traits. The baby is not clearly boy or girl, and the swan with its phallic neck and round soft body combines masculine and feminine. Turtle and Eagle, Poseidon and Mermaid are clearly masculine or feminine, paired opposites that may represent potential development of their cooperation in forthcoming sandplays (Figure 7.7).

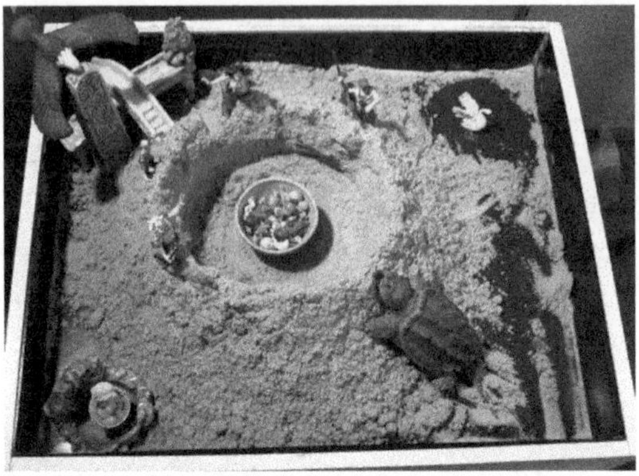

Figure 7.7 *Helena: Kiva, babies, Poseidon and Mermaid, Turtle and Eagle*

May 2, 2009: First Self-tray: Oak tree in the center of five concentric circles, four corners

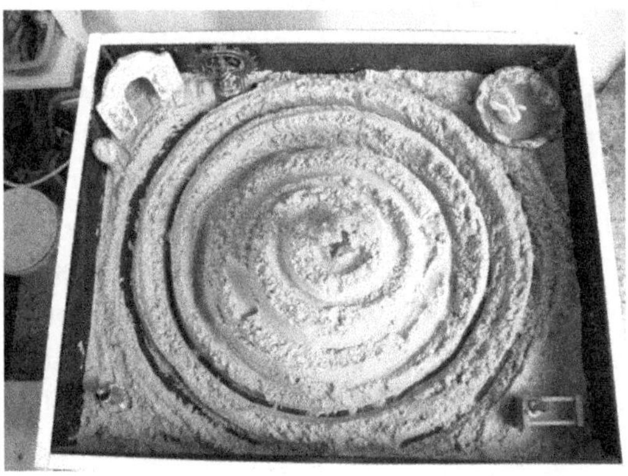

Figure 7.8 *Helena: First Self-tray, Oak tree in the center of five concentric circles*

Eleven sandplays later, in the sixth year of therapy, a strong oak tree grows from the center of a group of five concentric sand circles. With objects in all four corners, this is a first clear image of a Self–Ego axis. Helena enjoyed her creative vitality, letting her sculpted central sand mounds evolve into structures, and enhancing their themes with imprints and figurines. In the far-left corner, a strong but gentle diagonal movement emerges from a portal that invites entry from beyond the sandtray. A dancing Shiva and a Madonna and Child stand guard on either side of the portal's opening. The diagonal moves through the central tree and reaches the front-right corner, where a baby in a crib faces center. A second diagonal quietly balances the first, and again a swan faces outward from the far-right corner, but she is now contained in the pond that held the baby in a bucket in Figure 7.7. This diagonal reaches down to the front-left corner where a Native American woman with a papoose faces outward. Again, the objects on this diagonal, the swan and woman, can't see the center or portal or whatever might enter (Figure 7.8).

September 28, 2009: Anastasia: butterfly symmetry

"Anastasia," a figurine of a young positive adult feminine, presides over objects with interiors that can be opened—a treasure chest, a wind-up clock, a large house and a stove. In several early sandplays, Anastasia's role was not clear, but here she seems to hold the key that opens the deep gnawing childhood traumas of the little girl in the red dress, and support and protect her when they are together. The two empty metal chairs in the front area may be a preparation for Anastasia and the little girl to reflect each other. Two chairs also suggest the therapist and Helena reflecting together on her past, present and future. The flat "butterfly" symmetry of this sandplay emphasizes communication between left and right sides, and between Helena's unconscious and conscious. Her aesthetic sense enhances the beautiful symmetry and stabilizes and strengthens her, integrating sand forms, selected miniatures and the deep blue color of the sandtray bottom. This same balance and reflection of left- and right-sided symmetry, has another potential, to open a door to dark monsters that will emerge from underworld twilight into the light (Figure 7.9).

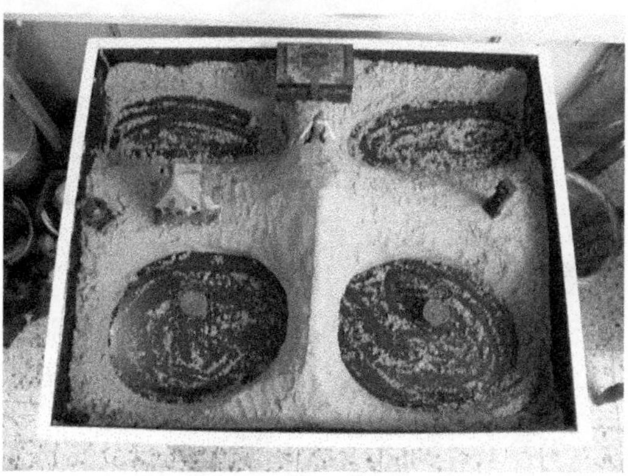

Figure 7.9 *Helena: Anastasia, Butterfly symmetry*

July 6, 2011: Handprint, triple spiral, musical instruments, green dragon and little girl

A handprint of Helena's left hand, the hand that encased her sense of self in shame, that she was forbidden to use as a child, is now proudly impressed on the central peak of a round mound. Her handprint is anchored on its palm by a round triple spiral, a red drum on the thumb, a red flower on the second finger, a dark green fir tree on the middle finger, a French horn on the fourth finger and a violin on the pinky finger. The sounds of each musical instrument vibrate differently: the drum is struck, the horn vibrates from the passage of air through its labyrinth, and the strings of the violin vibrate when played with a bow or plucked. The three interconnecting spirals may mirror these three types of sound, an orchestral interaction, like that of the body, soul and spirit. The handprint supports integration and relationship within the Self. The little girl stands on a long green dragon, observing from above. The round mound itself is enclosed on the blue surface by two concentric circles etched out by a rolling crystal ball on the right, whose transparent clarity may signify a divine wholeness, the Self moving in a circular orbit to create form. The corners are empty. The color red in three objects reinforces the life energy of the girl. Red, the color of blood, heat and life flow, contrasts with green, a stable color of plant energy, taking form as a dragon rather than a whale (Figure 7.10).

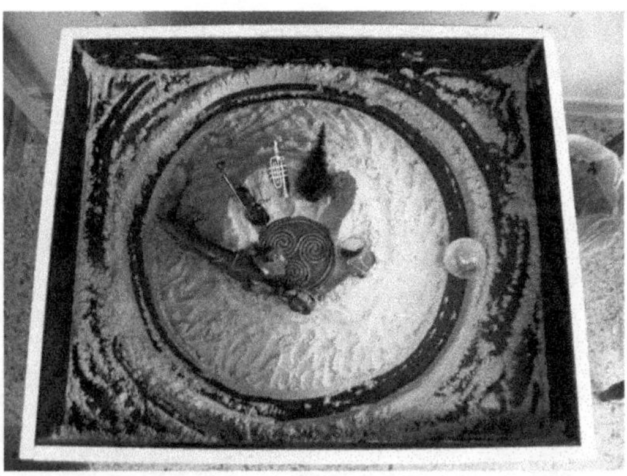

Figure 7.10 *Helena: Handprint on mound, triple spiral, musical instruments, green dragon and girl*

Phase two, the following eight years

In the next eight years, Helena came when she needed to sculpt in the sand, spontaneously but precisely, her deepest, most painful issues. Her relationship with her ex-husband and with their children was good. She moved with her dog and cat to an apartment with a small garden but still struggled to define her true self.

November 19, 2015: Phoenix and Firebird

At end of her twelfth year of therapy, a circular mound became a bird shape "with wings," crowned at the last moment by a miniature firebird. The sand firebird and miniature phoenix have similar shapes and symbolize death and resurrection through fire (Cooper, 1978). Helena placed a small nest below, with a chick that she thought was wounded, like one of her children who now needed her nurturing and love. She felt a chest pain as she observed the phoenix and sensed death as well as power. The phoenix self-immolates and rises from the ashes. Helena's psyche had presented her with this image to heal herself and the relationship with her child. Four small sea shells in the front-left corner are receptive containers for new life (Figure 7.11).

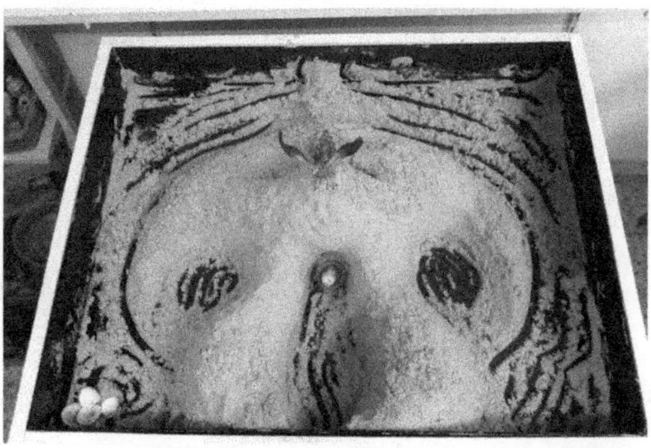

Figure 7.11 *Helena: Phoenix and Firebird*

January 16, 2016: Tree of Life, Poseidon and Mermaid

Helena felt anxious. She remembered a dream where she lived in a world with no sky, covered with a disc, ruled by a man who looked nice but was not, and who would electrocute her if she revolted. Her hands moved in opposite directions in the sand, filling the entire sandtray with a symmetrical Tree of Life with a strong trunk, a crown that covers almost half the tray holding all the sky powers within it. Its roots seem to reach the center of the universe. A Cretan snake goddess presides in the far center above a tiny uroboros like a third eye on the forehead. The uroboros reminded her of her dog who bites her own tail. Under the left side of the sand tree, Poseidon, a symbol of masculine control seemed unfamiliar to her but not threatening, as if she need not be afraid of new things in reality. On the right, a mermaid represented the feminine, life, music, song and art. The masculine and feminine do not face each other, but she knew they were connected and part of the same whole (Figure 7.12).

In the next few months, Helena attended a dance class, held family dinners and hosted several new friends. She was amazed at her dog's natural instinct, giving birth to several beautiful puppies, cleaning them and eating the afterbirth. She planned a trip to Europe with an old friend. Several symmetrical sandplays featured sand sculptures of positive feminine animals such as a whale from whom she could learn (recalling the first whale nine years ago) and a cow, for nurturance.

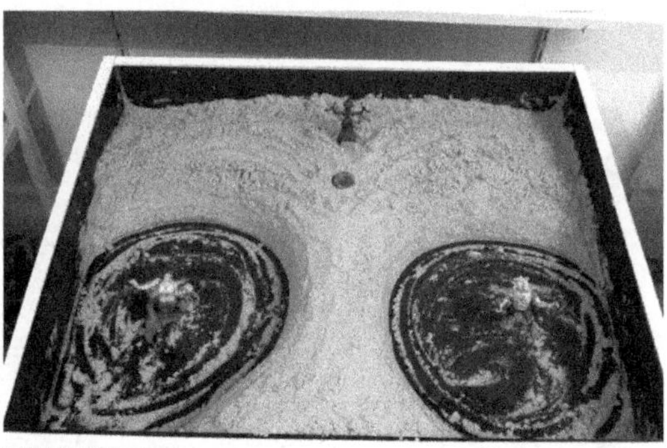

Figure 7.12 *Helena: Sculpted Tree of Life, Poseidon and Mermaid*

September 20, 2016: A battle with a wicked witch who wants to steal a baby

Helena was stressed. She had co-led a group of difficult adolescents and felt as if she had "disappeared" and forgot all her abilities. She held many objects in her hands before touching the sand and talked about her "steel" grandmother who ignored her if she didn't do exactly what was expected. A great battle ensued in the sandtray around a wicked witch who intended to steal a baby. Helena felt compelled to give the baby to the witch, but she resisted and moved the baby figurine to a pool in the front-left area, near a mermaid on a rock, backed by the Venus of Willendorf. In the far left, she placed two examples of protective parents who hold their babies safely in their arms, a Neanderthal couple and a Madonna. To help defeat the witch in the far-right corner, she flanked the witch with several powerful feminine goddesses and a Native American hunter. The Great Turtle approached the witch on a diagonal from the front-left corner and toppled her. Helena felt deeply attached to the mermaid and the baby (Figure 7.13).

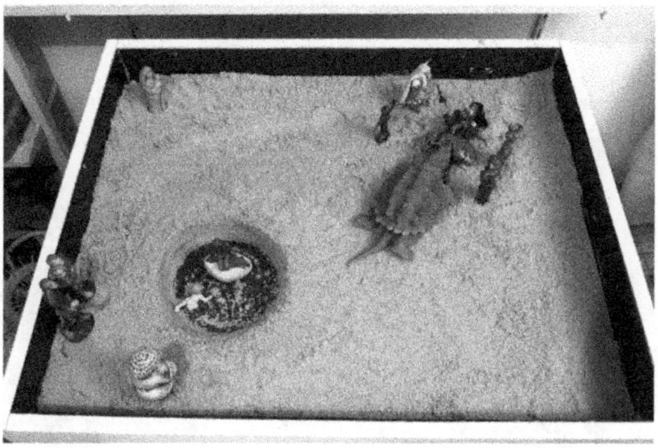

Figure 7.13 *Helena: Battle with a wicked witch who wants to steal a baby*

September 28, 2016: Kiva cleansing, a performance in an unsymmetrical sandplay

Childhood memories surfaced—climbing trees with her neighbor and friends, and unclear sensations regarding her father. She wanted to bury a large skeleton to represent fear, abuse and everything connected with it. The thought of her father made her feel penetrated and nauseous. But he was the only one who showed feeling for her. She loved him and could not be angry, because of his terrible mental state. Her mother beat and cursed her, and told her to shut up. If she could feel compassion for her parents, she might be able to let them go. She wanted the fire of life to return to her, to be able to live without fear. In the sand, she arranged many objects into three groups around a low, round central mound similar to a Kiva and enacted a "performance." On the mound, a gypsy dancer watched over the "fire of life." Nearby, she blessed a large, closed shell with water. In the far center, she buried the skeleton under a washtub while the witch watched from the far-right corner. She left a container of water there as witches are afraid of water and the emotions that water releases. Two groups observe: on the near-left edge, the little girl in her red dress and her dog stand in a boat, and in the near-right corner are the baby in a bucket and her mermaid. Helena remembered how she anticipated her grandmother returning home from work and switched on the light just as she came in, so that she would know that Helena had thought of her. In her body, she felt a flow of energy connecting her throat and the organs of her lower body. The little girl was stronger now. Helena placed a blue starfish and blue fish near her in the blue water. The healing energies of fire and water work together (Figure 7.14).

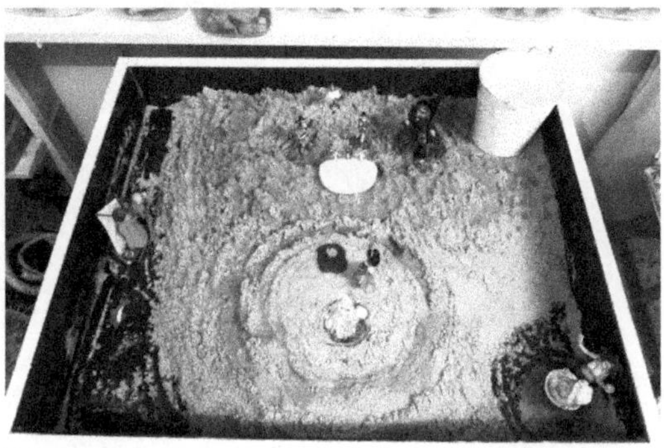

Figure 7.14 *Helena: Kiva cleansing, a performance, an unsymmetrical sandplay*

October 19, 2016: Cow Skull symmetry and the entrance to the underworld

A week later, Helena said that her life was going well, her relationship with her ex-husband was pleasant, and she was studying Jungian psychotherapy and tarot. Yet she was flooded with tears for the wounds of the generations before her—father, mother, grandparents and their ancestors. At the session's end, she went to the sandtray and made a small deep central hole, drew symmetrical spirals around it. It became a monster who needed horns. She placed a large cow skull in the far center, an oyster shell in front, and sprinkled water and sat. The small central hole pulled her inside "like a deep hole that you must enter for advice, like Tiresias advising Odysseus from inside the underworld, as if inside there was something that illuminates, like Theodor Reich who discovered energy in darkness that can illuminate. The shell is like a mirror" (Figure 7.15).

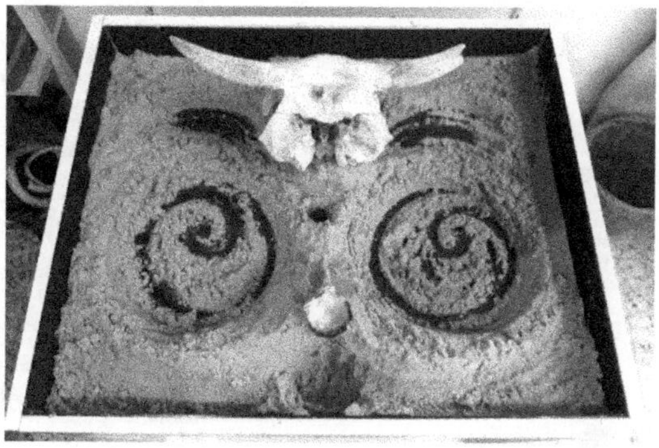

Figure 7.15 *Helena: Cow skull symmetry, entrance to the underworld*

February 27, 2017, The girl in the red dress joins Anastasia in a boat

Helena felt uncomfortable in two groups, in her Jungian group and at work with groups of children. I imagined her "inner child" trying to learn how to accept boundaries and feel protected. With large symmetrical rounded hand movements, she formed a strange face in the sand, carved round blue lines on either side and made eyes filled with turquoise sea glass. Where a nose or mouth might be, she placed a boat and put the little girl in the red dress and "Anastasia" with her, both in the same boat, both with oars for steering. Helena liked their relationship—a young girl and a woman riding the waves of the unconscious in a boat. The beige sand waves curve like the face of the sea, their light color emphasizes the contrast between the blue "eyes," and warm reds in the boat, a collaboration of water and fire as in Figure 7.11. In past sandplays, boats floated on the edges of Helena's blue symbolic waters. For the ancient Egyptians, a boat conveyed the sun each night over the "abysmal ocean of darkness toward sunrise and rebirth, just as consciousness is conveyed over the nether seas of sleep" (Ronnberg and Martin, 2010, p.450). Here, in a rowboat in the front center, the girl and the woman navigate together on a whale-shaped "wave" mound, the evolution of the little girl alone on a whale's back in Figure 7.6. This boat in the waves, but close to shore, brings with it inner unity after a long solitary odyssey, a homecoming. The "whale-shaped wave" also recalls the whale's role as dark container of psyche, and ancient mother from whose belly a soul is rebirthed into life, expelled, like Jonah, onto dry land (Figure 7.16).

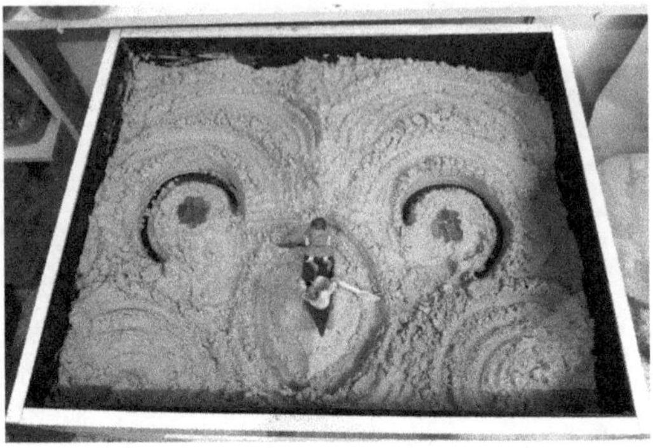

Figure 7.16 *Helena: Little girl in a red dress together with Anastasia in the same boat*

June 7, 2017: Steel Grandmother's tears

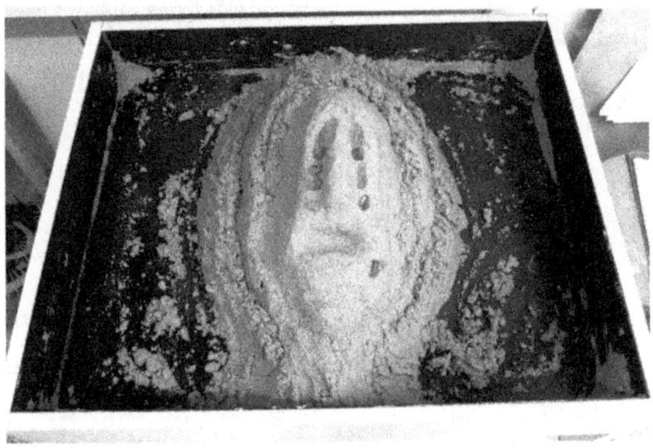

Figure 7.17 *Helena: Steel grandmother's tears*

Helena's sixtieth birthday was near but she did not feel like an adult. Her garden was lovely, her dog and cat got along, she had friends and she dreamed about her mother sitting and waiting patiently, radiating light like an angel. She made herself a good breakfast and felt she could love herself. It was time to bid farewell to suffering. In a series of sandplays, she placed clusters of positive objects on central mounds with nothing in the corners. At work, she was wary of people who might hurt someone to protect themselves, or who made her feel undervalued. Today she saw her mother's face in the sand, and said: "She wants to save herself and can't see me. She always accused me of something bad, lying. She saw that I suffered, but said that she suffered because of me. Fear of others completely paralyzes me and I disappear." But the screaming face she sculpted became her paternal grandmother, who told her she was bad, with whom she had to plead for forgiveness. She added tears of sea glass to soften her steely evil character and recalled a dream where she had to hold her sky father and earth mother apart. This exhausted her but did let in the light. If she stopped, they would merge and darkness would return (Figure 7.17).

In the next year, five centered and stable sandplays helped Helena resolve issues of boundaries, merging and aggression, so she could navigate relationships with more control. She enjoyed singing in a choir. In her dreams, a young girl went to places with her. She made another sandplay where the little girl and Anastasia rowed together in a boat in the front-right corner, like a family. She still felt that her masculine side was weak and undeveloped like her father, and consciously chose male figurines for their positive potential. A mermaid was "real, naked and unafraid." But stomach pains, fear and guilt made her aware that she may have "merged with her own children" as her father had with her. She began to identify causes of anger between herself and them. A Buddha gave direction. Images of the positive feminine increased. Babies, children, young women and mothers emanated warm, feminine instincts. She felt as if part of herself had returned to her, healed. She left one job where she had difficulty with staff hierarchy.

October 21, 2018: Elephant, death hiding, dramatic symmetry

In a dream, she saw her body from above, floating face down in an underground water channel like a nymph in nature, but dead. She felt dried out from work and from helping her children. In the sandtray, she pulled the sand into a central "spine" with four spiky "ribs" extending to each side. She wanted to symbolize death, but not confront death itself, and placed a lightning cloud in the near center of the spine and added large bones that formed a cross. In the rear center in front of a black sun, a mammoth and elephant clash tusks. She hid the death figurine that frightened her behind a mask in the far-left corner, added a skeleton playing a violin nearby, and a ladder on the sand. In the front-left corner, a small baby rests in an open ceramic sarcophagus. In the far-right corner under a black torii, the little girl, a dog and a cat observe. A sundial in the front-right corner points to the center. Helena's body ached near her heart. She said: "The little girl has the optimism needed to live, even though she sees the world of death. As a child I had to protect my father from death. He loved music and sang, but I lost my own music. There is no place for joy inside me. Someone strong enough has to mourn, the elephants are big enough to do that. I must allow myself to mourn, to part with something" (Figure 7.18). This image is a dialogue between the beauty of Helena's images and her suffering, now on its highest level of communication.

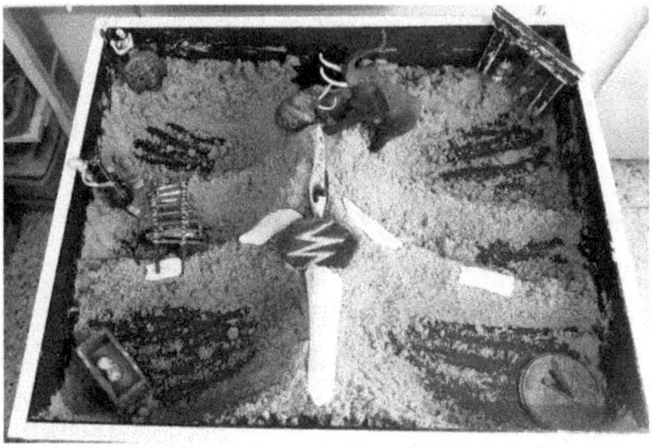

Figure 7.18 *Helena: Elephant, death hides, dramatic symmetry*

November 22, 2018: Howl

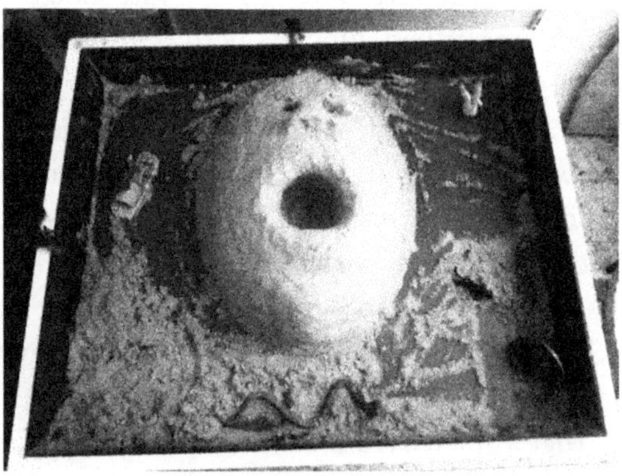

Figure 7.19 *Helena: Howl*

One month later, due to an electrical power failure in the studio, Helena worked by candlelight. A large central mound with a hole in the center metamorphosed into the screaming face of an old woman. She formed the open mouth, placed stones in the eyes, made nostrils and added snakes, dinosaurs, a wolf, a swan, a metal Roman helmet and a black raven, to protect the old woman who howled with pain. "The snakes protect and support her; when will all this suffering end?" Helena held the sand head between her hands and cried and said she really felt this woman (Figure 7.19).

January 22, 2019: Reading together, everyone wants to hear the story

She found it easier to speak in creative groups that she enjoyed, in writing, ceramics and music. As she impressed her fingers and handprints deeply on this low, heart-shaped mound, she recalled a dream in which an eagle pecked at her. She placed a sitting eagle on top, inserted her fingers even more deeply into the sand and added Anastasia, the little red-dressed girl, a baby, a little boy, several tiny animals and a book for Anastasia to read to everyone. She commented that this was so nice, if only it could stay this way without reality intruding. Even so, the strong Eagle would protect everyone. She then thought that she could read, maintain contact with reality and feel what was happening without fear. In the author's experience, repeatedly inserting fingers deeply into the sand can signify deep anguish, irreparable heartbreak and regret for a troubled relationship or for a deceased person. This idyllic scene of harmonic relationships is built on silent mourning, letting suffering sink into the earth (Figure 7.20).

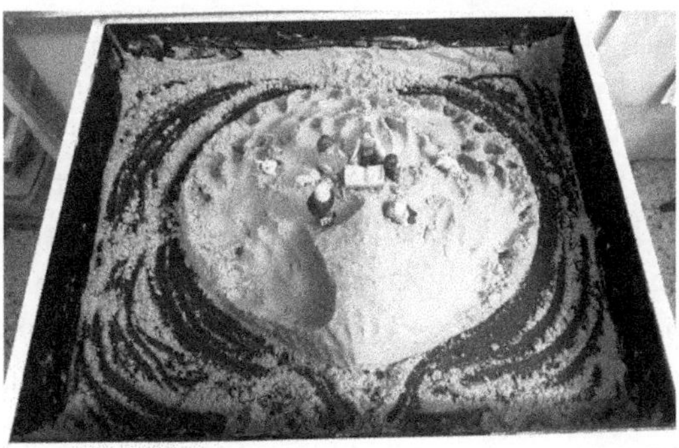

Figure 7.20 *Helena: Reading together on the mound, everyone wants to hear the story*

July 15, 2019: Healing underneath the mound, connecting to reality above the mound

Six months later, Helena dreamt about a depressed adolescent girl who wanted to die by suicide, supported in this by her mother. She formed a strong central sand mound, excavated a deep cave on its left side and inserted a boat with Anastasia, a young peasant girl and two oars into the cave. At the cave entrance, the Venus of Willendorf and the little red-dressed girl looked inside. Helena began planting trees on the hilltop, and placed a cat, snake, butterfly, roses and a dog. But the cave was not deep enough, and she removed sand several times. She moved the little red-dressed girl to the top of the mound to "take charge of what happens." A bridge on top leads to the right far corner, to consciousness, a "reality" of earth, trees and houses extending down the entire right edge. Above the cave entrance, she placed a butterfly-shaped metal box with a red stone and a white stone in its blue interior. She poured water into the box and seemed calmer. She pushed the boat deeper inside and cried: "I don't have an inner container. I close things too quickly. It is hard to see at the same time what's happening inside the cave, and what's happening outside. The young adolescent girl is very angry, I left her, she believes in trees, when I am sad or distressed, I go inside myself. I must close the cave opening, this is an internal ceremony." She hung two blue and brown cloths over the entrance and held them in place with the butterfly box and said: "Something important is happening inside. My adolescent girl, I suffered so much, I ran away from her, tried not to see her pain, her suffering. One must accept suffering, but I constantly tried to escape from it. My body became weak. Now there are two women inside in the boat, the mother and the girl, there is a growing closeness between them in the dark, despite all the problems that exist between what I am able to do and her ability to trust me. On the hilltop the little girl, who was brought up by the grandmother, calls for an emergency meeting to figure out how to help. The animals are thirsty, the butterfly takes nectar from the flowers and will enjoy life. The snake understands things between death and life and watches over the balance, how much poison to take, to live in all the worlds. In the (far-right) corner there is a place for a relationship with myself and with other people, a house, children, grandchildren. Most essential is to live in harmony with nature. It was hard to build this place. The Great Mother is watching over it all, is accompanying me from the beginning, and there is a bridge from reality to what lies inside" (Figure 7.21 photographed from the vertical left side of the sandtray and Figure 7.22).

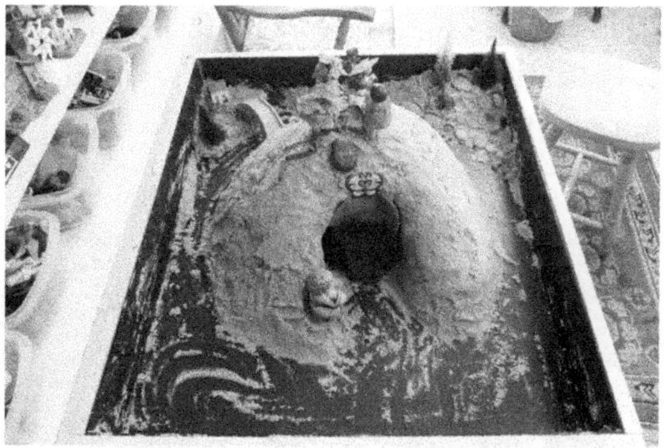

Figure 7.21 *Helena: Healing ceremony under the mound, connecting to reality above*

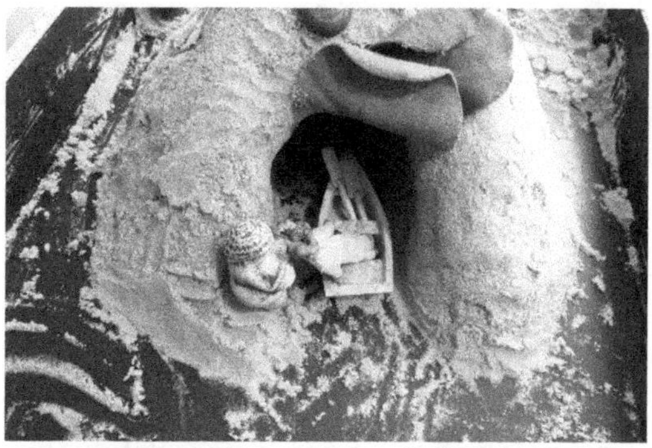

Figure 7.22 *Helena: Under the mound*

October 2, 2019: Final sandplay, a sand nest or a hollow, for eggs in a mound of flour

Three months later, Helena planned a trip to her childhood home. She ordered airline tickets and found a room next to the house where she had grown up. She intended to use the visit to focus on seeing and hearing things differently than she had as a frightened child. A dream of a man with a visible phallus, who didn't see what he had, confused her, as if she could not differentiate between father and lover in relationships. She made a mound in the sand and smoothed the insides into a central hole, like a nest. It reminded her of her mother making bread, putting eggs in a hole in the center of dough and kneading. The sand structure of this final sandplay resembles Figure 7.5, in which a mother duck and several eggs fill a central hole or nest, observed by an Eagle who could have stolen the eggs, symbol of new life potential, pretending to protect them, like her father, who merged with Helena and "devoured" her. In this empty "nest," her memory shifted to her mother, preparing bread dough, with eggs in a hole of flour (Figure 7.23).

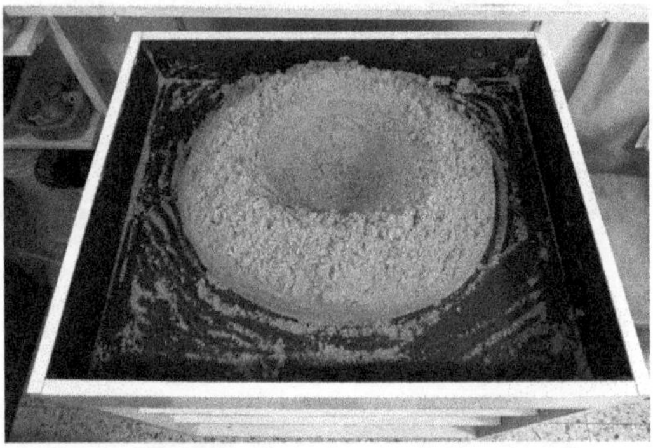

Figure 7.23 *Helena: Final sandplay, A sand nest, or a hollow for eggs in a mound of flour*

Conclusion

The sandtray center was a continuous and stable anchor for Helena throughout 16 years of sandplay therapy. Her first central mounds were independent, surrounded by emptiness, like a fortress without the dangers inherent in relationships. After several years of gradual integration of positive symbols, in a transition from isolation the center became a place of relationship between Self and Ego where the first Self–Ego axis could appear. Balanced symmetrical sand structures had kept Helena's center stable and secure. This gave her freedom to choose varied objects and place them asymmetrically. Helena's symmetrical center suggests her inner dialogue between the left and right lobes of the brain, between logic and instinct, consciousness and the unconscious, a dialogue that began in conflict and transitioned to reflection of each other. Being born left-handed and forced to use only her right hand had been traumatic, but was now healed. Jung says: "The idea of creating a symmetry would thus indicate some kind of climax in the task of accepting the unconscious and incorporating it in a general picture of the world" (1953, para. 226). Helena had continually gathered herself together in life, just as she continually gathered sand into independent mounds until she was no longer in peril of being devoured by monsters lurking in her dark unconscious. Later, her fear of death, the evil feminine and agonizing pain but also deep unconscious sources of healing could manifest as elegant sand forms in the reality of the sandtray. She accessed a healthier, more balanced way of living for herself and in her relationships with family, friends and work colleagues. Winter (1999, p.91) writes that when the ego, the center of the personality, locates itself in the center of the sandtray, it "reflects the Self's desire to incarnate into ego form and the ego's desire to be connected to the Self."

8

Signposts and Symbols on the Path of the Sandplay Journey

Symbolic signposts, paths, stages and maps of the journey: Where am I?

Getting lost on a journey is usually preventable by consulting maps (or electronic applications) to guide us through roads, villages, towns and cities with numbered streets, and signposts showing distances to further destinations. But unmarked paths, a paved stone trail ending in the wild, a worn footpath through the woods, or a centuries-old animal track also beckon. A beautiful flower lured Kore-Persephone into a field where she was abducted to the underworld, planned by Hades and his brother Zeus, God of Olympus. The sandplay path, like the path of Persephone, Psyche, or Odysseus (see Chapter 11), has no signposts to point a client towards a destination. Only in retrospect does a review of the sandplay process reveal an orchestration of its stages, as if prescribed in advance by mysterious gods, or by the unconscious. In each stage, the symbols evoked are appropriate to that client and to their location on one's inner path. From the outside path towards a sandplay clinic, one cannot know what will transpire on the other side of the door.

Leaving "home," but is there a path?

One must first have an image of "home" before leaving it. The first sandplay image, the current inner "home" of the sandplayer, can provide diagnostic and prognostic information. It is also a portal for a sandplayer to enter remote unmarked regions of the psyche, new inner landscapes, and hidden pitfalls. Jung viewed the inner path as an autonomous powerful guide, coming alive when an individual steps on it and begins to move (Jung, 1997, p.1226). In 1933, he wrote in a letter to Frau V. that the individual way is

> the way you make for yourself, which is never prescribed, which you do not know in advance, and which simply comes into being of itself when you put one foot in front of the other. If you always do the next thing that needs to be done, you will go most safely and sure-footedly along the path prescribed by your unconscious. (Jung, 1973/1992, pp.132–133)

Some symbols on the sandplay path

In a first or second sandplay, some kind of path constructed in the sandtray with sand and specific objects might represent a prognostic map of the sandplay journey. Once the client intuits that there is a path, albeit as yet unknown, the unconscious provides symbolic support at appropriate moments and turning points in the journey. In an early sandplay, a "hamsa," an imprint of one or both hands in the sand decorated with marbles or crystals, symbolizes divine help. The hamsa is worn in the Middle East to avert the evil eye, as is the color blue which is painted around openings such as doors and windows. The blue sandtray bottom may be uncovered as an unconscious request for a blessing during the therapeutic journey. Ritual purification and cleansing in preparation for descent into the unconscious might manifest by pouring water or sculpting a circular Kiva. Changes in color, transformations from black, white, yellow and red, are alchemical stages coordinated by the psyche that indicate the stages of the process (Ehlers, 2022). Objects such as frogs, butterflies and grasshoppers can indicate stages of metamorphosis and transformation, and may be placed in a sandplay unrelated to anything else in the tray. Keys and bridges can predict movement from one state to another, as might diagonal movements from the front-right corner towards spirit in the far-left corner, or from the front-left corner towards the world in the far-right corner. At a later stage, a pyramid or dolmen might appear as a portal for a soul passing through the underworld preparing for ascent into rebirth. A labyrinth in the sand that circumambulates the center throws the sandplayer back and forth, but although the path is slow, the center is reached. Spiral sand paths to the center may appear towards conclusion of a process. A fisherman may also appear, indicating the ego's ability to hold the tension between opposites (Steinhardt, 2009).

The sandplay genie, "the spirit of past wounds"

In the air above the sandplay, there may be an invisible "smoke-like" presence made by a large genie released from a very small bottle. A genie who is freed after a short imprisonment may gratefully grant three wishes. But after a long imprisonment, as happens with adults who begin sandplay later in life, frustration may have festered. The genie, representing the "spirit of past wounds," will be angry. In the *Tales of the Arabian Nights*, a fisherman who had released a long-imprisoned vengeful genie was able to re-imprison him in his bottle through cunning (Lang, 1898/2017). Another option to delay a genie's revenge is to distract him by telling a story that does not end, with twists and turns, chapter by chapter, like chapters in a sandplay journey guided by the unconscious. Images of wounding are unexpectedly coped with, healing images access new understanding of relationships in outer life, and the genie's anger is transformed into fascination. At some point, a centering mandala appears, and archetypal support is internalized and indelibly absorbed into the psyche. In the end, the sandplay genie may no longer be preoccupied with revenge and will happily grant three wishes and go on his way. The client has attained emotional freedom and discovered positive potential and the self-awareness to live an authentic life.

First sandplays with no path

In many first or second sandplays, like a symbolic map predicting the path of an unfolding journey, an actual path is intuitively constructed within the sandtray. But some early sandplays have no discernible path and resemble a scattering of undifferentiated pebbles and shells thrown up by the sea onto a beach, exposed on the sand. This scattering can resemble a pre-ego unconscious "uroboric" state between an infant and its mother, from birth to three months, intended by nature to provide an experience of merging and unification, a "Participation Mystique" without differentiation or boundaries, with no object and no subject (Neumann, 1973/1988). Three brief examples of "uroboric" sandplays presented below begin with an age-appropriate sandplay of "Oron," a young boy. Two similar examples of scattering in an adult's first sandplay, of "Bella" and "Rose", might mirror a sense of early abandonment or lack of containment.

> **Oron**, a boy aged two years eight months first scattered many small figurines in the front area of the sandtray, and then raked a large containing

semi-circular "womb" around them (Figure 8.1). His first sandplay is age-appropriate, still in the matriarchal realm. Until the age of six, he played spontaneously in the sandtray and progressed through natural developmental stages until other creative activities began to interest him (see Oron, Chapter 10).

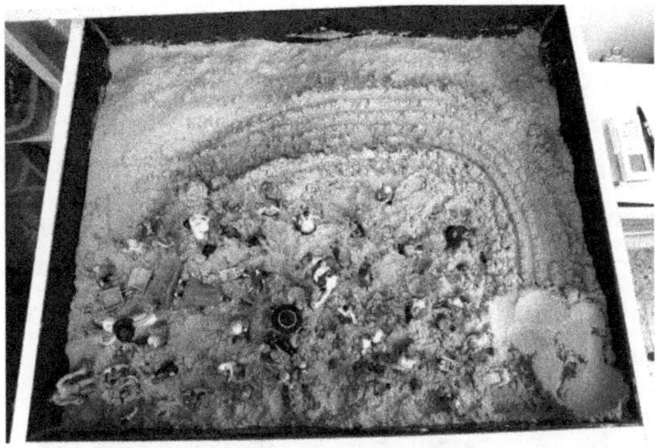

Figure 8.1 *Oron: Age two years eight months, First sandplay, Uroboric*

Bella, a devoted mother and an accomplished artist, was adopted as an infant. In her first sandplay she dispersed many small pieces of sea glass and a few tiny objects in the front sandtray area. They seem nameless and insignificant, an inner unprotected state of maternal rejection corresponding to her early abandonment. One tiny dark stone in the center of a barely noticeable circle of sea glass in the front center might represent her, enclosed in a magic circle that protects its contents from the frightening glare of a row of figures leaning on the far edge (Figure 8.2).

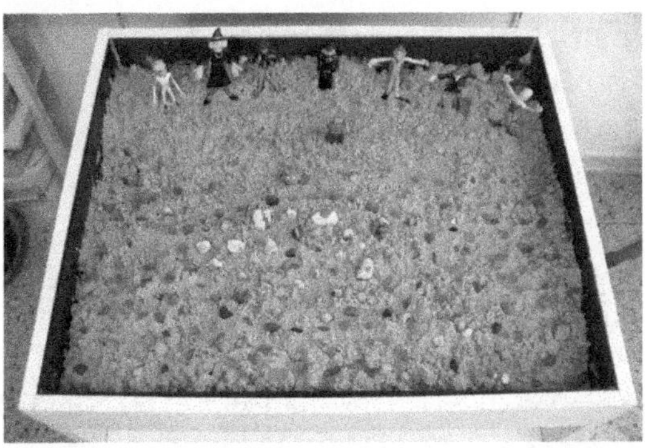

Figure 8.2 *Bella: First sandplay, Abandoned at birth*

Rose, a mother of young children, scattered pebbles, shells and glass in the "feminine" front area of the sandtray, suggesting a lack of holding and inner fragmentation. In the far masculine area, a group of sea creatures, mermaid, fish and crabs seem to passively observe. Rose reinforced the front-left edge with a flat stone wall, and the far-right corner with a large abalone shell creating a diagonal movement. The stone wall prevents her from falling out of the sandtray into the collective unconscious, or prevents entry of frightening forces which might mirror her early childhood experience of lack of containment. The large abalone shell whose inner spiral structure can symbolize development seems contained by the sandtray's far-right corner, near where the therapist sits. The sandtray and the shell as therapeutic holding containers, are a place for her self-nurture and development, until she can begin to walk an inner path alone (Figure 8.3).

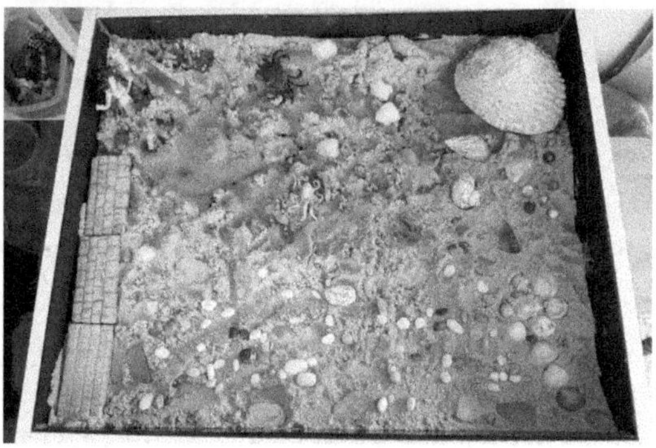

Figure 8.3 *Rose: First sandplay, Fragmentation, a need for containment*

Sandplay paths in a first or second sandplay: a blueprint for the journey

The five paths described below were intuited by each client's psyche as if to present a preview of the ensuing sandplay journey. The first sandplay paths of Aya and Jana mourn the untimely death of a parent. Blocks in the first sandplay paths of Ziva and Grete were resolved in later sandplays. Sandplay paths "above and below" of "Blissful Tara" close this chapter.

Aya was in her late teens, depressed and silent. Since the death of her mother, she ran the household, cared for her father and siblings, and kept up her grades in school. In her creative therapeutic process, her loss and longing for her mother was expressed in drawings, painting and sculpture and sandplay. In her first sandplay, a gentle wavy line meanders like a slow river, in a diagonal path between the far-left corner and the front-right corner where it is deeply incised. The "river" divides the sandtray into two triangles, a large far area and smaller near area. Turquoise sea glass "tears," embedded in high sand in the far left, seem to flow back to the unconscious. Stuck in the front-right center of the river are a mother duck and ducklings. This symbol has recurred in several sandplay processes of children orphaned of their mothers, and may express longing from a young age. The river continues to flow towards a bridge, a pool and a fish. In the far right, a grave-like mound covered with a cluster of red roses is near an old house surrounded by trees and small animals. A sand path leads from the house to the bridge and across to the front area. There, seven small green trees, two cedar trees of the kind planted in cemeteries, and a dead tree stump make altogether ten, her age when her mother became ill. Tiny squirrels that store their food before hibernating in cold winters may mirror her emotional hibernation. Aya expressed her sorrow and loss in art and in sandplay, and was able to register for university to study a scientific profession (Figure 8.4).

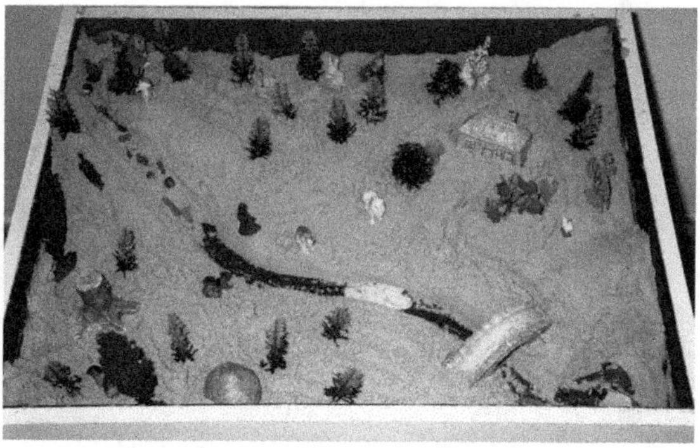

Figure 8.4 *Aya: Blue path of mourning*

Jana was in her early teens, at home alone with her father when he suffered a stroke and died. Now, as an adult, she carried a burden of guilt that she could not save him. In her first sandplay, a blue diagonal path flows in high and low loops from the far-left corner to the front-right corner. This "river" divides a seemingly calm country landscape into front and rear areas covered evenly with 11 green trees, farm animals, cars, eight buildings and five pairs of people, each with a man and a woman, scattered in both areas. The five couples stand close to each other like once her parents did. There are no figurines of children. There are 11 green trees but the twelfth, a silver-penny branch in the left-front center often symbolizes mourning. The front sand area's contour resembles two people, a pair joined together. Two pairs of sailboats on the river sail in opposite directions. On both ends of the narrow blue waterway, the water disappears before it reaches the sandtray edges. Six of the eight buildings are paired but stand apart from each other—two small houses, two lighthouses on opposite sides of the river, and two fortresses. The fourth pair contrasts the somber small house with a bright gingerbread fairy-tale house in the front area, perhaps an irreconcilable distance between Jana's feelings for her home before and after her father's death. The two different houses might also indicate a split between masculine and feminine aspects of her psyche. Jana's sandplay path progressed from grave scenes to sand mounds that resembled ancient burial sites to a sea journey on a whale, then to differentiation of the opposites, help from divine figures, a central mound and a return to the marketplace of life. She resolved her guilt for her father's death and mother's widowhood, and became decisive in her professional goals and in her friendships (Figure 8.5).

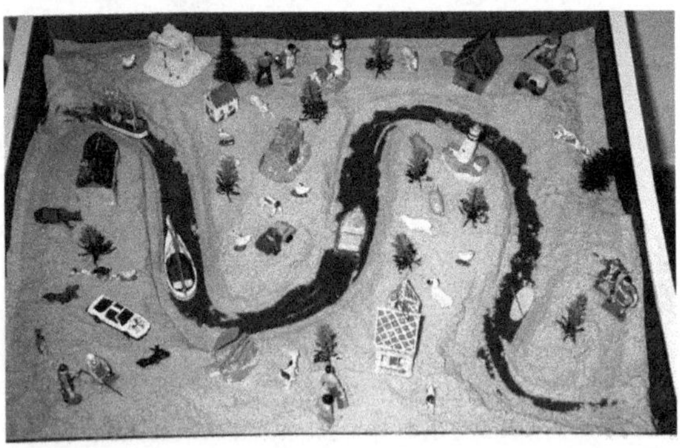

Figure 8.5 *Jana: Turbulence beneath a blue path of mourning*

Ziva was the only child of Holocaust survivors. She felt stuck in her work and in her life. A friend suggested she try a non-verbal therapy. Her sandplay path alternated between life-affirming images, grave scenes, sudden violent devastation and then rebuilding, a mirror of her parent's tragic history and loss. In her first sandplay, everything seemed hopelessly blocked. A high bridge standing horizontally in the front center as if over a chasm has no connection to a land road on either side. On the bridge, two cars face each other, blocking each other's passage. From a dark closet in the far center, a vertical sand ridge leads towards the bridge and divides dark objects on the left side from fantasy objects on the right. A large boat on the right cannot pass to the left through a tiny tunnel under the ridge. A lighthouse stands on the left side without water (Figure 8.6). In her second sandplay a water path from the far-right corner descends diagonally towards a clay goddess in the front left, giving some hope. After several sandplays with graves, a sandplay with a serpentine path of cars and a family of turtles seemed to be moving towards a "home" corner in the front left, but then violence erupted with an arsenal of metallic weapons surrounding a central blue pistol shape in the center. Happily, four months later a miraculous birth appeared. A woman giving birth in the far-right corner is supported by several Buddhas, goddesses and other numinous figures, protected by a dragon in a pool in the front-right corner, and by turtles, frogs, a sphinx and two pyramids as well as three monkeys who face the front-right corner and do not intrude (Figure 8.7). Soon after, Ziva sculpted a sand ferry and dock on the entire left side of the sandtray, opposite an open sea on the right. Passengers leave the ferry on a sand path towards the shore, predicting the end of therapy. At our final session, Ziva said that sandplay was very beautiful, even if she couldn't understand the language (Figure 8.8).

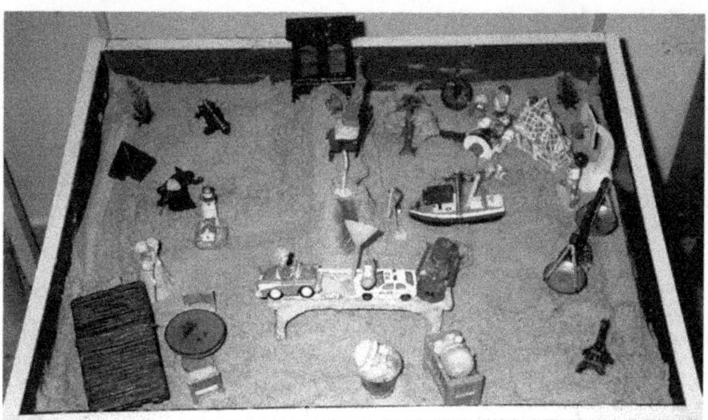

Figure 8.6 *Ziva: First sandplay, A dead-end path*

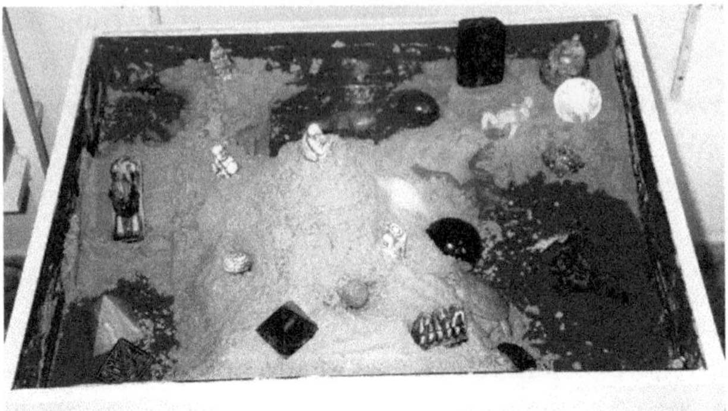

Figure 8.7 *Ziva: Sandplay 16, A birth in progress*

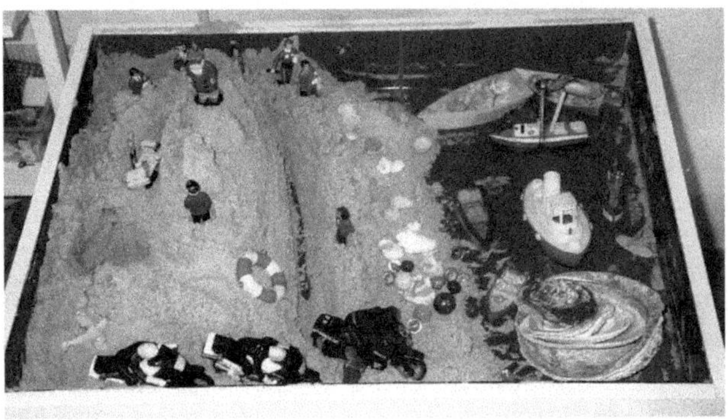

Figure 8.8 *Ziva: Final sandplay, Leaving a sand ferry after a voyage*

Grete planned to visit the country where she was born, together with her grown-up children. In her first sandplay, she meticulously arranged a path of small and large white shells and stones along the front edge, like a beaded necklace on a string connecting the left and right corners. It may have symbolized a connection between her original home on the left and her present family on the right. A Little Mermaid, perhaps her age when she left her home near the sea, sits on a coral, gazing outward at swirling blue paths drawn lightly with sand on the "patriarchal" space of the far area (Figure 8.9). In her second sandplay, another path like a string of prayer beads of turquoise sea glass and pebbles leads from four witches in the far-left corner and moves in the shape of a small rectangle and large triangle whose diagonal crosses a large "ocean" pointing to a small African male god in the far-right corner. This construction seems superimposed over a geometrical sand construction that divides the tray vertically. Both sandplays map potential connections between undeveloped or negative feminine entities and illusive but controlling or weak masculine entities. I recalled the two paths of Hansel and Gretel, two abandoned children, whose first pebble path shone in the moonlight and led them out of a dark forest to their home. Abandoned a second time, they scattered a path of breadcrumbs that were eaten by birds. They wandered in the forest and came upon a gingerbread house where they were in danger of being devoured by a wicked witch. They survived by making a transition from helplessness to conscious control, eliminated the negative feminine by fire, strengthened both the young feminine and young masculine, and returned "home" as individuals (Grimm Brothers, 1981). In her eighth sandplay, Grete gathered all the sand into a powerful mound that juts into the blue bottom of the sandtray from the front edge and is encircled by concentric water paths around it. An archetypal feminine blue Cretan goddess stands above on the front center, complementing the archetypal masculine presence of the mound. This numinous pair bonds Grete to the goddess, to the mound and the paths that have opened in the blue unconscious sea (Figure 8.10). Before our final session, Grete placed four large round stones from my garden in the front-right corner of the sandtray, solidly anchoring her to her present home. They rise diagonally towards a large abalone shell in the far-left corner, which contains many shells, some mine and some hers from her country of origin. Stones are timeless, but the containing abalone shell can symbolize potential rebirth. Its location here may point more to the rebirth of spirit, of creativity, and her innate connection to Nature's beauty and mysterious intent (Figure 8.11).

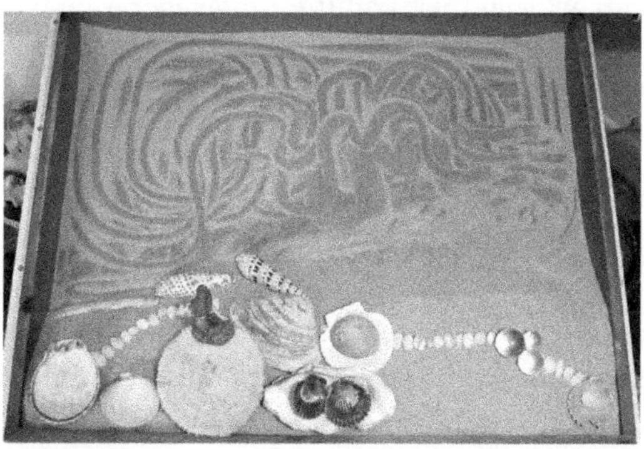

Figure 8.9 *Grete: First sandplay, A path of pebbles*

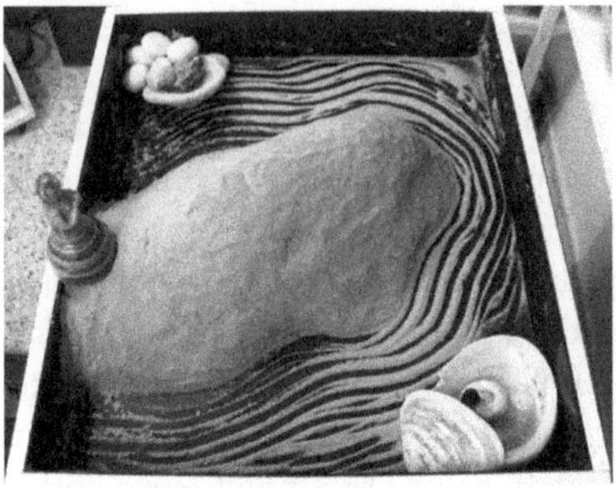

Figure 8.10 *Grete: Sandplay 8, Paths in the unconscious, feminine and masculine archetypes*

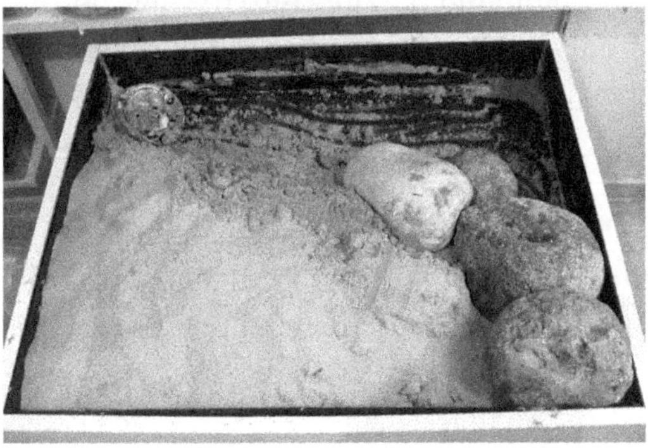

Figure 8.11 *Grete: Final sandplay, Path from stones to shells, spiritual rebirth*

BLISSFUL TARA, a spiritual sandplay process: center, place of origin and of return

Tara was an art therapist and life-long vegetarian who had practiced meditation for many years. In my studio, our easy professional relationship changed for me when she began to work in the sandtray. Instinctively, I distanced myself so the space around her, the trays and objects would be hers alone. A sculpted symmetrical sand base in Tara's first sandplay became the pattern for sculpted bases in each of her 21 sandplays. A second pattern was equal representation of masculine and feminine, as men and women or as male and female divinities. Multiple paths in her second sandplay became a theme that was resolved in her twentieth sandplay with a round central pond as the origin of many paths. I will briefly summarize several sandplays whose paths were resolved in her two final sandplays.

Tara reported a dream where a lion in a field of wild animals ran towards her. She was unsure if he wanted to eat her. She wondered why she never chose aggressive figurines such as a witch or dragon to represent evil. Actually, just once, in her first sandplay, the two objects she placed first were a tiny horned demon in the far center, hiding behind a spinning wheel. They were followed by a vertical sequence of round objects towards the front center, a table with lit candles, a triple spiral and a piece of white coral in front on which a blue goddess stands, facing front. This vertical axis is intersected by a horizontal mud river with two sailboats facing each other, forming a cross. On the left and right sides of the sandtray, Tara balanced male and female gods, men and women, figurines of fire and water, trees, small houses and dwarfs; she called this a "community" (Figure 8.12). Weinrib (1996, p.24) states that the "critical element" of the cross is to hold the center together, usually after the constellation of the Self, supporting the ego so that it can withstand the tension created "between powerful opposing personal values." The presence of this cross in Tara's first sandplay rather than at a later stage might reflect a mature self-knowledge and understanding of her personal values, gained in verbal therapy and in her work as a non-verbal therapist, previous to actualizing her sandplay process.

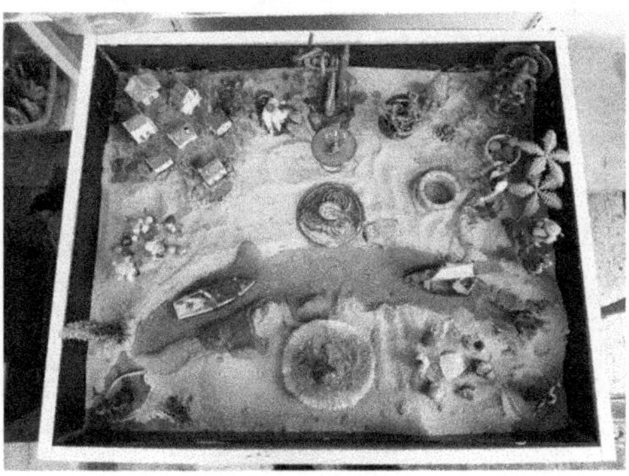

Figure 8.12 *Tara: First sandplay, Home*

The space of her second sandplay is filled by a symmetrical butterfly-shaped form, again organized around a central axis with steps and paths formed by objects made of hard materials—ceramic, stone, metal, glass and shards. The apex of the axis is a grey ceramic cave imprinted with a triple spiral. Inside the cave, a small open round metal treasure box contains a gold ring with a blue stone. A ring as a symbol can mean union, power and the cycle of life (Cirlot, 1971/1996). This ring is a treasure calling to be found, guarded by a samurai on the left and Ishtar, a blue metal fertility goddess, on the right. The cave faces a ceramic bridge between the left and right sides. White stone steps lead under the bridge to a lower level where water flows forward and branches out into two lung-shaped areas of muddy water with some blue showing through. In the right water area, a man in a sailboat with a tiny lifesaver faces a canoe on the left side, with a Native American woman carrying a papoose and three brass jars. His hand reaches towards her, but her hand does not respond, as if each must travel an individual path first. At the front edge, a ceramic flat round triple spiral mirrors the triple spiral on the cave above, inferring a vertical connection between far and near. Their placement in the sandtray recalls Jung's words "as above, so below" (Jung, 1971, p.136). The spirals recall spiral movement in nature and in the universe. A triple spiral can symbolize the perpetual intertwining of "past, present and future," "life, death and rebirth," "sky, sea and earth" and the therapeutic sandplay relationship—"therapist, client, image" (Steinhardt, 2009). Green glass steps on the left invite ascent from the water to a white pebble path. On the right, red ceramic shard steps lead up to a wide turquoise sea-glass path. The two paths encircle the axis on opposite sides, continue upwards and meet on either side of the bridge, implying opposites of consciousness and the unconscious, or mundane and spiritual, or that masculine and feminine opposites must first walk individual paths and then meet on the bridge and obtain the treasure together. Tara had balanced several life roles—mother, wife, therapist, artist, spiritual person and seeker of knowledge—and walked these paths simultaneously. She placed an equal number of feminine and masculine human figurines with a few divinities among them, noticed the two wells and was pleased that the two triple spirals closed the central vertical axis above and below. In her next session, she remembered with pleasure the sensation of constructing stone paths and inserting green glass and red shards as steps in the sand (Figure 8.13).

Tara intended to continue last session's theme in her third sandplay, but her psyche had other plans. A large sandwoman appeared, sitting cross-legged, adorned with crystals, dried pods and a pearl as a central navel. In her next sandplays, she chose small houses, palm trees, flowers and fruits, natural objects, boats, bridges, birds, fish, some bears and elephants, wells, fire symbols and sky powers, and a starfish that appeared five times. She sculpted a huge sand starfish in Sandplay 7 and in her final Sandplay 21. She continued to balance human and divine masculine and feminine figurines and sand sculptures. In Sandplay 17, a sculpted wise, gentle old man with three brown feathers and a red one on his crown chakra conveyed spirit. In Sandplay 18, a sculpted sea goddess with a necklace of three pearls and water-related objects arose from the depths of the sea and conveyed feminine benevolence. Sandplay 19 connects above and below with masculine and feminine divinities in the corners, a central vertical axis capped by a rainbow ending with Ishtar in a small round mud pool in the near center. In the near-right corner, two children contemplate the sky, protected by a blue ceramic goddess and white unicorn.

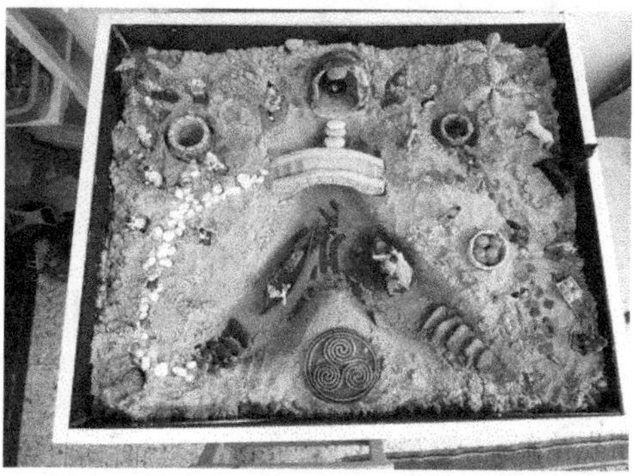

Figure 8.13 *Tara: Sandplay 2, Multiple paths*

In Sandplay 20, Tara opened a blue circle in the center and sculpted several low mounds around it like flower petals. She placed a Native American woman (for the fourth time), two musicians, ten houses, 14 women and 14 men, birds and about 13 flowers in a peripheral circle around the mounds and blue center. A businessman with a briefcase exits the far-right corner. In this return "to the marketplace," there are no divinities but there are three new objects—a boy striding on green grass with baskets of flowers, a small princess and a couple sitting by a table. In the central blue circle, a white swan (for the fourth time) is surrounded by six goldfish, an orange starfish, a white duck, and two sailboats that Tara thought represented the absence of ego. The objects seem to rise into visibility from the depths of the numinous blue water. Around the center, four paths between the sand mounds leave the center in semi-circular routes and seem to curve back to center. Each is made of one material—red cherries, white pebbles, turquoise sea glass (for the eleventh time) and marbles. Tara said that walking these low paths was joyful and less exerting than ascending to the higher paths in Sandplay 2 (Figure 8.14).

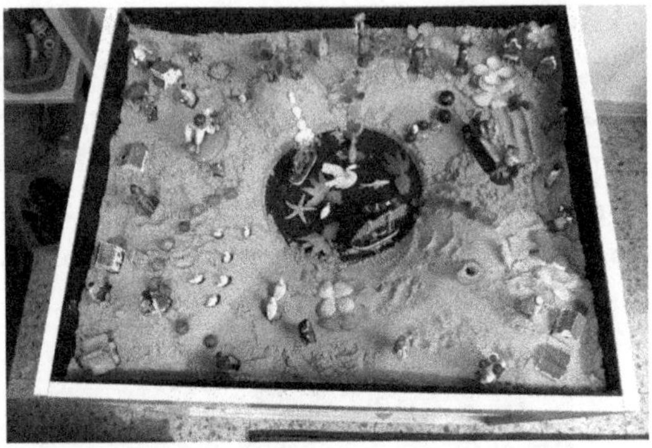

Figure 8.14 *Tara: Sandplay 20, Blue pool in center, multiple paths leave and return*

The elegant white swan, combining water and air elements, feminine purity and beauty holds the center of the round blue pool. Previously, the swan appeared in a central blue pond enclosed in a sculpted sand uroboros in Sandplay 8, and in the far and left areas of Sandplays 9 and 16. The swan is sacred to Aphrodite, Greek Goddess of Love, who rose fully formed on a shell from the sea, like the sea goddess in Sandplay 18. The swan's long phallic neck, its movement and soft round body point to a union of opposites and to satisfaction of a desire. The silent swan is said to sing a beautiful song before leaving, or dying (Cirlot, 1971/1996, p.322). Bachelard (1999, p.36) described the swan as integrating masculine and feminine traits:

> Like all images active in the unconscious, the image of the swan is hermaphroditic. The swan is feminine when brilliant waters are contemplated, but it is masculine in action. For the unconscious action is an act... An image that suggests an act must evolve in the unconscious from feminine to masculine.

Thus, the swan in this sandplay appropriately symbolizes the inner integration of the opposites, and signals a song of ending this process.

A celestial path in Sandplay 21 concludes Tara's sandplay journey and integrates themes from previous sandplays. A five-rayed sculpted sand star fills the tray, its apex pointing upward, two "arms" extended to each side and two "legs" resting on the front edge. Tara felt joy and sculpted smiling faces on four mounds in the corners like positive forces that exist in the world. They all face a small round yellow hut in the center. A white whirling dervish stands on the far-left mound, the delicate green jade Kwan Yin is on the far-right mound, and on the central apex a graceful white goddess holds the Scales of Justice. Paths of turquoise sea glass flow from these three objects and meet beneath the yellow central hut. Their path continues to small red objects at the tips of the left and right "arms" and below to the two lower mound portraits (Figure 8.15).

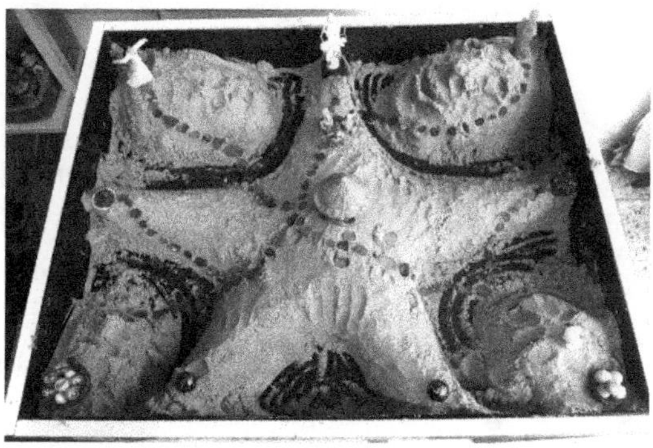

Figure 8.15 *Tara: Sandplay 21 (final sandplay), A celestial afterward*

In her review, Tara felt that Kwan Yin, Goddess of Compassion and "she who hears all prayers," was the source of all these paths. She said that Kwan Yin had made a clockwise round of all four corners, from Sandplay 5 in the far-left corner, Sandplay 12 in the front-left corner, Sandplay 15 in the front-right corner, and now in the far-right corner. The five-pointed sand star connects a celestial star and the sea starfish, reflecting different levels of a universal structural reality, and can symbolize man, with two arms and two legs and a head that coordinates them (Cirlot, 1971/1996). In Sandplay 7, Tara had sculpted a six-armed sand star with concealed underground passages below, while the same yellow hut marked the center. Now the hut stands openly in the center of this final five-point sand star and turquoise sea-glass paths flow visibly like a celestial map, connecting masculine and feminine, upper and lower worlds, divinities and humans. Tara's symbolic sandplay process had ended and she returned to a material world. The yellow hut signaled a need to renovate her apartment, and renew other things in her life.

9

Jasmin, 13 Sandplays: from Divination to Archetype

Introduction

In 2019, at the ISST Congress in Berlin, I presented the three-year sandplay process of Jasmin, a 32-year-old woman whose hands touched the sand as if guided by an unconscious memory of an original maternal loving touch in 13 sandplays, almost without objects. Yet her first sandplays revealed her original painful relationship with her mother and family. In a mid-stage of therapy, images of the good archetypal feminine appeared, and in a later stage she created an Ego–Self relationship, sifting sand into a high hill in the center of the sandtray and placing one large house and six mud balls on the left of the tray. We ended therapy with a review of her artwork but not her sandplays. Twenty years later, I remembered her spontaneous hand movements and symbols in the sand and reviewed my notes and photographs of her work. I contacted her and she immediately gave me permission to use her sandplays in a presentation, but she had no interest in seeing her work. After the conference, I called her again about an article based on the presentation. This time she was curious to know what interested me, and we met in my studio. She looked well, and was happy with her work, children and family. We reviewed her sandplays. Some evoked clear memories of traumatic family situations. We agreed to include her comments when relevant, to change details of her history and to call her "Jasmin."

Sand, mounds, mud balls and pre-conscious memory

For Jasmin, the sand was generously compliant, able to fulfill a yearning to arrive at a form through touch and movement. She felt the qualities of sand alone, its color, texture, and its infinite granules that sparkled in the light. Mounds and mud balls were part of her sand vocabulary. Mounds are large and can be attached to the sand surface sometimes with blue areas around them. Mud balls are small, wet, round and independent, a primal object molded in the cupped palms of the hands and taking their shape. Older children at the beach prepare an arsenal of mud balls to throw or to roll. Three mud balls, one on the other, form a rudimentary person.

Margaret Lowenfeld, the originator of sandtray and the World Technique (1993), and D.W. Winnicott were contemporaries, and were in contact in the late 1920s (Davis and Walbridge, 1989, p.192; Davis, 1992). They widely agreed about the nature and function of play in children, and both crystallized their ideas by observing and writing. Lowenfeld wrote *Play in Childhood* (1935/1991), emphasizing that the experience of play was therapeutic and helpful in adaptation to life. Winnicott practiced listening carefully, and recorded minute observations of case histories of mothers and their babies in ongoing sequences of actions, in the stages between absolute dependence and independence. He focused on the significance of early infancy and even pre-birth, and formed theories about the pre-verbal history of the individual, and its influence on emotional development and the total life of human beings (Davis and Wallbridge, 1989, p.31). Winnicott's concept of primary maternal preoccupation and holding also seems to apply to a child or adult sandplayer, gently and sensuously forming the sand as if guided by pre-conscious memory of the mother's body (Davis and Wallbridge, 1989, pp.93–100; Winnicott, 1971). An infant held securely, touching the mother's body, feels supported and plays with the breast while nursing. For Winnicott, "playing...was that which gives quality to life. It covers the whole of an individual's contact with the phenomena of external reality, and is manifest in the whole history of our cultural evolution" (Davis, 1992). Sand is a pure, ancient element in nature that represents universal as well as personal memory. For Jasmin, sand form unfolded into an unconscious reincarnation of the original lost object that could be caressed, entered, its depth explored.

JASMIN, a princess in distress

I will introduce Jasmin as if in a fairy tale, a princess in distress who was rescued by a wonderful prince. He brought her to his kingdom, they married and had a son, and they lived happily with his warm, loving family. But Jasmin had distanced herself from her own father and mother. Her parents came from two very different cultures and both had suffered traumas of different kinds during their early lives. Later, they met and married as adults in Israel. And like a fairy-tale king and queen, they may have imagined that marriage and giving birth to a child would magically heal past wounds and ensure a happy end. Their child, Jasmin, was much loved by each of them. But both developed psychiatric illnesses, and they divorced when Jasmin was eight years old.

Jasmin's father was from a Yiddish-speaking Eastern European culture, from a land of forests covered in winter with white snow. He worked in the family business from a young age. Her mother came from an Arabic-speaking North African country, a hot land full of color and the smells of spices. As a child, Jasmin's mother and her family had witnessed violent attacks on the Jewish population, which forced them to flee their home and leave all their possessions behind. Jasmin's mother, as the eldest daughter, was allowed only basic education and her traditional role was to raise her younger siblings. She was the only one of her siblings who married, but there was no happy end for her marriage. After her parent's divorce, Jasmin and her mother moved frequently from house to house. Her mother's large extended family and grandparents were influential, although she never lived with them. At family gatherings, meals usually ended by divining the future, reading Turkish coffee grounds. Jasmin may have viewed her sand creations through this cultural lens, reading the sand to find her fortune. She was very pretty and charming, and she was a good student. After her army service, she met and married her prince, and gave birth to a son. But to protect her new family from her unstable parents and her mother's family, she avoided all contact with them. One day, her young son asked who took care of her when she was a child, and she began to cry. She began a three-year art therapy process and made 13 sandplays spaced out between her paintings.

Jasmin usually began a sandplay on the vertical axis of the tray, continued working from the other two or three sides and then returned to the vertical view. With both hands, she moved sand back and forth, and sprinkled it above the tray until a mound was formed, or just sprinkled it like a blessing from above. She combined forms and broke them up into new forms. She would also turn the sandtray itself, to work or observe from multiple angles. While she worked, she spoke about her present family and friends, and brought up memories of her Ashkenazi father and her Sephardi mother. Two sandplays done on the horizontal axis of the sandtray accessed the feminine nurturing archetype, bestowing inner strength to manage her relationships with her parents and build her own happy home. Jasmin's pattern of movement could have been acquired in childhood, witnessing the different cultures of her parents, abruptly leaving different homes, viewing the world from different houses and neighborhoods, being abandoned by either father or mother, and she abandoning them now. Freedle (2019) describes the organization of behavioral patterns around somato-sensory rhythms based on what is stored in the brain from previous experience. These activate body-based memories and associated neural pathways, and mediate "the symptoms we want to change and at the intensity required for change" (Perry, 2006, in Freedle, 2019, p.93). I usually had to photograph her sandplays from several points of view.

While doing her second sandplay, she briefly mentioned her mother's family tradition of fortune-telling by reading Turkish coffee grounds (tasseography, or tasseomancy). In many Middle Eastern families, it is common cultural practice to read fortunes in coffee mud, and to rely on talismans to invite divine protection for various aspects of life. As I reviewed my notes, it seemed possible that her movements in and around the tray, to work and to observe, might have been influenced by this family tradition, reading the sand-like coffee mud, to find a better fortune and future. I briefly researched the coffee-reading method of divination. As with other types of divination, the setting is structured according to precise rules, in contrast to the unplanned patterns or symbols that emerge in the leftover coffee mud. The coffee must be boiled correctly and served to the client in a special cup. The client drinks most of the coffee, leaving just a little liquid in the cup. The saucer is placed over the cup. This is overturned and the cup is swirled around and returned to an upright position. As the mud drips down, it forms symbols inside the cup, such as paths, mountains, animals and objects. The reading begins with the cup handle as the front-center point. Then the inner space of the cup is divided into sections of left and right, far, near and central areas, as well as into top, middle and bottom areas. The coffee-reader is considered to have a special gift for interpreting coffee-mud symbols and is called to do a reading when bad omens or worries arise concerning love, wealth and health (www.instructables.com/Turkish-Coffee-Fortune-Telling).

Interestingly enough, Ammann's map of the inner space of the sandtray uses the tray's horizontal front center, like the cup handle, as a fixed point of view. Similar to reading coffee drips inside the cup, the sandtray space is divided into right, left, far, near, center and corners. Ammann also considers height, surface and depth. Meaning is attributed to the location of things. In a sandplay, the left side is regarded as less conscious and the right side is considered closer to consciousness; the area closer to the body may reflect feminine aspects, and the far area reflects masculine aspects (Ammann, 1991, p.47). Although Jasmin worked more on the vertical axis of the tray and less from the horizontal front view, Ammann's schema was helpful for me at that time for providing a spatial understanding of her sand forms.

Jasmin's abrupt changes of position around the sandtray seemed disorganized. Yet the number of a sandplay within her process sometimes coincided with the archetypal meaning of that number (Eastwood, 2002). In each of her first four sandplays, the number two appears as pairs of sand forms in conflict. In a second stage, from Sandplays 5 through 8, there is a sequence of numbers as forms, from the number two as a harmonious pair, to numbers three and four as hills, culminating in many archetypal hill forms. Jasmin's last five sandplays, 9–13, constitute a third group with a conscious goal of building her own warm home. Yet, unconsciously, the sandplays in this group visually express differentiation and then unification of masculine and feminine energies, and the creation of the Ego–Self axis. Jung considered numbers as autonomous entities, organizing factors in the unconscious that function as archetypes of order. He wrote: "Number helps more than anything to bring order into the chaos of appearances" (Jung, 1960). Jasmin's sandplays are presented in three stages, amplified through archetypal cultural connections, numbers and Jungian interpretations.

Stage One

Jasmin wanted to build a happy home with her husband and son. She loved her husband's family, but rarely spoke to her own parents or to her mother's siblings. She had recurring anxious fantasies that they would kidnap her child, or that she would be divorced, poor and homeless. In her first sandplay, she touched the sand as gently as a mother's hand stroking her first baby. The sand might have evoked an early loving relationship with her first object, her mother. Yet she renounced the objects on my shelves that could reflect the loss of her mother, or loss of childhood possessions left behind after her original home broke up. She may have learned to depend only on herself, and only what she made herself had meaning for her (Figure 9.1).

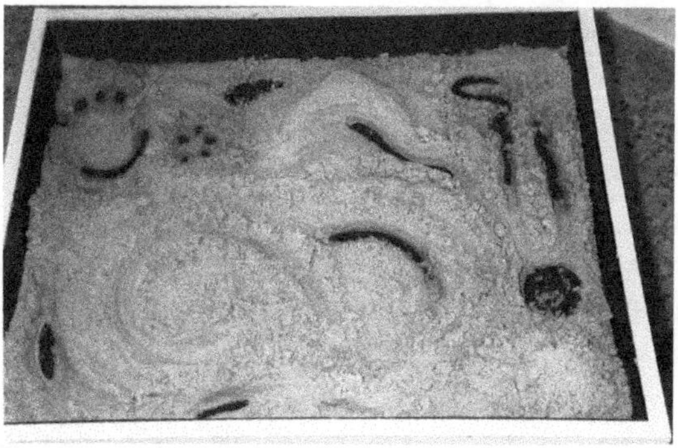

Figure 9.1 *Jasmin: Sandplay 1, Pairs, hamsa and cave*

Her soft touch on the sand contrasted with a series of abrupt transitions that she made between fairly distant areas in the sandtray. I mapped her journey in this first world with a blue line drawn above the sandplay landscape and numbered each stop (Figure 9.2). She began with a small hill in the front-right corner (1) and then jumped to the far center to make another little mound with a cave entrance (2). Moving to the far-right corner, she made two deep snaky lines touching the blue base (3). From this point on, she opened a small blue area in every place she worked, each like a small local oasis in a dry desert. This may indicate a readiness to go deeper into whatever issues are symbolized in these locations, but with caution. Behind the cave, she opened a small blue area (4), then moved to the far left and impressed her left hand strongly so that her handprint touched the blue surface (resembling a "hamsa," a talisman worn to ensure divine protection) (5). Near this, she imprinted the fingers of her right hand deep into the blue (6). She returned to the cave and gently stroked out a blue path leaving the cave towards the right (7). She opened a blue circle on the right edge and transferred that sand to the first hill in the front-right corner (8). Crossing over to the front left (9), she made a path with two blue areas and built a low barrier there (10). She incised deep lines in a central spiral and created a horizontal figure-eight with some blue on the right round line (11). She finished by taking sand from the front-right corner (12) and sprinkling it onto a lake in the opposite far-left corner (13).

As she observed the image, she spoke with similar abrupt transitions between memories and sudden emotional insights:

It seems like a tangle, a knot, but also yin yang. The cave reminds me of a painting in my grandmother's house, strange, I never thought of her as meaningful in my life. This reminds me of trips we took, one to a Mediterranean beach, a calm landscape, boats, sailing into peaceful coves. In Europe we went up a mountain with snow. It was hot on the slope. I hate lies. That's meaningful for me. It was so cold on the mountain top I stayed in the car and we left soon. This reminds me of places that are not scary. Usually I'm afraid of heights, but I took a parachuting course. On the right there is something like a snake. Three places on the right edge are connected. The mountain in the front-right corner is softer, the water is more rigid. Maybe the lake behind the cave formed when the sand moved. That print of my left hand is a hamsa. The circle of dots from my right hand is like an animal footprint. I arranged it like a flower. This is a desert that has water. I like a very hot dry desert. But the water isn't scary. To live in the desert, you need water. Just a minute ago, I felt like I was choking. The far-right corner is less pleasant. Cold and heat, like water and dryness. A childhood friend of mine has many hamsas in her home.

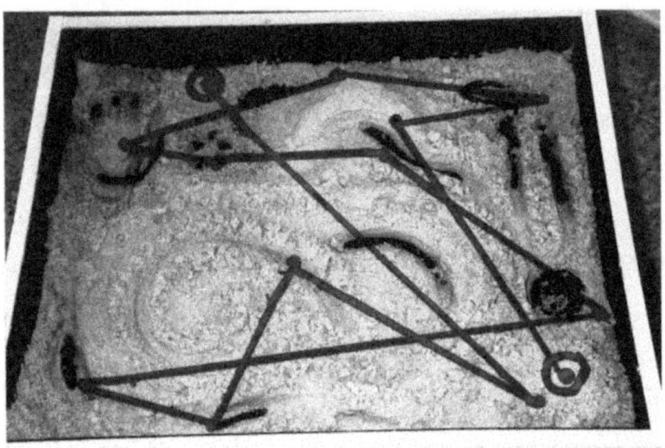

Figure 9.2 *Jasmin: Map of movement sequence in creating Sandplay 1*

Stability was represented by the cave, her grandmother's home, and by a childhood friend with many hamsas in her home who had a stable life and a "lucky family." Yet beneath this scattered assortment of forms, there is an underlying order of pairs, either similar and close, or separate: there is a horizontal division between the far masculine area, and the larger near feminine area; there are two hills although separate, two handprints together, two snaky movements, two breast forms enclosed in the horizontal figure-eight sculpted center, which is also a sign of infinity, and two tiny lakes on the front left. But the single cave above the horizontal figure-eight is possibly a symbol for the one irreplaceable personal mother, or the One Great Mother. The number eight was also her age when her family disintegrated.

Jasmin invited divine protection into her first sandplay with the hamsa she made with her hand in the sand. This talisman is used to avert any potential threat caused by people or circumstance. The need for divine protection is also a universal need. Many cultures use magical objects, oracles, horoscopes, cowrie shells, wishing on a star, tarot cards, tea-leaf reading, coffee-mud fortune-telling, and even sand divination. In the Chinese method called Fuji Writing, a forked tool (a planchette) is held in the hand of a certified medium and "allowed" to inscribe Chinese characters in the sand as if by itself, which are then interpreted. In my childhood, children wrote wishes in the sand at the beach, and watched the tide carry the words away to some divine power that can make a wish come true.

One month later, Jasmin began her second sandplay standing on the vertical left side of the tray, opposite and most distant from where I sat on the right side of the tray. She moved sand from area to area, sprinkled it and built a mound. She worried about how her father lived without money, yet she had not spoken to him, or to her mother. She was afraid of feeling pain in therapy. She mentioned friends getting divorced or widowed who couldn't get along. She covered blue openings near her but left just a little blue visible (Figure 9.3). Moving to the front, she said: "I see a head, myself, and an embryo, and now I see my mother in the same figure. In the culture I come from, my family read fortunes in coffee grounds...at first you see nothing, no clear person." She returned to the vertical left side of the tray and said: "From here it shows my activities, maybe a pregnancy, work, my plans, my daily life."

At that time, I saw the image as a person lying down, divided in half into a top and bottom. But 20 years later, her comment about coffee fortune-reading struck me as a key theme. The beginning of the sentence—"In the culture I come from, my family read fortunes in coffee grounds"—could hint that she observed her sandplays through the lens of her maternal cultural history. The second part of the sentence—"at first you see nothing, no clear person"—may have embodied her hope to discover a better image, a brighter fortune; now it motivated me to look more deeply into her sandplay process.

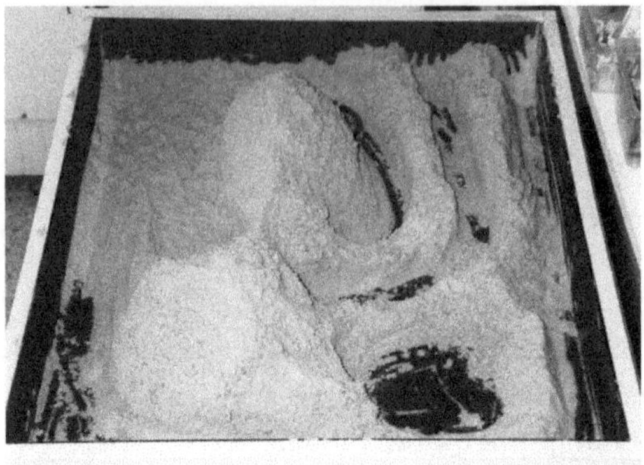

Figure 9.3 *Jasmin: Sandplay 2, Person, womb, daily life and Turkish coffee fortune-telling*

Five weeks passed. Jasmin said that she had spoken to her mother, who complained that Jasmin's husband doesn't respect her. She and her husband both work late. It annoys Jasmin that he falls asleep when she talks to him about her mother. But he doesn't discuss his work with her any more, and she is not really interested in that anyway. If a girlfriend tells her about her therapy, she is interested. She began her third sandplay on the left opposite me, then moved to the front, and then very near me, constructing a high mound separated from the front blue area by a long horizontal ridge (Figure 9.4). She said that the entire mound was herself, her husband and child and the future. Observing from the left side, she said: "The front-right blue area is my mother, I built the ridge to block her off from my family, but it is not strong. I like the center." She observed the image from all four sides. But from any angle, this sandplay shows a pair in conflict: a high mound with a defensive wall, protecting it from a small empty blue corner.

Two weeks later, Jasmin thought she might be pregnant. As she worked on her fourth sandplay, she remembered asking her mother, "What are people made of?" And her mother would say, "From sand from the sea shore and from water, that god packs together very tightly." Then she continued with the difficult present relationship with her mother:

> Lately I have begun to call my mother, just to talk. I just had a birthday, 31. My mother called. I told her that it made me so happy that she called. A week later, my aunt called at 11:30 at night, hysterical, she said, "Your mother

wants to kill herself because of you. Don't say I didn't tell you." I replied, "You're responsible too." I gave the phone to my husband who told her that they put us through hell for five years, that I would not visit my mother with my child. I finally took the phone and told my aunt not to call anymore.

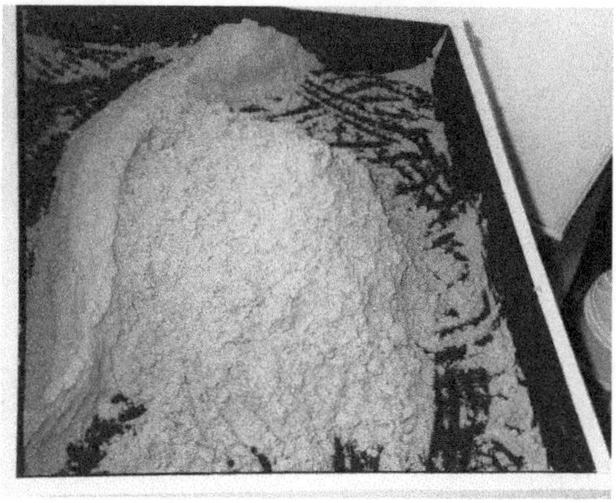

Figure 9.4 *Jasmin: Sandplay 3, First mountain and defensive ridge*

She turned the sandtray on a diagonal and stood at an angle to me. On top of a hill, defended by an outstretched horizontal barrier, is a small piece of turquoise Roman glass, the first object she added to the sand. This glass had been in the Mediterranean Sea for 2000 years at the site of an ancient glass factory. It is radiant, responsive to light, perhaps a tiny first symbol for a new emerging consciousness. She pointed to it, saying, "I am here." She named the large mud ball in the blue front area "Mother" and hoped the barrier would protect her family and enable her success in life. Again, two areas are in conflict: the mound holding the translucent glass, opposite the small mud mound and five unresolved mud balls in the front blue area (Figure 9.5).

Alternately, the turquoise glass sitting on the pinnacle of this mountain could symbolize a beneficial deity, a supernatural power on a site set aside as a dwelling place for the divine. Deloria (2006) describes a Native American concept of the universe, where invisible supernatural beings exist within the same time and space as humans and our natural world. A mountain peak can be a holy liminal space, a place between two realms. To honor the divine, people may approach a mountain top but not go on it. Jasmin commented in her first sandplay about not getting out of her car on the cold peak of a mountain.

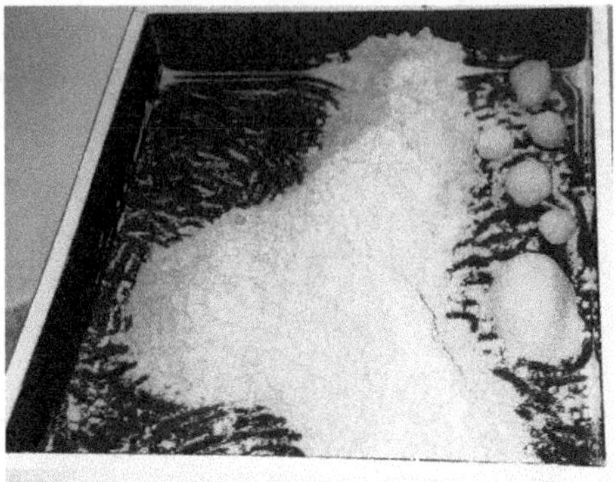

Figure 9.5 *Jasmin: Sandplay 4, Second mountain and sea glass*

Stage Two

Tragically, the price paid for Jasmin's survival was to distance herself from her mother and family, a loss of mother and of her roots. Jung writes that:

> it is the body, the feeling, the instincts which connect us with the soil. If you give up the past you naturally detach from the past; you lose your roots in the soil, the connection with the totem ancestors that dwell in your soil. You turn outward and drift away, and try to conquer other lands because you are exiled from your own soil. (Jung 2002, p.73)

In the second stage of her process, the psyche had begun to tend to her psychological exile from her roots by providing inner archetypal feminine support. Jasmin's images were now deeply personal, but also contained universal themes that hinted at wider sources of amplification, such as myths that are meaningful for me.

Jasmin began to work on her fifth sandplay on the vertical axis. She confirmed that she was pregnant and had trouble eating, but she was happy. She moved to the horizontal, sprinkled sand and continued moving back and forth (Figure 9.6). She observed the work from all sides and said with surprise:

> This time it looks to me exactly the same from every angle. Two fish, a big fish and a small fish. I feel like the big fish, pregnant. The big fish is familiar, the little one is not, but I know that it came from the hollow space in the big fish. She is a great teacher. Every stage in pregnancy is preparation for the next stage. Nature has given me time to understand, to feel. This looks

> like after the birth. I am the comfortable big fish. Fish have no hands. They can't hug each other. I think the little fish feels good... When I pick up my son in kindergarten, he first tells me everything that happened and then he smiles and comes to me. For me, transitions are still very difficult.

The number two is now resolved as a symbol of harmonious relationship in an unconscious sea. Fish symbols are thought to protect against the evil eye (Steinhardt, 2013).

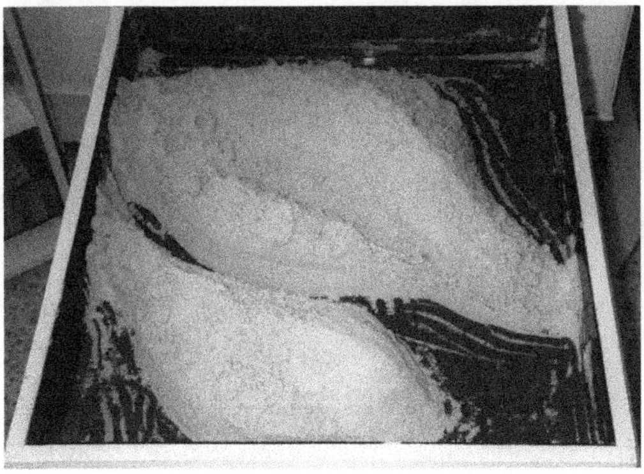

Figure 9.6 *Jasmin: Sandplay 5, Two sand fish in harmony*

Jasmin is now five months pregnant. She visited her grandmother during the Passover vacation, but not her mother. She works vertically opposite me, pours water but keeps the dry and wet sand separate. She draws a long serpentine line from the top where I sit to where she stands, and creates two mounds. Then she moves to the horizontal front center, returns to the vertical side and adds a third hill. She adorns the hills with a purple amethyst, green glass, a rose quartz, a glass pear and two blue stones, and sprinkles sand on them from above. She likes this sandplay, says it is light and flowing, like spring. Here, in her sixth sandplay, there are six partially hidden crystals and stones, and three hills with two tiny mud balls on them (Figure 9.7).

Edinger (1972, pp.184–185) describes the number three as a trinity, a totality of various dynamic phases of a developmental movement in which a union of opposites produces the third. Edinger adds that "feminine trinities seem to derive from the categories of the natural, biological-growth process, such as birth, maturation and death, while masculine trinities seem to relate specifically to the development of the psyche or consciousness." Some well-known feminine trinities are the Triple Goddess of Maiden, Mother, Crone, and the Three Fates. A well-known masculine trinity is that of three brothers, the Greek gods: Zeus, who rules from heaven, Poseidon, who rules the sea, and Hades, ruler of the underworld.

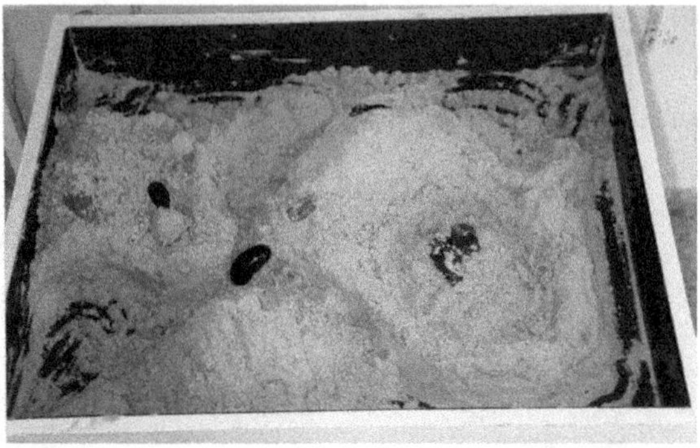

Figure 9.7 *Jasmin: Sandplay 6, Three hills and six jewels*

These six precious stones on three mountain peaks are positioned in a place where they could catch the rising sun's first rays, like a growing rainbow of consciousness. They could also resonate with certain Native American customs, myths and beliefs recorded by Lakota scholar Vine Deloria Jr. (2006) in his book *The World We Used to Live In*. He described large "sacred stones" on the mountains of North Dakota that served as oracles for the people. The spirit of the place directed birds to sketch out messages, or pictures, on these stones, which predicted "events to come." Lakota religious leaders went to these stones in the early morning to read their messages, and to act accordingly on them. An Episcopal minister recorded an incident in 1919 in which several Native Americans told him that lightning would strike someone that day, for a picture on a holy rock described this. And lightning did strike and nearly killed a woman. He remembered other predictions that foretold events to come but could not explain this. Hopefully, Jasmin's crystals are oracles of favorable events to come.

Jasmin had headaches during the pregnancy but they passed if she ate enough. She began Sandplay 7 opposite me, creating horizontal and vertical furrows, and mountain peaks separated by walls. She felt a strong physical urge to move to the horizontal axis of the tray and destroy the walls between the mounds. She moved sand from the walls to the four peaks and center base to strengthen them, leaving blue lines around the edges (Figure 9.8). This sandplay was restful for her. She saw the four mounds as her family with the unborn baby. Her previous image of three hills has transitioned from a trinity that expresses the totality of psychological experience in its dynamic, developmental temporal aspect, to a quaternity that expresses the totality of the psyche in its structural, static or eternal sense (Edinger, 1972, p.182). These four mountains comprise a symmetrical unity of left and right sides, unconscious and conscious, and far and near levels, which reflect and balance each other. They could represent integration of Jung's four functions of the psyche—feeling, thinking, sensation and intuition—or reflect other groupings of four, such as the four elements, four directions, four winds, four seasons and four phases of the moon. The square or rectangular shape of four is associated with responsibility and stability. This image could be a Self-tray, with four mounds surrounding a center that accesses the presence of the positive feminine archetype and an inner permanence.

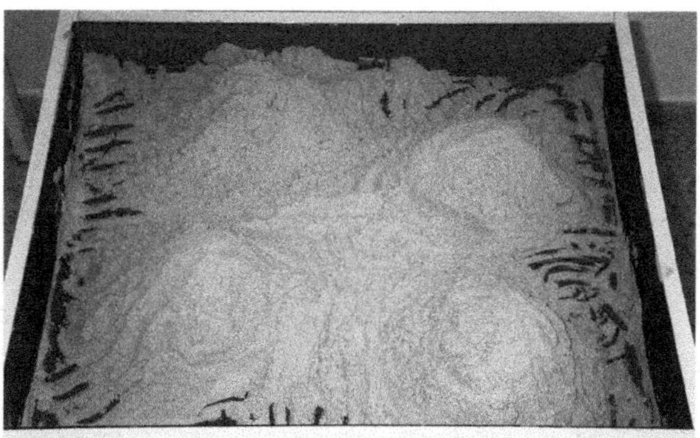

Figure 9.8 *Jasmin: Sandplay 7, Four hills and center*

But these four mounds also resemble four actual mountain peaks which delineate the boundaries of Native American Navajo tribal land. Jasmin was probably not familiar at all with Navajo cosmology and did not intend to sculpt holy mountains. But Sacred Mountains do exist around the world. The Navajo say that The Holy Ones placed all the peoples on the earth where they were meant to be. They believe that The Holy Ones gave the Navajo Four Sacred Mountains that outline their territory. They are described in a clockwise circular motion that follows the light and cosmic scheme of the rising and setting sun. Each mountain is represented by a color, time of day, a specific animal, a direction and a masculine or feminine figure (Carey, 2015). Blanca Peak in the east is first, associated with the color white and "Dawn Man," referring to sunrise. Mount Taylor in the south is associated with the color blue and the "Horizontal Blue Man," referring to daytime. The San Francisco Peaks in the west are represented by the color yellow and the "Horizontal Yellow Woman," associated with the setting sun. Hesperus Peak of the La Plata Mountains in the north is represented by black and associated with "Darkness Woman," representing the night-time. The attributes of each mountain create balance and equality in the whole, between masculine and feminine, and in transitions between light and darkness, Jasmin has been guided to place herself in this kind of center. This sandplay is a supportive archetypal image that will remain intact in her psyche (https://en.wikipedia.org/wiki/Four_Sacred_Mountains_of_the_Navajo).

Jasmin is six months pregnant. In her eighth sandplay, she makes small mounds, sprinkles sand on them and cries about her cut-off relationship with her mother. She recalls her lost childhood home and says:

> My mother lives now in the house I was born in. After my parents divorced, we changed apartments every few months for three years, no place was home. Today her house is run-down, the entrance is filled with junk. Someone asked me about my mother and I began to cry.

She breaks up the mounds into smaller units, again sprinkles sand on them. I notice that she is working again from the front horizontal feminine axis of the tray (Figure 9.9).

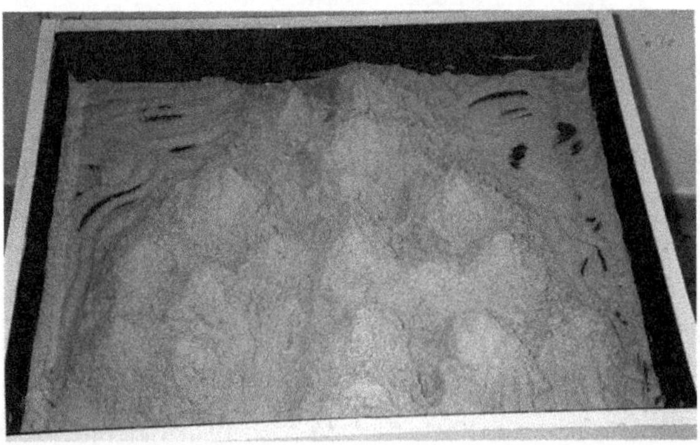

Figure 9.9 *Jasmin: Sandplay 8, Many hills and feminine abundance*

In her last sandplay, she accessed archetypal support when she moved to the horizontal, feminine axis of the sandtray. Jung states:

> the archetypes are, as it were, the hidden foundations of the conscious mind...the roots which the psyche has sunk not only in the earth in the narrow sense but in the world in general. Archetypes are systems of readiness for action, and at the same time images and emotions. They are inherited with the brain-structure—indeed, they are its psychic aspect. (Jung 2002, p.198)

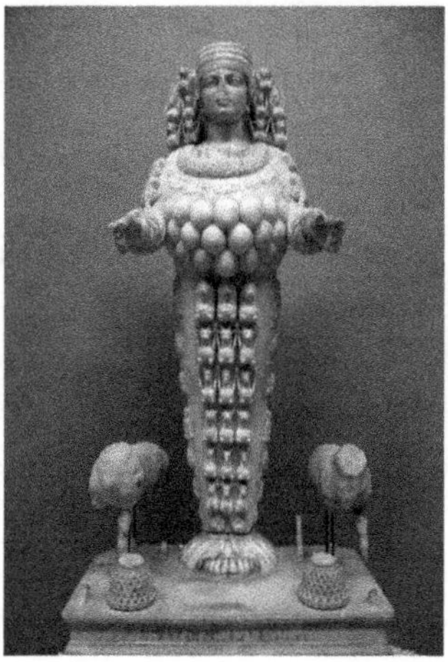

Figure 9.10 *Artemis, the many breasted goddess, Ephesus*

Jasmin has broken larger mounds into many small more manageable hills. The original unified archetype is now divided into multiple parts, which can be assimilated each at a comfortable pace, into human reality (Edinger, 1972, p.140). When we met 20 years later, these many hills reminded Jasmin of the enmeshed relationships in her mother's extended family. For me, they resemble sculptures of the Greek Moon Goddess Artemis in her temple in Ephesus, portrayed with many breasts, like these many hills (Figure 9.10). Artemis is a virgin goddess, independent and unmarried. She acquired her role as nurturer and protector of all newborn children and animals when she herself was just born. Her mother, the Titan goddess Leto, had become pregnant with twins—Artemis and her brother Apollo, the Sun God—by Zeus, God of Olympus. Hera, the jealous wife of Zeus, condemned Leto to wander the earth in labor and in pain and never find a place to give birth. Zeus then secretly created the floating island of Delos where Leto gave birth first to Artemis. But Hera prevented the Goddess of Childbirth from helping in the second birth of Apollo. Thus, baby Artemis had to become midwife to her mother Leto. Artemis is also Goddess of the Hunt and can kill with her bow and arrow. The opposites in her character, as in nature, protect new life and can bring death (Graves, 1955/1960). Artemis is associated with the abundance of the number eight, the number of this sandplay (Eastwood, 2002) which might resolve the figure-eight in Sandplay 1.

Stage Three

After Jasmin's last sandplay and the strong presence of the archetype of the nurturing feminine, she seems to have the strength and confidence needed to manage her relationship with her unstable real parents, and to build a house and happy home in reality. The five sandplays in this last stage, Sandplays 9 through 13, are sculpted in sand alone, with one large house placed in Sandplay 11. Sand is a component of deserts and wilderness, places associated with themes of alienation, emotional exhaustion and depletion of inner resources, but also with eventual revelation. Jasmin carefully left open tiny areas of water throughout her process that could symbolize potential renewed contact with the instincts, the nourishment needed to heal the dry desert alienation, to integrate masculine and feminine and the unconscious and consciousness (Edinger, 1972, p.50).

Jasmin's baby is five months old. Her conscious goal is to plan and build her own house and a warm home. Sandplay 9 is the only sandplay done in dry sand, and there is no visible blue. From the front of the tray she built two hills, connected them, but then leveled everything with a rake, leaving traces of circular and straight lines in the sand (Figure 9.11). An interim period of nine months between Sandplay 8 and this sandplay may have constituted a psychological pregnancy. This culminated in a symbolic birth of two types of basic lines, unresolved masculine and feminine elements, like the "fraternal twins" in the mythological births of Artemis and Apollo. Meanwhile, she had told her son more about her parents, who had fought and separated and never again lived together. She knows she must find a way to visit her mother with her family.

Three months passed. She had visited her mother and had also spoken to her father but didn't tell him she had seen her mother. She had differentiated between her parents in her psyche, and now could relate separately to each one in reality. She began Sandplay 10 from the left vertical side of the wet tray, sculpting rounded shapes and a rectangle and sprinkled sand on them (Figure 9.12). Here, the lines of the previous sandplay grow into three-dimensional forms and show better integration of masculine and feminine energies. In this image, she saw an eye, a head, a person, rounded hands in a state of rest, a tree and roots, and also a key. She said:

> I saw the figure as if lying down. I felt the back, the base. The blue lines are like tree roots. If it were standing up the hands would make a wide movement. If the hands were above the head it needs to be sure that no one will punch him in the stomach.

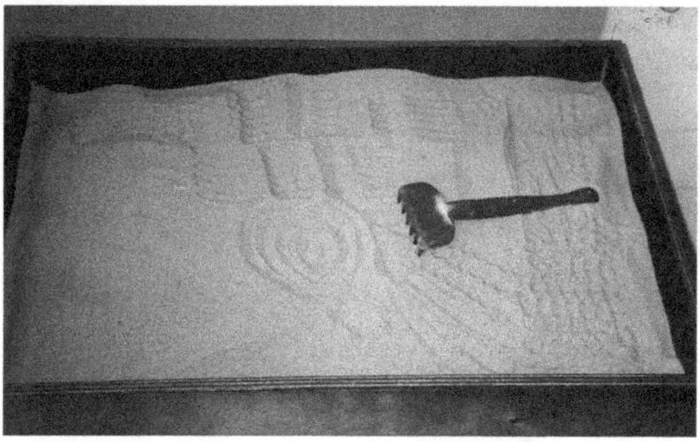

Figure 9.11 *Jasmin: Sandplay 9, Thoughts of building a house*

She saw a real human being, resting, standing, extending its hands, yet still not completely secure. If this was a key, it could open her inner doors and release imprisoned energy into positive action; perhaps she had already done this when she visited her mother. She also saw tree roots, new symbolic roots growing in her psyche.

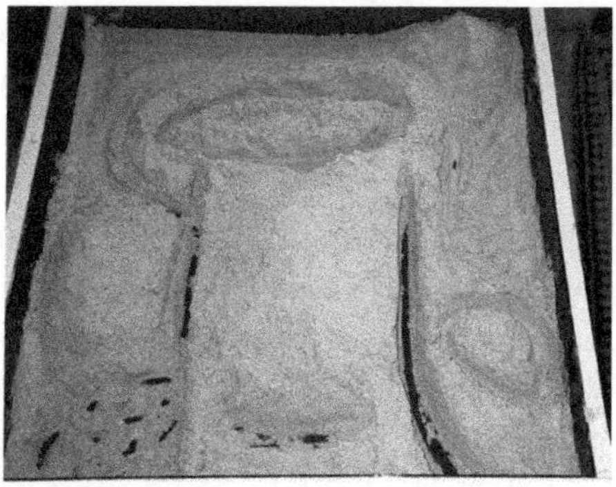

Figure 9.12 *Jasmin: Sandplay 10, Tree, tree roots, a person, a key*

Three weeks later, Jasmin happily tells me that she and her husband are buying a house in a rural area. Standing on the left vertical side, she makes many forms in the sand and then flattens everything completely. I am surprised when she chooses a very large red-brown house, a first object with a clear identity, as if the strength and balance of Sandplay 7 has metamorphosed into a stable house in her psyche in Sandplay 11. She places the house on the vertical far left, then continues to sprinkle sand in the center until it rises high into a mound, that she says represents good things (Figure 9.13). She adds mud balls to the front-left side and says: "The mud balls are unfinished, there are five—why? They look like falafel, oriental food, why?"

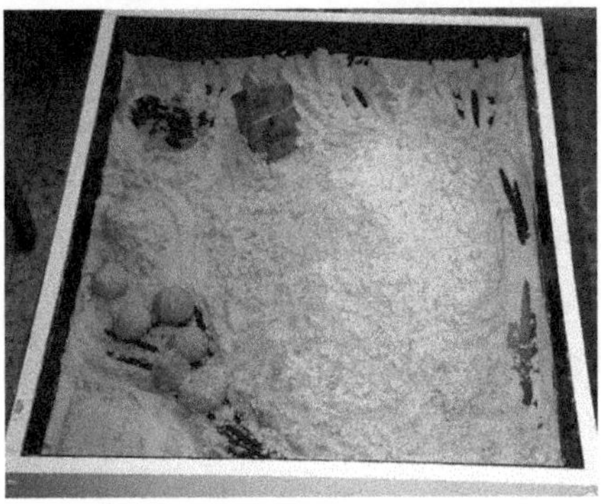

Figure 9.13 *Jasmin: Sandplay 11, House beneath the hill*

The house has a strong presence. It stands at the rear-left base of the mountain, not on the peak, like a respectful Ego that is relative to the Mound as nature and Self. The Ego–Self relationship is symbolized with One House as Ego, standing at the base of One Mound as Self. Jasmin counted five mud balls on the front-left side, but there are six—three wet (feminine) and three dryer (masculine). The number six now balances masculine and feminine opposites with six mud balls. Behind them is a small, unresolved hill merged into the surrounding sand. These mud balls may resolve and transform the five mud balls plus the Mound representing her mother in Sandplay 4. Geometrically, the number six can form a Star of David: two overlapping triangles—one masculine, pointing to Sky, one feminine, pointing to Earth, a union of opposites.

Another nine months have passed. She and her family live in their new home. Sandplay 12 begins from the vertical side. Jasmin smooths and gathers sand into a small mound and draws long vertical lines. She discusses women she would like as friends, but not too close. One friend told her about her difficult childhood and she replied that sometimes it's better to be far from parents. Then she felt she revealed too much of herself. She moves closer to me, makes a hill and talks about a divorced friend who gets along but has an inner sadness. She moves even closer to me, and makes one big hill that fills the sandtray (Figure 9.14). She says:

> I don't want relationships with sad people. I don't want my children to reach the age of 14 and realize that they have an aunt or grandmother that they knew nothing about. I want to tell my children about my family without tears. I want to stop being afraid that I will suddenly meet my relatives somewhere. I want to walk around Tel Aviv with the children tomorrow, but I won't because once I met my uncle or my aunt there.

She turns the sandtray at an angle and asks me to photograph it from the vertical side. She said, "It looks to me like a person, a Native American.".

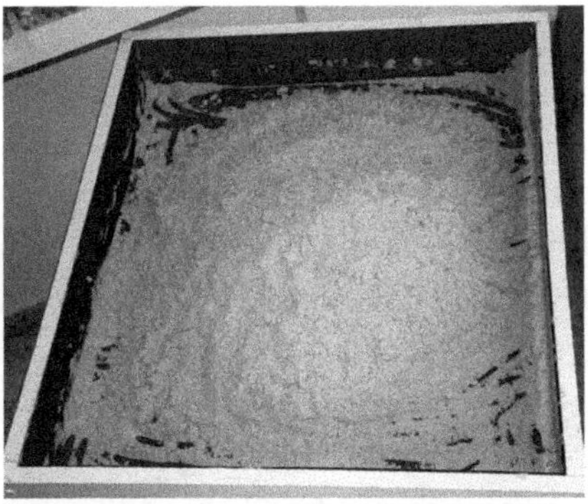

Figure 9.14 *Jasmin: Sandplay 12, One big hill*

Jasmin's final sandplay was similar to Sandplay 12 done two months before. From the left vertical side, she used both hands to make sand handprints and symmetrical finger spirals that looked like two ovaries. She moved to the front but then turned the sandtray so it faced her vertically. Suddenly, she became dizzy and nauseous and felt like fainting. She recalled being so sick after her parent's divorce that she almost never went to school. She turned the sandtray again to face her horizontally, calmed down and smoothed the sand. She said: "I am not interested in finding out what is wrong with me, I just want it not to be." She made one mound, talked about having more children, split the mound in two, and then unified it again. She said her mother was now getting help from all the family. A few sessions later, she felt ready to end therapy. Jasmin accepted that relationships with her original family would be limited or remain unfinished for the meanwhile.

Conclusion

We met again 20 years later. Jasmin was surprised that I had researched Turkish coffee-mud reading and that I thought it might be important. She laughed and told me that every morning she looks at the mud in her coffee cup to see how her day will go. If she doesn't like what she sees, she doesn't pay attention to it. She also was surprised to hear that in my experience people usually do sandplays from a frontal horizontal point of view without moving all around the tray or moving the tray itself. She developed her career with caution, but her strength, sense of humor and independence, like Artemis, enabled her to make her own decisions. Her father died several years ago. She calls her mother periodically but rarely visits her. She, her husband and her children are all pursuing personal goals. She did not take home any photos of her sandplays, although she has kept all her paintings. Jasmin absorbed many forms of knowledge in her life, being born into a particular convergence of genetic history, family and social-cultural concepts, landscape, style of communication and the social norms and opportunities of her own particular generation. I was privileged to witness Jasmin's call to do a sandplay and to follow her carefully paced process, while accepting the intervals between sandplays that her psyche had determined. I will remember her touch on the sand and the constant movement and change that culminated in numinous landscapes and finally revealed her psyche's underlying direction and purpose, towards her healing and growth.

10

Developmental Spontaneous Sandplay of Boys and Girls

Introduction

My work as an art and sandplay therapist has taken place in a small one-room studio in a garden behind my house for over 30 years. The studio has also been a creative play space for children visiting with their family and parents. While the adults converse in the house, the children can play in the studio, in art or in sandplay. They call me to photograph their finished work, or to help reach an object on a high shelf or sometimes just for me to be present for a while. Several boys and girls who visited frequently with their parents could be safely left alone in the studio from about age two and a half. They engaged in sandplay whenever they wanted and for as many years as they wanted. Their natural relationship to play in the sandtray enabled a merger of creativity, life events and memory. They might play in the studio several times in one week, or take a break after a period of intense involvement. The boys were interested in sandplay until age six or seven, and then transitioned to other creative options. The girls enjoyed sandplay until about age 11 and also dictated stories which I wrote down and read back to them. I dated and filed the photographs of each child's sandplays with their title and story, if there was one, and prepared a gift album for each child when they were over 18 years old.

As I organized the photo albums, I noticed that these long natural sandplay processes developed according to the stages and goals described by Neumann (1973/1998) and also corresponded to Jones's 1986 research on stages of play with sand and water in the sandtray according to age and sex (Mitchell and Friedman, 1994, pp.91–94). Neumann's stages, Jones's research and the Greek myth of Theseus and his "hero's journey" (Campbell, 1949/1973) are briefly summarized below as a theoretical background for the developmental sandplay processes of three children, Oron, Ben and Maya. Each child played freely in the sandtray for several consecutive years from about age two and a half, with no predetermined goals, without being evaluated for the results and without clean-up. Sandplay was a familiar activity in which they could cultivate personal expression in the sandtray and tell stories with symbolic elements which unconsciously mirrored their relations with their parents, siblings or friends. Their sandplay constructions were consistent with their emotional, cognitive and creative growth over a much longer time span than that of most children in time-limited, fixed therapeutic settings, either public or private. Thus, all the sandplays of these children, boy or girl, progress through several developmental stages. This opportunity to observe the flow of guidance of the psyche of each child reveals how themes are represented by symbols that change, and by symbols that remain throughout the process over years.

The therapeutic ambience of my studio, designed for a relationship between therapist and client, may have supported the inner relationship of these children to the sequence of their sandplays over time, without the presence of a therapist-witness. Their innate capacity for healing of their relevant issues was activated by play in my studio, which was secure and familiar. The material setting itself, the sandtrays and abundance of objects offered infinite possibilities for self-expression, letting the psyche determine if things happened "now" or at a later time. Less obvious invisible factors such as the containing space of the studio, subtle boundaries, stages of ego development and the "sandtray map" itself probably reverberated in each child's psyche in relation to their images with no need to explain their imaginary worlds. Forms, unintentionally imbued with content, emerged in a gradual, unconscious process reflected by the image in the sandtray.

Neumann (1973/1998), Campbell (1949/1973) and Jones (1986)

The boys and girls who played spontaneously in my studio with sand, water and objects from a very young age continued this activity for years until they lost interest. Two boys, Oron and Ben, stopped sandplay just around age six and a half to seven. Several girls continued after age seven, but came less frequently and sometimes decided to work in pairs rather than alone.

The sandplay processes of Oron, Ben and Maya all invoke themes around which each child might invent stories relevant to their current life, which they dictated to me to write down. The boy's sandplay processes were especially intense between the ages of four and six or seven, an age which corresponds to Neumann's "Magic Warlike" stage of "Early Childhood II, a Play Age." Their sandplays expressed the transitions from a young child's attachment to the good "Great Mother" to the ego's need for independence and transition to the patriarchate. The myth of Theseus and his hero's journey is especially relevant for boys. Theseus begins his journey when his mother revealed that his father's sword and sandals awaited him under a large boulder. These two symbols galvanize the separation from the mother, as the ego moves towards independent consciousness in the patriarchate (Campbell, 1949/1973). For Neumann, the stages of development of the feminine ego required separate consideration, and excerpts from his earlier works were added to the final chapter of "The Child" (Neumann, 1973/1998, pp.203–205). In his book of essays, *Fear of the Feminine*, he delineates the challenges of a young girl's ego development in a patriarchal society (1994), relevant to the sandplay process of Maya, from age three to 11. Jones's research and criteria for measuring sandplay behavior in six age groups (1986, in Mitchell and Freidman, 1994, pp.91–94) supports the age-appropriate use of sand, water and objects, space and boundaries, and clarifies some differences between boys and girls.

Erich Neumann (1973): Five stages of ego development in the lives of children

Neumann delineated five stages in a child's ego development from birth to 12 years old and beyond, focusing on gradual cognitive and archetypally determined growth that is commonly seen at each stage as a child matures. The mother of the primal relationship is the "good Great Mother," the foundation of the child's physical and psychic existence, providing security and enabling life. Her unconsciously directed "motherly" behavior coincides with the Mother archetype, an image common to all humans (Neumann, 1973/1988, p.21). From birth to four years old, the child lives within the matriarchate, and progresses through a succession of phases of ego development. "Infancy I," from birth to two years old, begins in the first three months of life, the Uroboric stage symbolized by a snake holding its tail in its mouth. This is a pre-ego stage with no object and no subject, an unconscious state without differentiation or boundaries in which the child and mother experience a unitary reality called "Participation Mystique." The Mother's presence equals the Child's Body, Self, and the World. The child experiences the Self through the body, and through the mother and her body.

The Phallic-Chthonian stage from three to 14 months is divided into two phases. In the first "vegetative" phase from three to seven months ("Infancy I"), the ego is still passive to a high degree like a plant attached to the earth. In the second "animalistic" phase from seven to 14 months ("Infancy II"), the child is able to sit and stand. At around 12 months, an integral ego consolidates and becomes the base for the child's individual Self although the child is still dominated by the "matriarchal power of nature and the unconscious." This is the child's psychological "second" birth and the beginning of the creation of a positive integral ego that can integrate frustrations that stem from fear and anger, pain, cold and hunger, etc. (Neumann, 1973/1998, p.139). For the child, the mother represents the role of the compensatory Self, as she insures that negative factors will not continue for too long a time, and is able to replace them with positive experiences. The child begins to develop his own positive integration and tolerance of the world and of himself with the mother's example. The ego controls his autonomic action through which he interacts with the world.

The ego will become more active and independent in the following two stages, the "Magic Phallic" stage of "Early Childhood I" from 14 months to four years, and in the "Magic Warlike" stage from age four to seven years old, "Early Childhood II, a Play Age." In the "Magic Phallic" stage, the ego is fairly active, and in the "Magic Warlike" stage it begins to overcome its dependence on the matriarchate in transition to the patriarchate. "The ego is still in the process of formation, consciousness and the unconscious are beginning to separate into different systems, and the ego has not yet assumed its central position in consciousness" (Neumann, 1973/1998, p.141). Language and symbolic ability develop, accompanied by magical fantasies or an imaginary friend. The child is very creative; his active ego directs him towards becoming independent of others, and independent in himself. The ego is focused on awareness that is consistent and inner-directed, no longer subordinated to the unconscious and to the world. The world begins to be experienced as an organized system in which times of day, people, activities and storytelling provide stability and continuity to the ego (Neumann, 1973/1998, p.147). This centering is the pre-condition for the ego's successful functioning in adulthood. The Ego–Self axis begins to polarize, yet the child still lives in a matriarchal world, and his consciousness is still not secure. This stage is analogous to the Son-Lover of the Great Mother. In the developing ego stages of the matriarchal phase, the ego is still guided by the unconscious as companion of the Great Mother, the goddess of vegetative and animal life and of human life as well (Neumann, 1973/1998, p.150). The active ego gradually overcomes its dependence on the matriarchate, confronting the world more boldly, progressively strengthening the ego and gaining the independence and sturdiness that will enable the transition to the patriarchate. After the formation of the Ego–Self axis, the aware Ego, and not the Self, is the initiator and executor of the vital will of the personality. A sense of control crystallizes, internally and externally. Within the male group, the tendency towards resistance to the feminine principle is intensified, and masculine supportive groups are formed (p.157). "The ego is released from the matriarchal, moon-dominated consciousness whose negative aspect is fear of the demonic world which for the male ego is a world determined by the feminine and the unconscious" (p.162). An active ego develops in both sexes, possessing a phallic masculine character. In this stage, the Mother archetype is symbolized as a dragon that threatens to devour the progressive ego, and thus must "be slayed," connoting the terms "Slaying of the Dragon," "Separation of the World Parents" and "Birth of the Hero" as the psychic events of the developing consciousness of the Magic Warlike stage from age four to age seven (p.179). From the ages seven to 12, children chronologically enter Neumann's fourth "Solar Warlike" stage of ego development, "Middle Childhood," leave behind their earlier dependence in the matriarchal stage and transition to identification with the qualities of the patriarchate, the "Great Father."

Theseus, an orphan destined to become a hero, and King of Athens

In Greek myth, Aethra, daughter of King Troezen, is impregnated twice on the same night, first by Aegeus, King of Athens, a guest in her father's house, and then by the Sea God Poseidon, who summoned her in a dream to meet him in a small inlet close by. Both Aegeus and Poseidon are absent fathers (see Chapter 11). Theseus is reared by a single mother, unaware of his dual human and divine paternity, until the age of 16 when his mother reveals to him that King Aegeus left him a pair of sandals and a sword under a huge boulder. He lifts the boulder, dons the sandals, takes the sword and sets off for Athens to meet his father, choosing a dangerous land route rather than a sea route where his divine father Poseidon would protect him. On the road, he outwits and kills six criminals who block his path, proving his heroism. In Athens, King Aegeus recognizes the sword and sandals that he left under the boulder years ago, and joyously greets his son. Yet he soon sends him to Crete, to kill the Minotaur who lives in a labyrinth, and devours seven young men and seven young women from Athens every seven years, payment of a debt owed to King Minos of Crete. Theseus accepts the challenge and sails to Crete with the 14 youths destined to be devoured. In Crete, Ariadne, daughter of King Minos, sister of the Minotaur, falls in love with him and consults with Daedalus, architect of the labyrinth, who gives her a flaxen thread to help Theseus find his way out of the dark confusing passages. Theseus promises to marry Ariadne and take her away from Crete. After he kills the Minotaur, Theseus, Ariadne and his crew sail away, and, with the hubris of triumph, stop at the island of Naxos to celebrate. In the morning, Ariadne awakens alone, abandoned on a beach. Theseus has sailed for Athens and forgotten his promise to marry her. He also forgets his promise to his father to hoist a white sail if he succeeds. King Aegeus sees a black sail and, believing that Theseus is dead, jumps into the sea. The old king is dead, and Theseus becomes King of Athens. Campbell (1949/1973) terms this a "monomyth" that expresses the universal theme of a hero's journey. He writes that just as the flavor of the entire ocean is contained in a droplet of sea water, the smallest fairy tale and the symbols of mythology "are not manufactured; they cannot be ordered, invented or permanently suppressed. They are spontaneous productions of the psyche, and each bears within it, undamaged, the germ power of its source" (1949/1973, p.4). The germ power of a boy's archetypally determined need to separate from dependence on the mother, establish an independent ego and become a hero, as Theseus has done, is a theme in the sandplays of Oron and Ben.

L.E. Jones (1986)

Jones used a fixed set of criteria to observe the development of structure and expression in initial sandplays of children in five age groups in a traditional sandplay setting, from birth to age 18 (Mitchell and Friedman, 1994, pp.91–94). The age groups were 0–1, 2–4, 5–7, 8–12, and 13–18 years old. She used six criteria to measure sandplay behavior for each group, matching the results to Piaget's cognitive and developmental principles. Her criteria included: early scattering, moving later towards cohesion and world view; ignoring sandtray boundaries or awareness of them inside and outside the tray; the non-use of sand or its use for burying, unburying and building; and choice of figurines, their placement and the relationships between them. Her sample population of five boys and five girls at each age level was limited to Caucasian middle-class and upper-middle-class families, and her research did not follow any single child's sandplay process or any use of water in sandplay, all of which should be addressed (Lowenfeld, 1935/1991, p.31). However, applying her criteria at each developmental stage does provide some insight into the construction and evolution of children's sand worlds, from early ages 0–4, to the more coherent, dynamic and cohesive sand worlds of older children. Jones recorded similar results for boys and girls, except that boys created fewer bodies of water than girls and no islands, and fewer boys used the sand between the ages of seven and 13, a period of peer identification, when operational thinking begins. Jones proposed that the process of separation from the mother might be more difficult for boys than for girls, as sand relates to "Mother Earth," instinct, nature and the feminine. Between the ages of two and seven, boys tended towards more dramatic aggressive play with miniatures, while girls tended towards cooperative dyadic relationships and family interactions, notably from ages five to seven and later. Jones's study was consistent with Piaget's and Jung's belief that there is a central organizing principle which determines the development of the human psyche.

A synopsis of helpful criteria for observing children's sand worlds

- Sand worlds develop from scattering and fragmentary worlds, at younger ages, into images with more cohesive and comprehensive themes and perspectives, at more advanced stages.
- Sand is at first used unintentionally and may be thrown outside the tray, advancing to more deliberate burying and unburying, and later to the creation of inner boundaries and structures.
- Wet or dry sand can be chosen intuitively at any stage. From about age five, water may be added instinctively to the sand, with control or with lack of control (flooding).
- Sandtray boundaries are not consciously noticed until approximately age four, when the sandtray edge, specific areas in the tray and creation of inner boundaries defined by grouping of objects, sand structures and vertical or horizontal divisions become part of the work.
- Figurines are deliberately chosen at early ages, from one or two years old, but their use and placement might at first be indiscriminate. From about age two, objects may be oriented with more intention, leading from random to meaningful relationships. From about age three and a half, and in later stages until adolescence, cooperation between figures, dramatic play and more complexed grouping increases.

Spontaneous sandplay processes of Oron, Ben and Maya

ORON, Eight sandplays from age two years ten months to five years eight months

From 20 sandplays that Oron made from the ages of two years ten months to five years eight months, I have chosen eight sandplays at approximately one-year intervals. They can be read as if inner developmental sandplay maps guided his sandplay process, of that day's work, of stages of the journey and of the form given to each sand picture within the sandtray. Oron began to play with miniatures on the floor of my studio at age two. Ten months later, he made his first sandplay in the sandtray. The sandplay setting offered him an experience of free and total expression, unconscious and conscious, and intuitive choice between the wet sandtray with its deep, cobalt blue color, and the dry sandtray whose lighter cerulean blue seems to bestow strength and support with less depth. Sometimes he used both.

Age two years ten months

Oron scattered many small miniatures of superheroes and ordinary men and women in the front sandtray area, and raked a semi-circle in the sand above to enclose them. This might portray a unitary reality, a first stage where everything exists within the initial uroboric relationship of mother and child from birth to age three months, with no differentiation. Neumann (1973/1988) writes that before creation there is darkness and a state of chaos. Creation psychologically implies the coming of light and the birth of human consciousness (Figure 10.1).

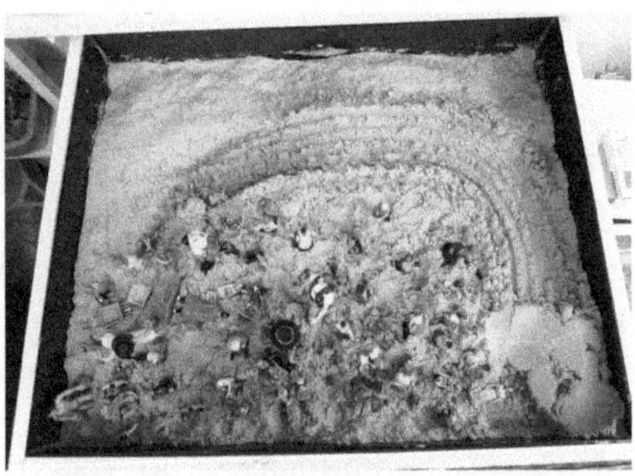

Figure 10.1 *Oron: Age two years ten months, Raked semi-circle and scattered figurines*

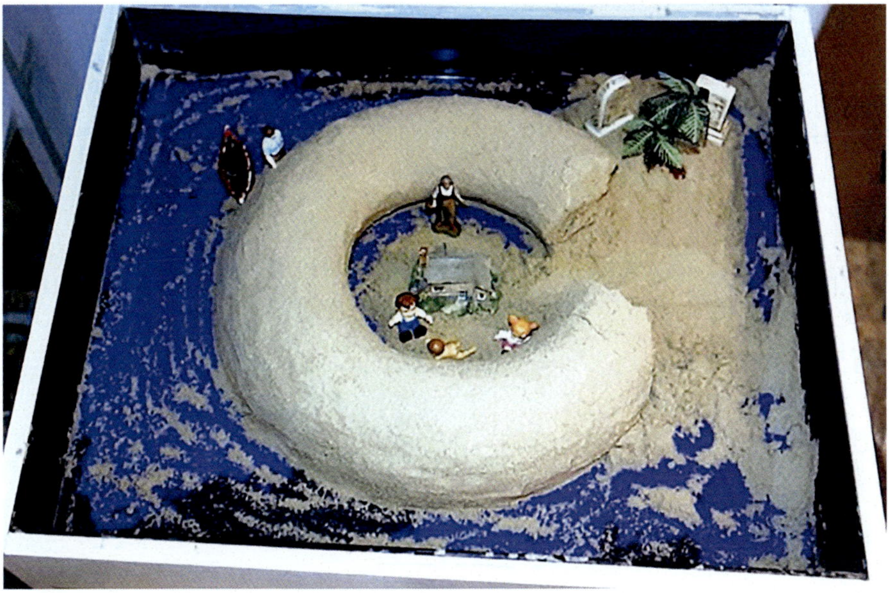

Plate 1 Helena: *After father's death*

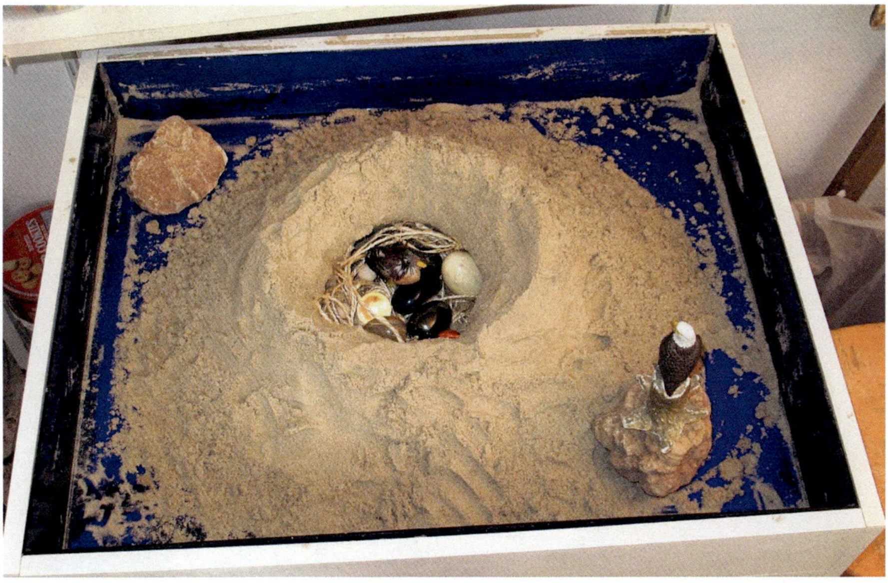

Plate 2 Helena: *Eagle, duck and eggs*

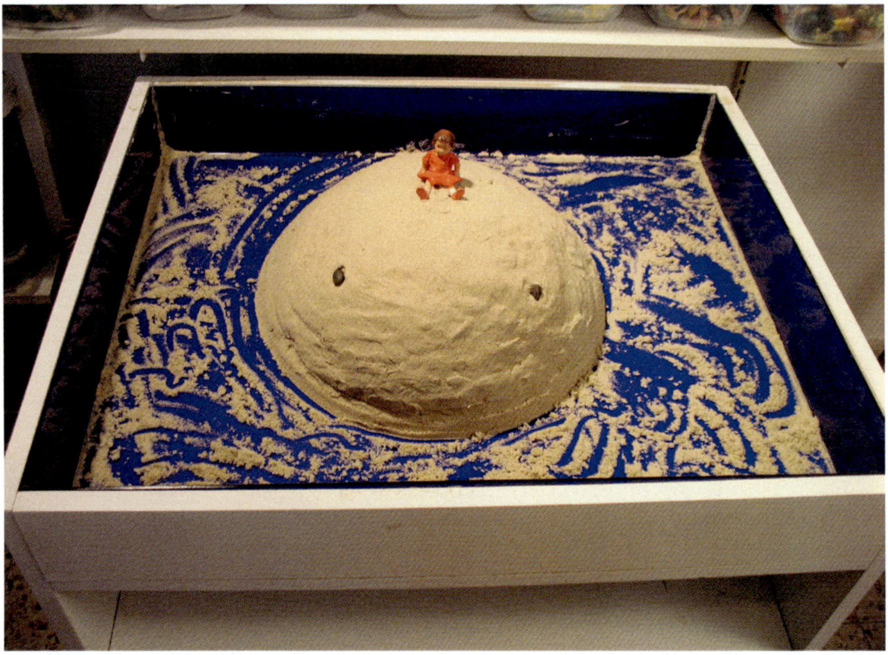

Plate 3 Helena: *Little girl in a red dress sitting on a whale mound*

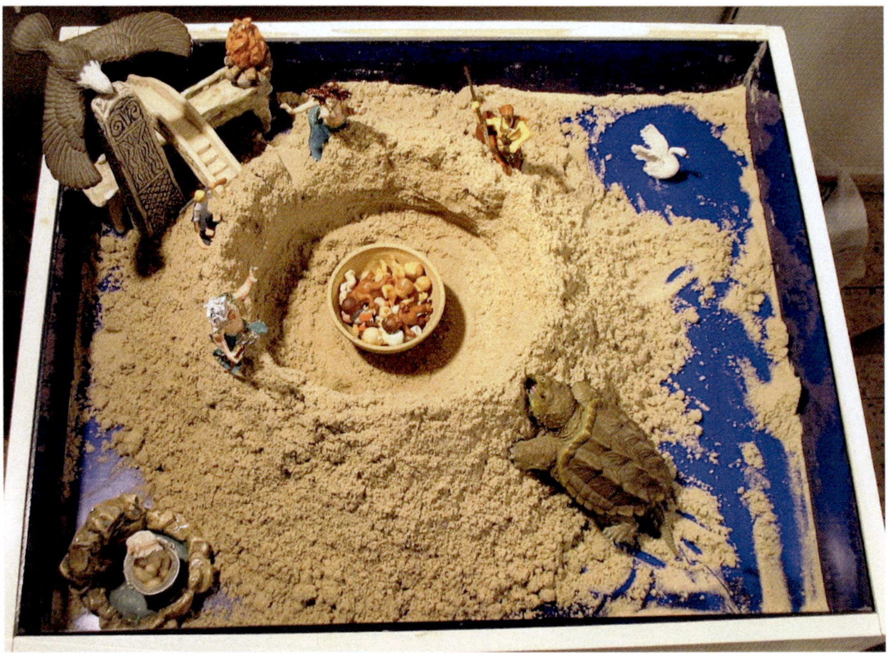

Plate 4 Helena: *Kiva, babies, Poseidon and Mermaid, Turtle and Eagle*

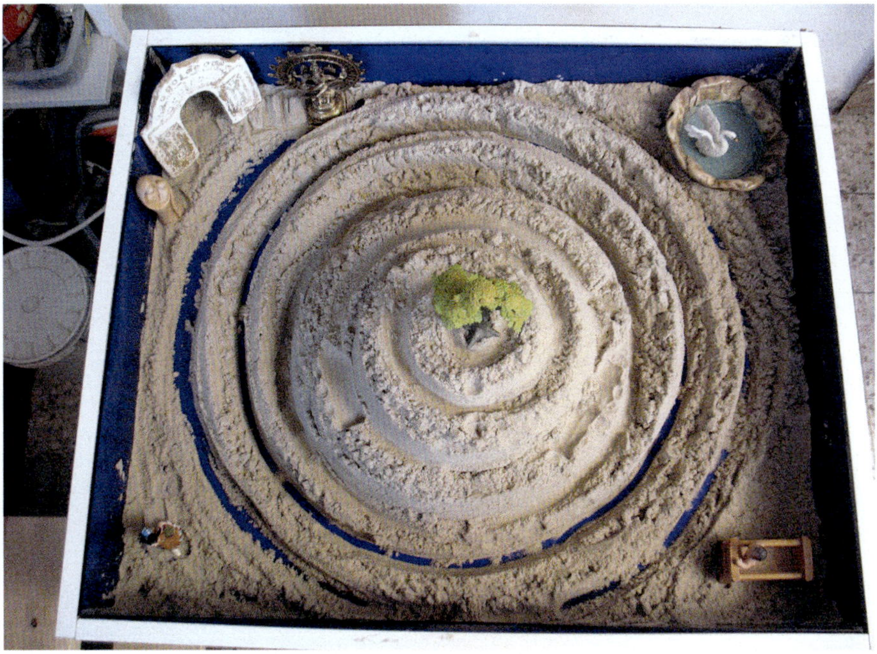

Plate 5 Helena: *First Self-tray, an Oak tree in the center of five concentric circles*

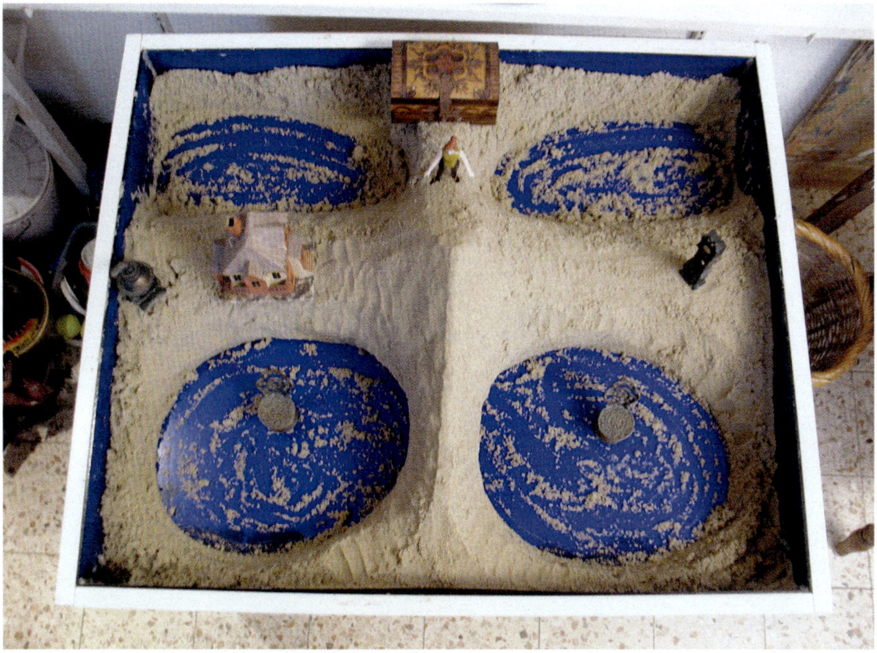

Plate 6 Helena: *Anastasia, butterfly symmetry*

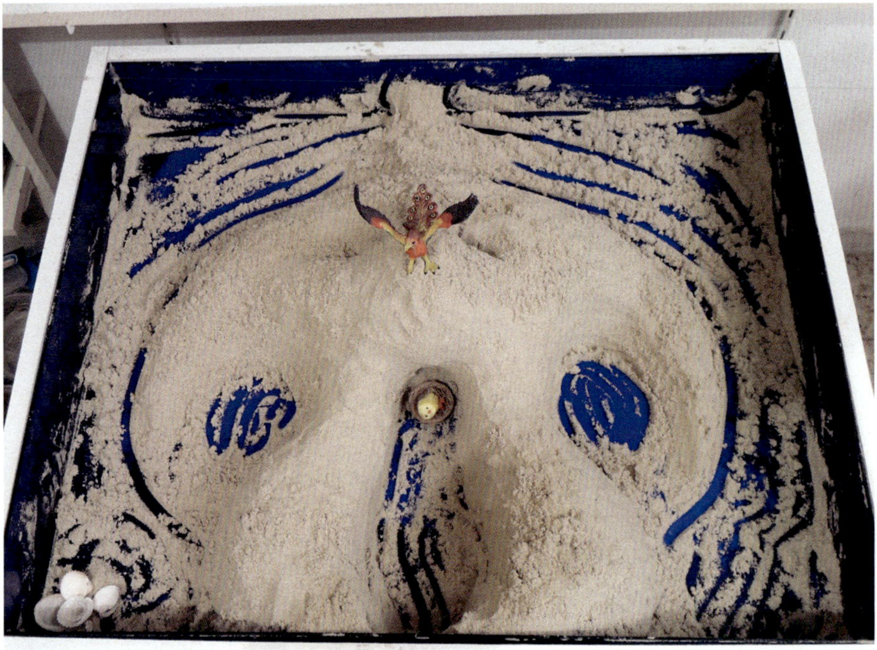

Plate 7 Helena: *Phoenix and Firebird*

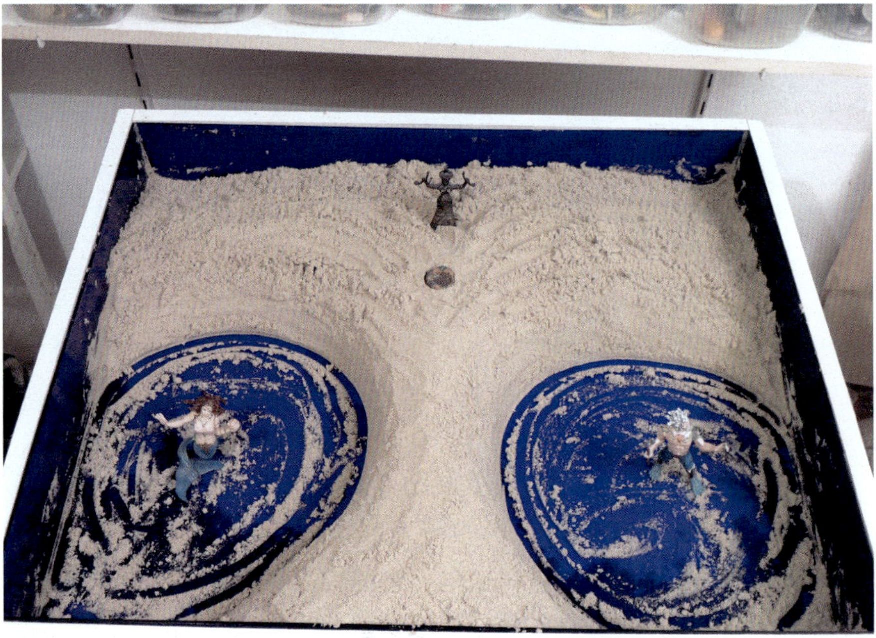

Plate 8 Helena: *Sculpted Tree of Life, Poseidon and Mermaid*

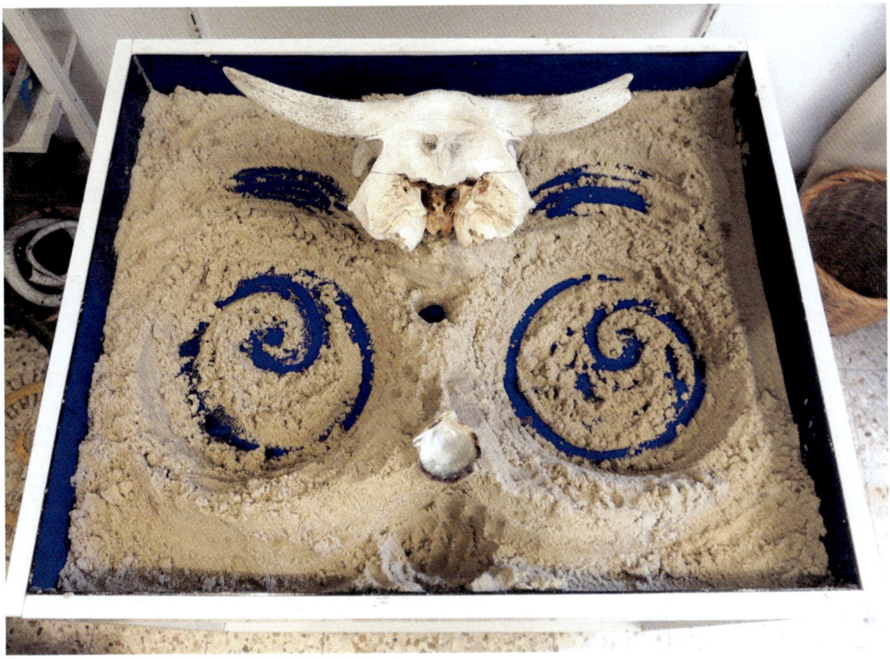

Plate 9 Helena: *Cow skull symmetry, entrance to the underworld*

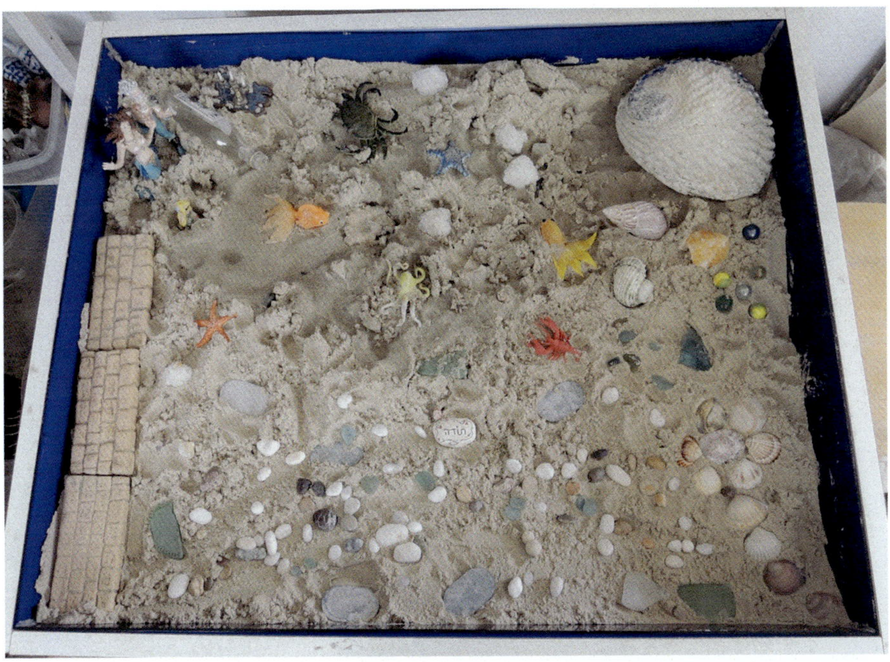

Plate 10 Rose: *First sandplay, Fragmentation, a need for containment*

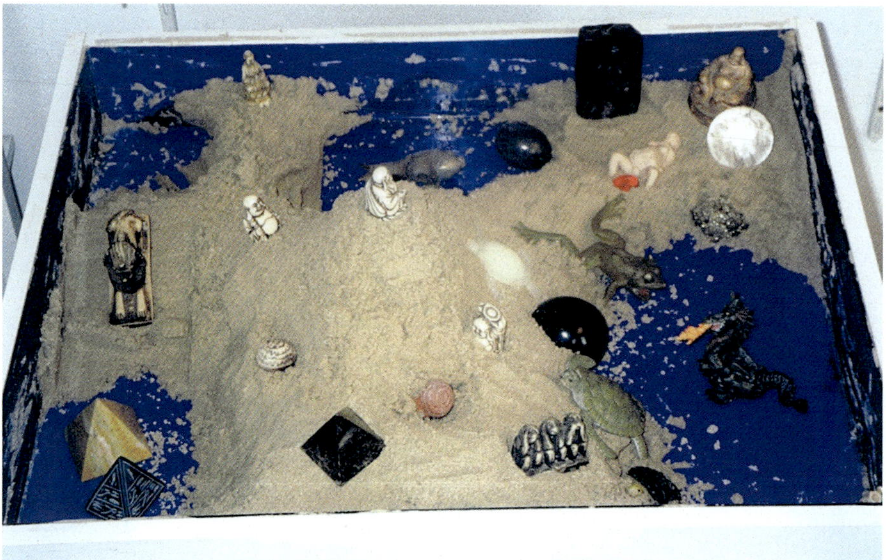

Plate 11 Ziva: *Sandplay 16, a birth in progress*

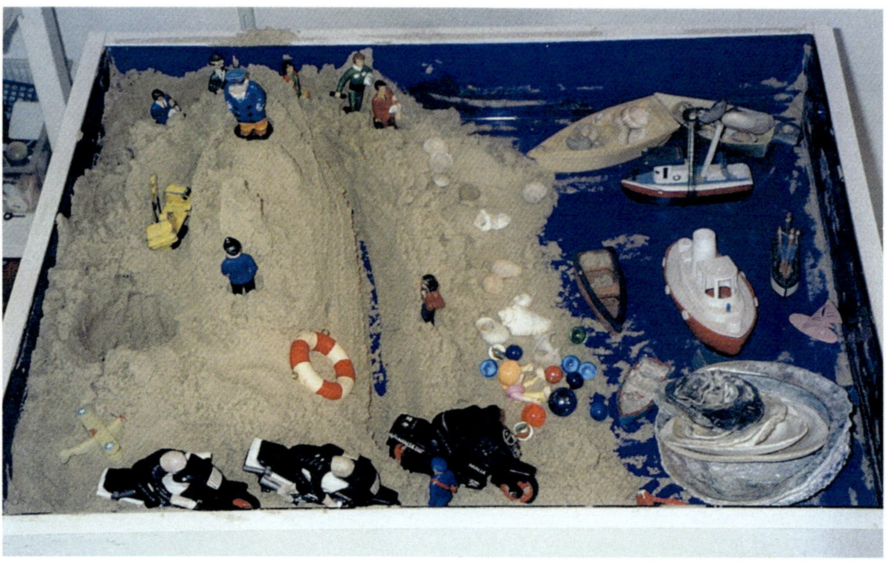

Plate 12 Ziva: *Final sandplay, Leaving a sand ferry after a voyage*

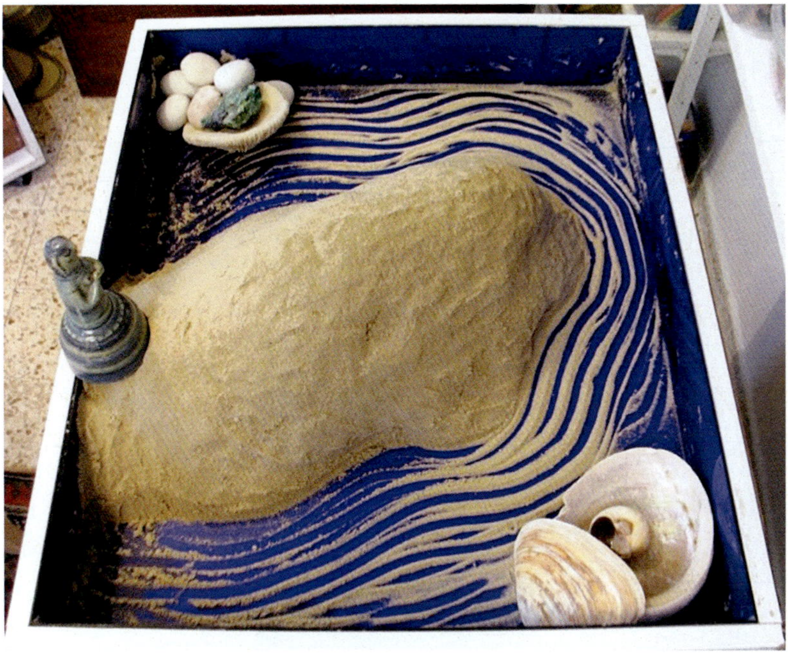

Plate 13 Grete: *Sandplay 8, Paths in the unconscious, feminine and masculine archetypes*

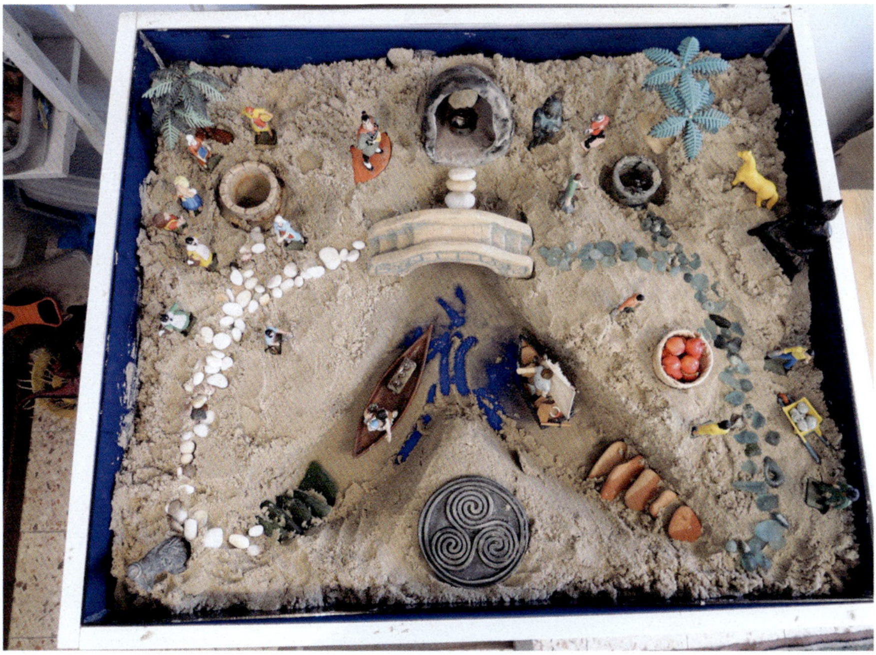

Plate 14 Tara: *Sandplay 2, Multiple paths*

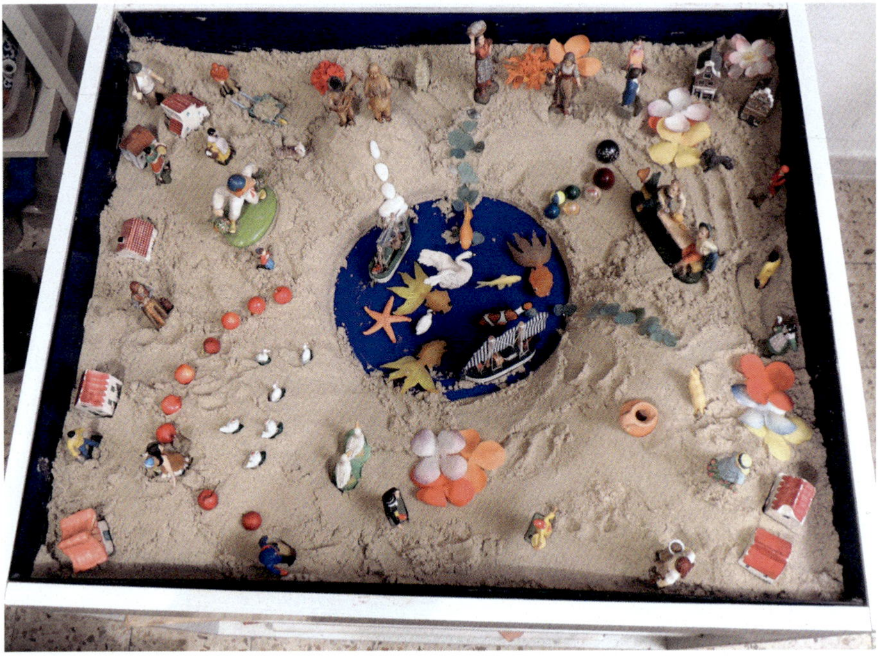

Plate 15 Tara: *Sandplay 20, Blue pool in center, multiple paths leave and return*

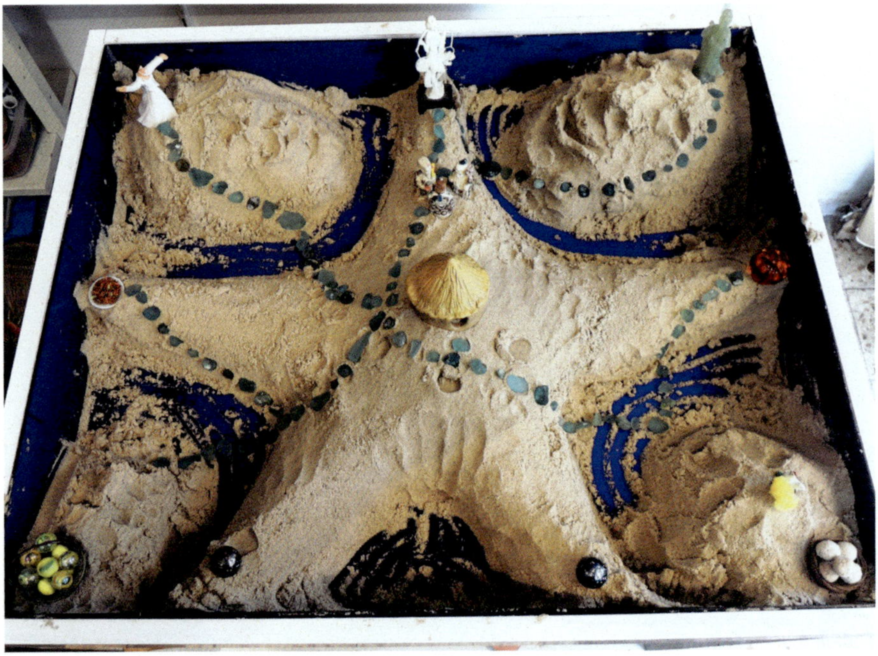

Plate 16 Tara: *Sandplay 21 (final sandplay), A celestial afterward*

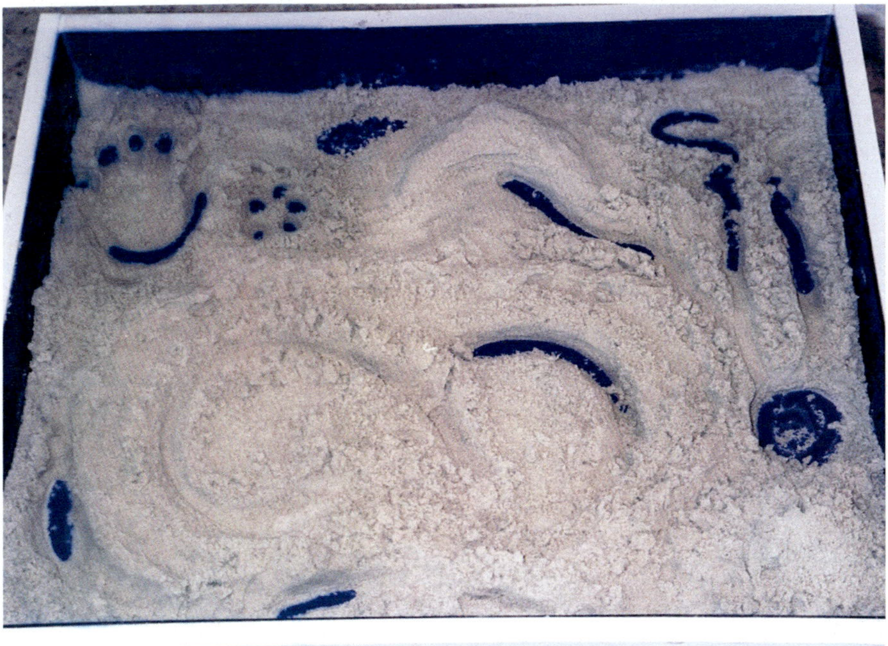

Plate 17 Jasmin: *Sandplay 1: Pairs, Hamsa and Cave*

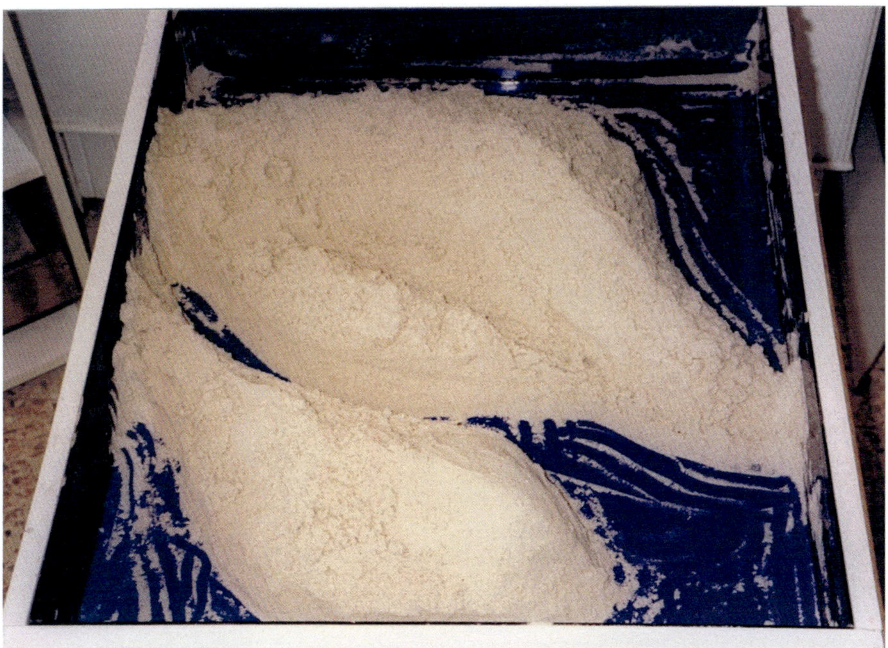

Plate 18 Jasmin: *Sandplay 5: Two sand fish in harmony*

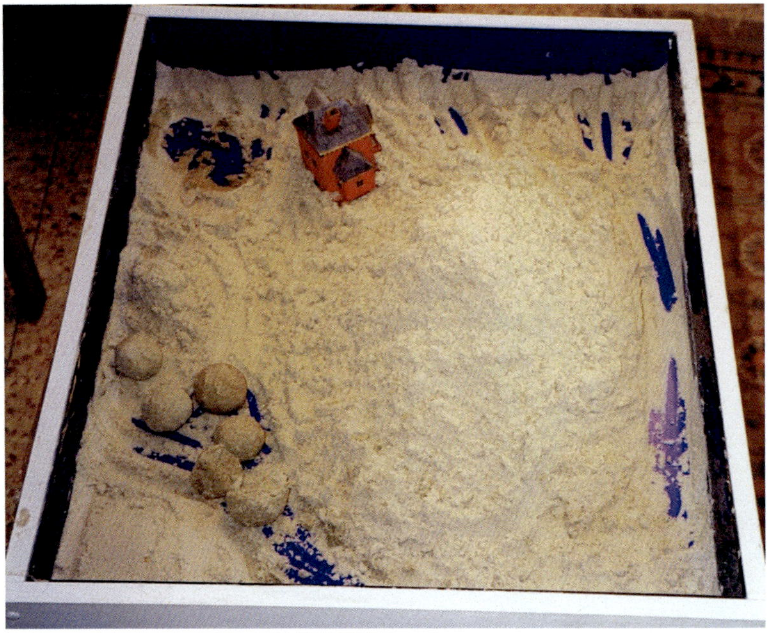

Plate 19 Jasmin: *Sandplay II: House beneath the hill*

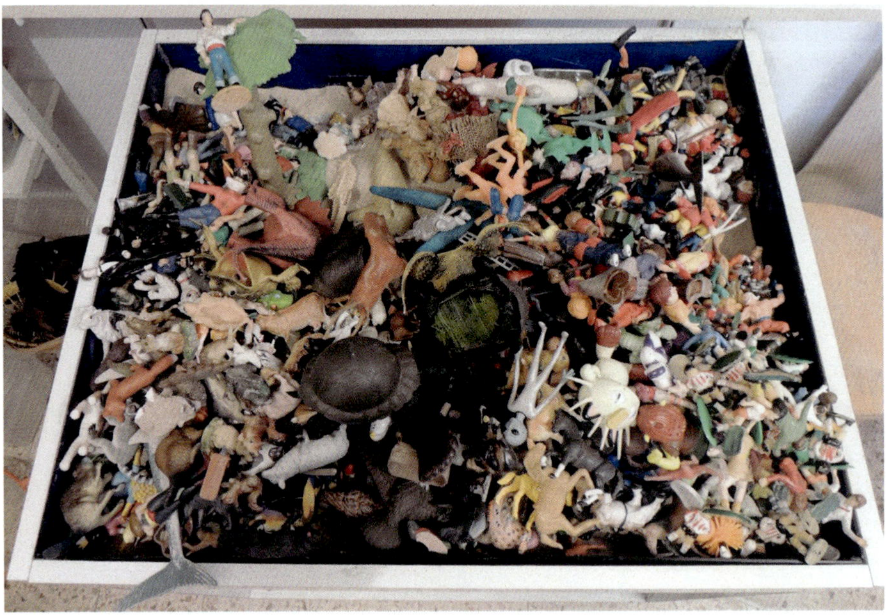

Plate 20 Oron: *Age three years ten months, High mound of figurines*

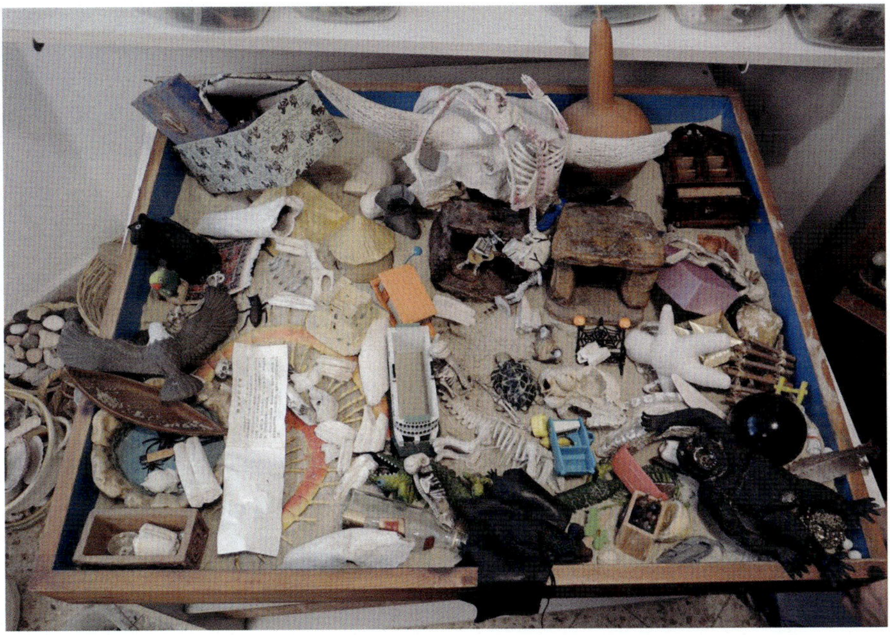

Plate 21 Oron: *Age five years seven months, Controlled upheaval, dark and light*

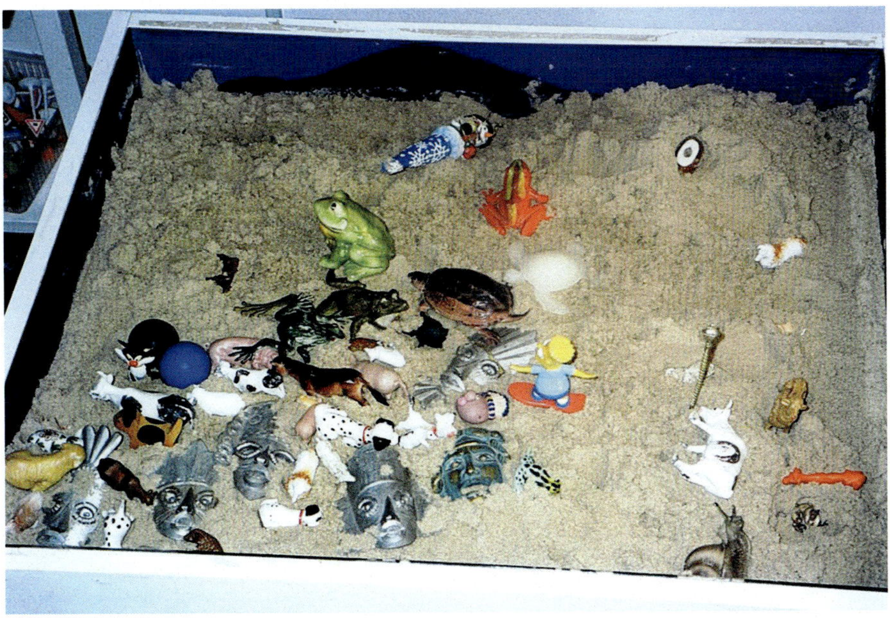

Plate 22 Ben: *Age two years five months, Masks*

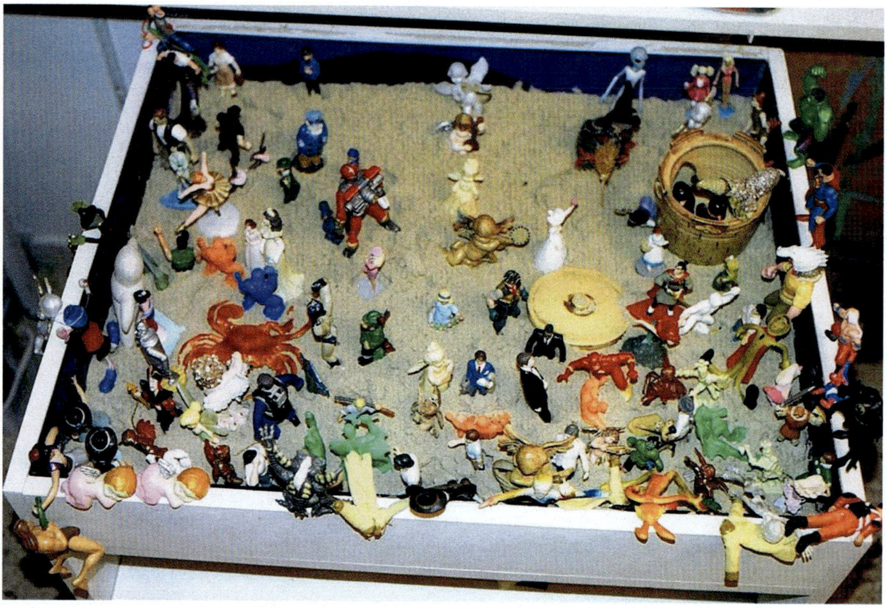

Plate 23 Ben: *Age four years four months,* Ice Age

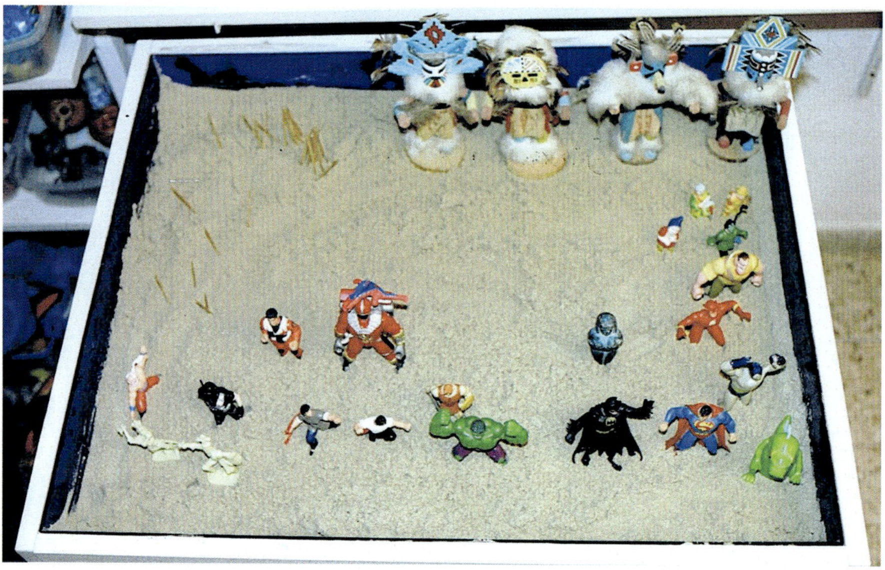

Plate 24 Ben: *Age four and a half, Sandplay 25, Kachinas, Ishtar and superheroes*

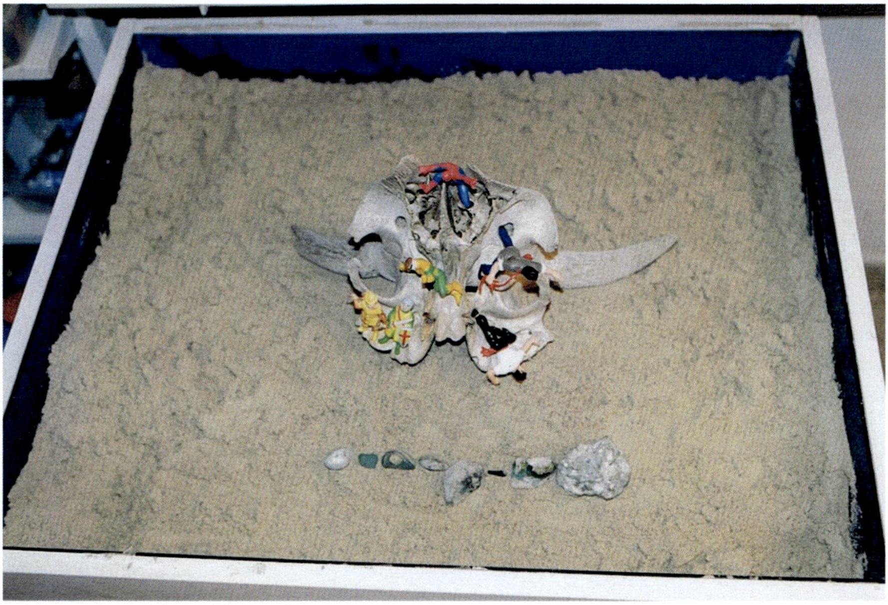

Plate 25 Ben: *Sandplay 31, Superheroes compete on the cow skull*

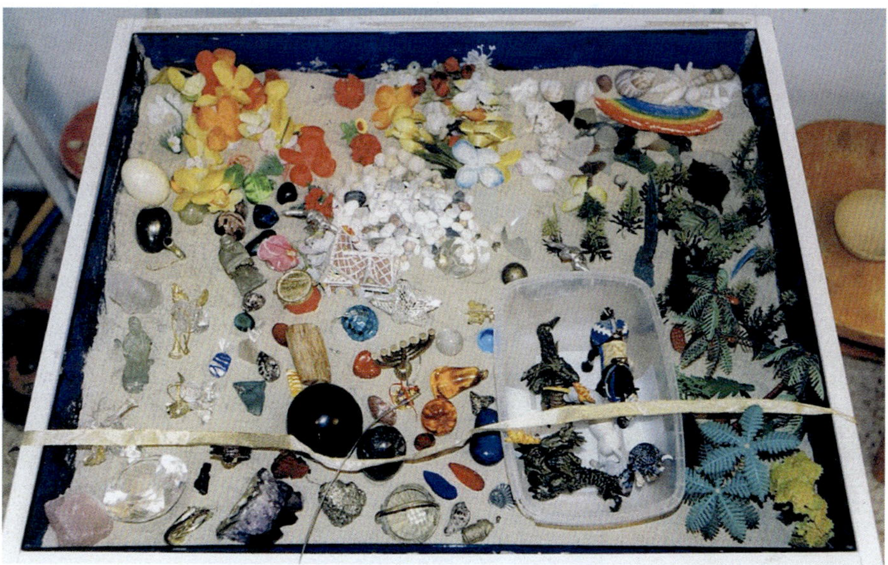

Plate 26 Ben: *Age five years 11 months, Sandplay 39, Shimenawa*

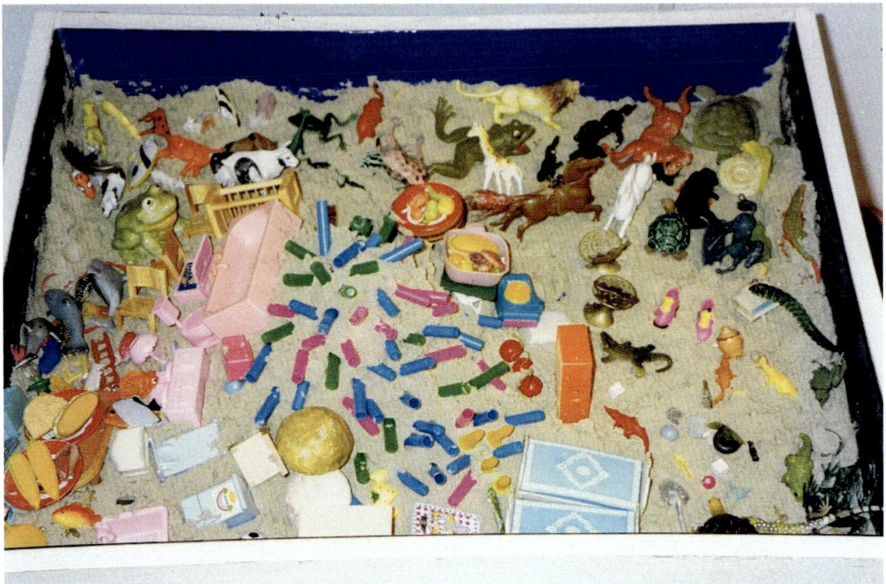

Plate 27 Maya: *Age three years eight months, Sandplay 3, Mound, pegs, wild animals, baby crib*

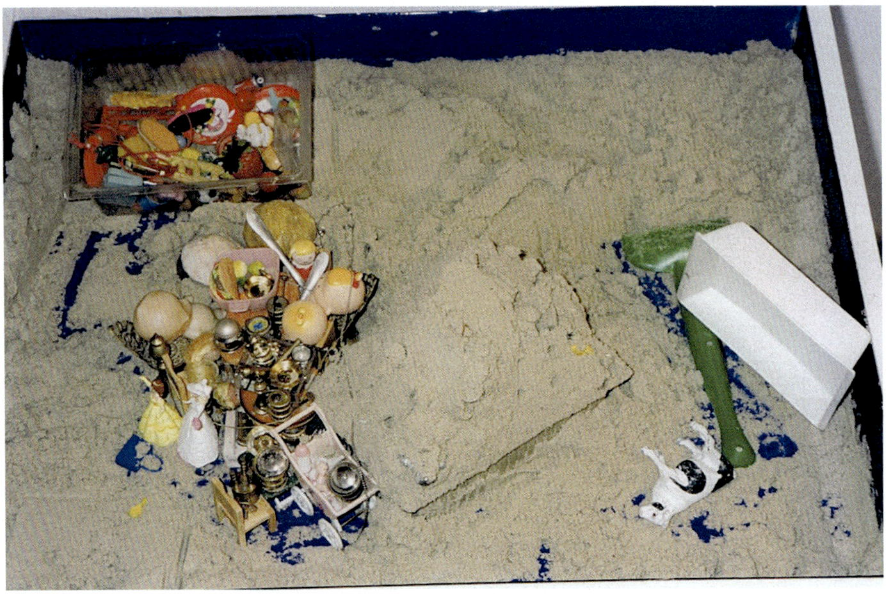

Plate 28 Maya: *Sandplay 5, Burying fear*

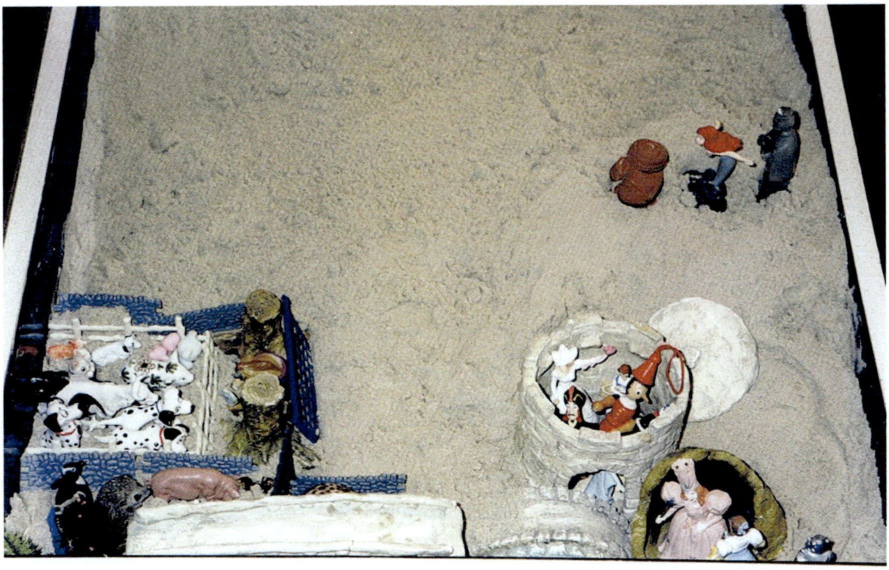

Plate 29 Maya: *Sandplay 9, Mermaid between godesses Kwan Yin and Venus of Willensdorf*

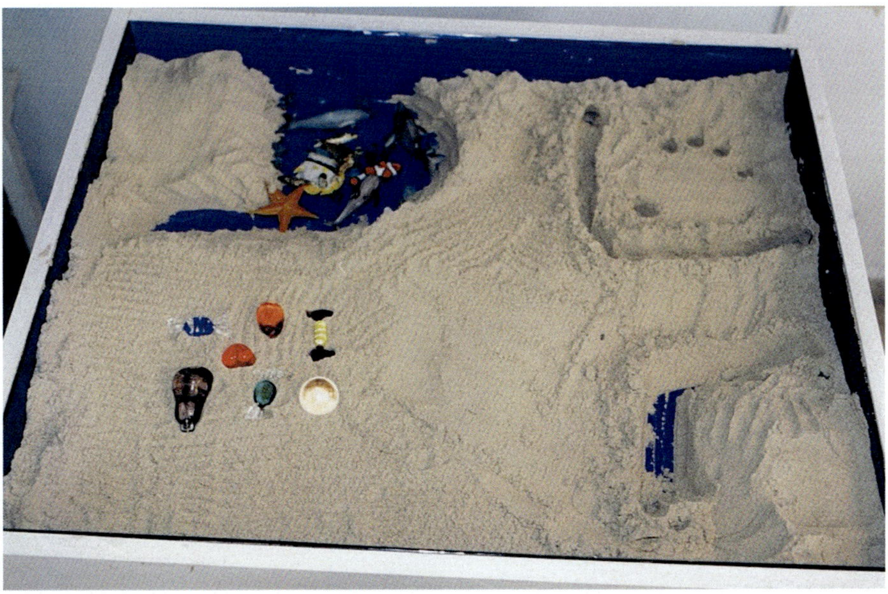

Plate 30 Maya: *Age nine and a half, Sandplay 24, Two black stones, two black eggs*

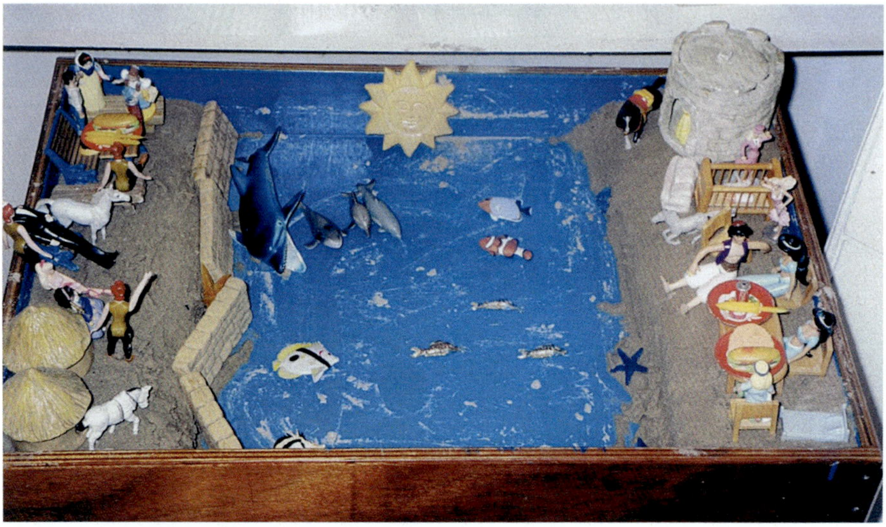

Plate 31 Maya: *Age ten, Sandplay 31, The war that makes love impossible*

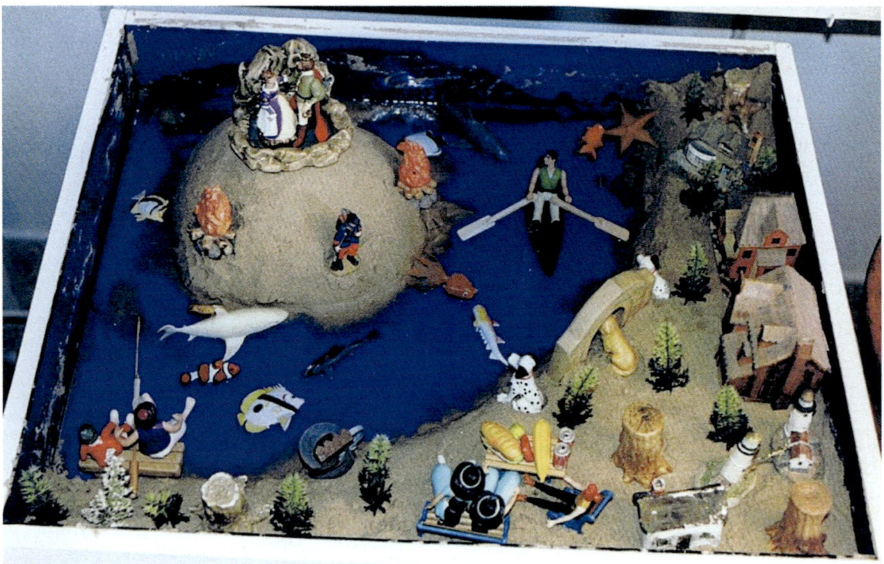

Plate 32 Maya: *Age 11 and a half, Sandplay 39, The Alchemical King and Queen*

Age three years and ten months

Oron said he wanted a lot, to build something very big, very high, a heap. He dumped several boxes of miniatures into the entire area of the tray, never doubting that the sandtray boundaries would protect this mass of objects. Looking closely at his heap, there is some order in his choices. The front-left area is full of large and small animals, the entire right side is filled mostly with various kinds of men and cartoon heroes. A box of women and a box of babies remained on the shelf. This kind of formless but contained chaos could represent an event of creation, birth and awakening, a beginning potential and preparation for ego consciousness to emerge into light and order. Oron is still embraced by the matriarchal but soon at age four he will begin the transition to the patriarchate (Neumann, 1973/1988) (Figure 10.2).

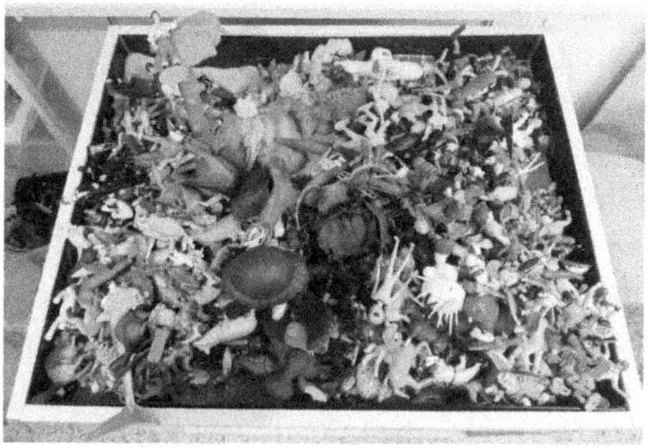

Figure 10.2 *Oron: Age three years ten months, High mound of figurines*

Age four years seven months

There is a clear separation between the left and right sides of the sand picture. Within each side there is a division of opposites in its content. The Great Opposites of Life and Death fill the less conscious front-left quadrant, with dinosaur skeletons and bones around a large Tree of Life. On the far-right side, a high sand ridge shaped like a semi-circle surrounds blue symbolic water. It separates four superheroes guarding the front boundary from the rest of the tray. In the far-right blue area, seven small dogs and three Smurfs meet near a globe. The sense of growing consciousness emerging in the far-right quadrant is protected by the raised sand and distanced from the powerful matriarchate on the left (Figure 10.3).

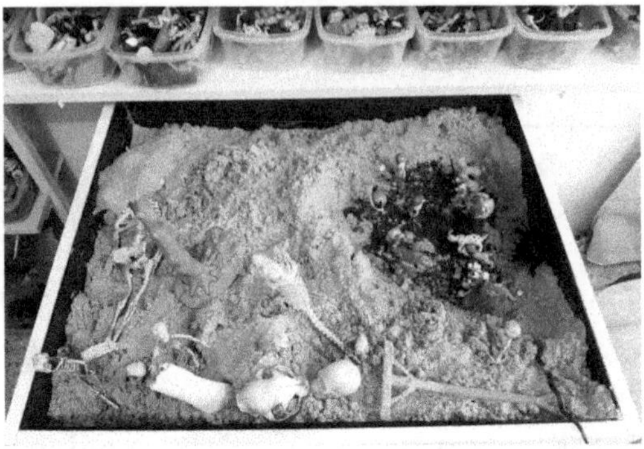

Figure 10.3 *Oron: Age four years seven months, Dividing the sandtray into opposites*

Age five years three and a half months

Oron completes two sandplays, one in the wet tray and the other in the dry tray. He calls me to help him move both trays together in the center of the room. He stands proudly behind his work, extending his hands to either side, for a photograph showing how big he and his sandplays are. In the dry sandtray on the left, the idea of row organization begins: large walls form a horizontal boundary in the front area that separates it from the much larger area in the rear. A long Chinese dragon is placed vertically towards the wall. Two rakes are left vertically in the far-right corner. A variety of masculine objects are scattered in both areas, but there are sandwiches on the left side—perhaps the masculine begins to provide its own nurturance unconsciously without a feminine presence.

The wet sandtray on the right seems organized into quadrants, with symbolic communication between opposite corners. For the first time, on the diagonal, the far-left area contains several trees and small household objects including a blue and pink camera, and the front-right area contains Pegasus, a colorful snake and a phoenix, hiding a small safari photographer, with a bathtub nearby. The camera symbol placed in a tree-filled environment and again between mythological creatures, may prepare the path from magical thinking to a growing rational capacity. The diagonal from the front-left corner contrasts two bridges and some trees, with a bridge, ladder, unicorn (fallen) and small superhero in the far-right area. The idea of communication becomes more conscious, leaving dependency on the matriarchal and preparing a move to the outside world while the superhero and unicorn wait. The center is left open (Figures 10.4, 10.5, 10.6).

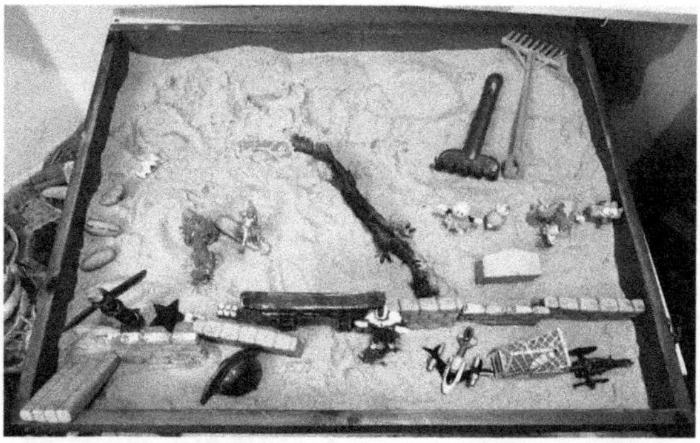

Figure 10.4 *Oron: Age five years three and a half months, Quadrants appear*

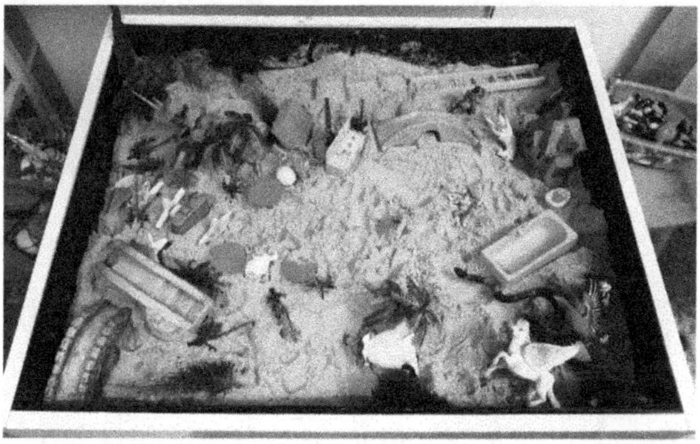

Figure 10.5 *Oron: Age five years three and a half months, Wet sandtray*

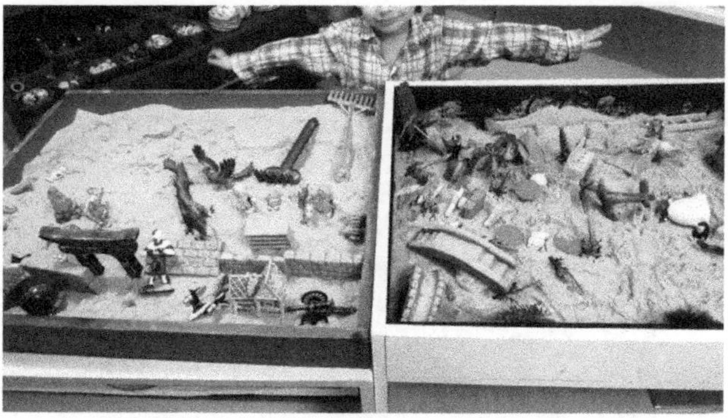

Figure 10.6 *Oron: Age five years three and a half months, Two sandtrays pushed together*

Age five years seven months

Oron chooses many dark and light large objects and animals and fills the dry sandtray, creating a general sense of controlled upheaval, quite different from Figure 10.2. Included are objects that may represent potential life (round huts, dried gourd with seeds), death (a large cow skull), rebirth (a dolmen) and independent survival (a small central turtle). An anonymous fallen white doll is the only human figure (Figure 10.7).

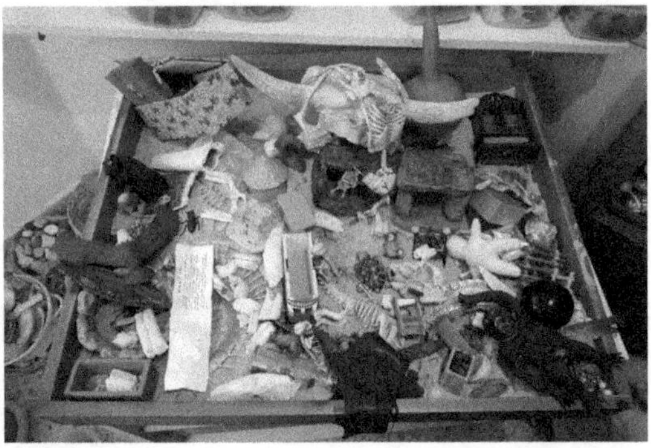

Figure 10.7 *Oron: Age five years seven months, Controlled upheaval, dark and light*

Two weeks later (age five years seven and a half months), a new phase of order begins. The dry sandtray is used to sort out rows of dinosaurs perhaps threatening a man in a canoe, with three large soldiers and a Native American chief around the area. The dry sand is a lighter color than the wet sand, and perhaps is chosen to prefigure the coming of light and order (Figure 10.8).

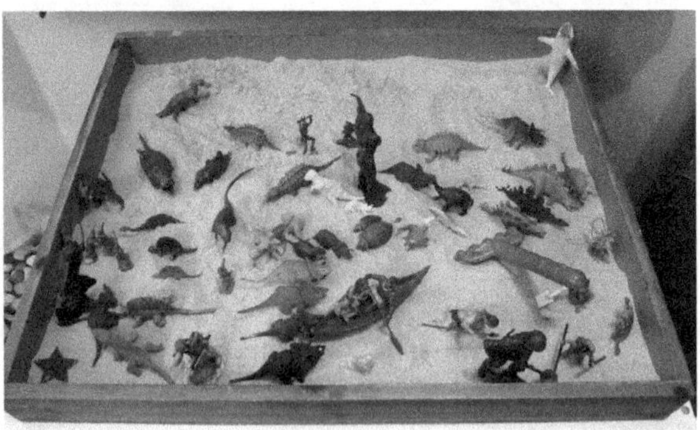

Figure 10.8 *Oron: Age five years seven and a half months, A new order, sorting, masculine dominance*

Age five years eight months

In the space of the dry sandtray, Oron arranges approximately 12 vertical rows of shells, animals, small masks, eggs, a black pyramid, a fisherman, treasure, a drum, sorted as if racing to the finish line where he stands. He called this "animal races." Nature, instinct, treasure, birth, death and rebirth stand together at the finish to collect the golden prize hung on the front-left edge of the tray (Figure 10.9).

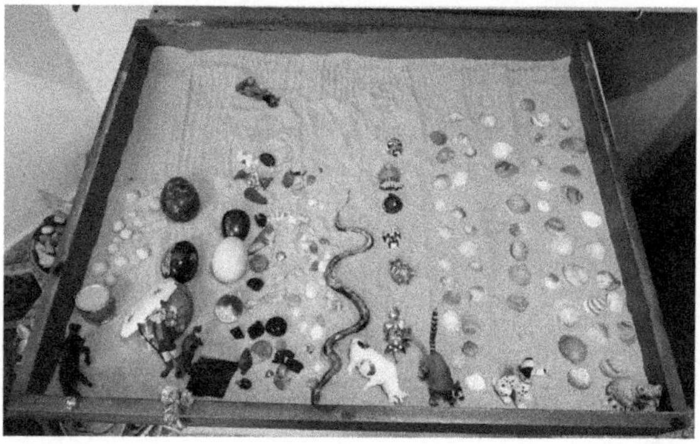

Figure 10.9 *Oron: Age five years eight months, Animal races*

In summary, the evolution of new developmental stages and structures is always accompanied by partial disintegration—devolving—of previous stages of development, letting go, letting once strong structures of attachment—such as those between mother and child—devolve and be replaced by evolving communicative structures.

BEN, A young boy's spontaneous sandplay process (two and a half to seven years old)

Ben was the eldest of his parents' two children. When he was two years and five months old, he began to explore my sandplay setting. He got to know the entire miniature collection in the studio by arranging on the floor whatever objects interested him, climbing on a stool to reach figurines on higher shelves. When he was tall enough to see over the sandtray edge, he began to place objects inside the tray in specific locations. Ben usually played alone and called me to photograph his work when he finished. If I asked, he would give a short title to each sandplay with an occasional short story. Ben was interested in sandplay for four and a half years. He completed 80 sandplays and then lost interest before age seven, completing Neumann's "Magic Phallic" stage of "Early Childhood I" (14 months to four years) and "Magic Warlike" stage (four to seven years old) of "Early Childhood II, a Play Age."

Ben's sandplays can be divided into six stages, each with a theme that resolved itself before a new stage began. He became acquainted with the setting in Stage One, from age two and a half to four years, and made nine sandplays separated by a few months between each. Between four and five years old, the start of a boy's transition from the matriarchate to the patriarchate, his need for sandplay and his identification with the hero greatly intensified. During this one year, he came 24 times and made 38 sandplays which are divided into Stages Two, Three and Four. Ben's need for sandplay lessened between five and six years old, Stage Five, with only six visits and nine sandplays. In Stage Six, from six to seven years old, he seemed to sum up his sandplay history in five visits to the studio and six sandplays. Twenty sandplays are discussed that together represent the stages, themes, continuity of symbols and quality of expression of his complete process.

Stage One: Exploring hierarchies of power (two and a half to four years old)

Masks, animals and Simpson, Sandplay 1

At age two years and five months, Ben made his first sandplay in the sandtray, juxtaposing an unusual assortment of figurines for a child of his age. Archetypal powers, large reptiles and farm animals are crowded into the front-left area, with one small human, Bart Simpson, on a skateboard in the near center, facing left towards frogs and turtles. His back is turned to a row of six metal Mexican masks in the front left, lying flat on the sand facing forward. Between the masks stand small farm animals and dogs, pointed in different directions. Opposite, small animals are dispersed on the right side. An upright gold staff stuck in the sand near the head of a large white cow lying on its side, facing left, and another dark cow also lying prone in the far left, perhaps reflect Ben's feelings about his mother, now that he has a younger brother. A red frog points upwards in the far center, near a flat snowman. Ben's choice of objects, their direction and placement on the left, right, far, near or center, alone or in groups seems deliberate (Figure 10.10).

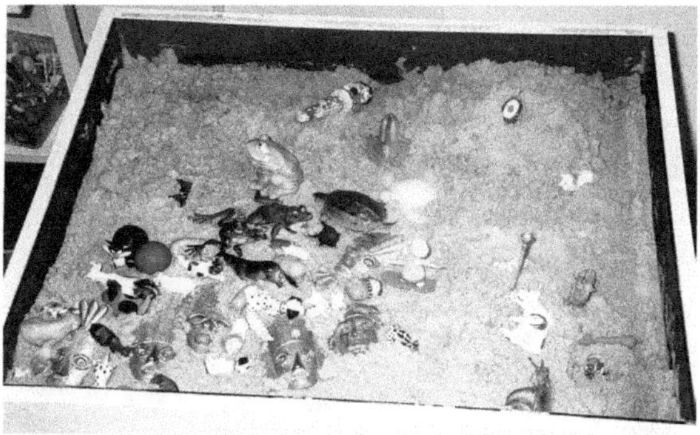

Figure 10.10 *Ben: Age two years five months, Masks*

Masks and superpowers, Sandplay 3

One year later, at three years and five months old, Ben placed the same metal masks in the same front-left corner, but now they stand along the edges, two covered with fabrics. These mask divinities surpass the powers of the superheroes and four human ninjas nearby. A tiny human cowboy aims a rifle at a yellow sun. A diagram of this sandplay could be divided into four quadrants, with a center encircled by two rows of objects, each row with a specific color family. The far-left quadrant is filled with a mass of oversize dark frogs, turtles, a snail, two lightning storm clouds, a rainbow and four small red fruits facing right, contrasting large and small, dark and red colors. The rainbow and fruits are also part of a prominent central area of three suns (two yellow, one black) and a red cloth with large red fruits. Encircling the central area are bluish and grey objects (covered masks, superheroes, lightning clouds, beige wooden objects and sticks) along the rear, left and front edges. The curve rises slightly on the front right towards six tiny white Jizo. In Japan, small stone Jizo statues represent beloved protective guardian spirits for children and travelers, and are found in cemeteries and on roads, to ease the journey to an afterlife of souls who passed away too soon. Here the Jizo stand in two rows of four and two, near the blue cowboy and his rifle, and close off a triangular area in the front-right corner. Four superheroes, Wonder Woman—the single feminine presence—and the six Jizo seem to focus on the yellow sun. Distant from the center in the far-right corner are another lightning cloud and a small Tarzan who may be leaving. Ben seems to sense a hierarchy of power, from divine masks, storm clouds, Jizo and giant reptiles, to superheroes and ninjas, to a cowboy. Wonder Woman may represent his personal mother, still felt as an archetypal powerful presence at his age. Ben points his figurines in specific directions, and contrasts opposites of left and right, divine and human, hidden and visible, large and small, dark and red colors, and pale blue or beige colors, in an almost mandala-like composition in the sandtray (Figure 10.11).

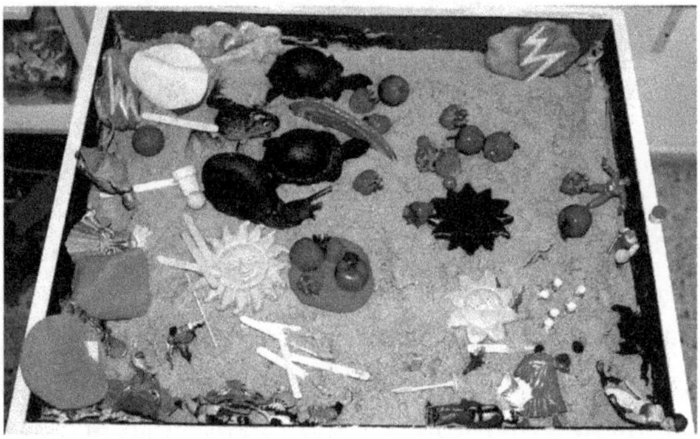

Figure 10.11 *Ben: Age three years five months, Masks, superheroes, Jizo and apples*

The rainbow bridge, Sandplay 5

Ben's sandplay two months later is balanced and cohesive. A small elf points to a central rainbow that bridges a crowded column of male and female figurines moving along the entire right side towards the front, and a few selected objects on the front-left side, a tall tree with a small elf on its green top, a partially naked girl and an elf prone on the sand, and a small green dragon and three adjoining wooden chairs behind the tree. The male and female figurines pass a glass gold-roofed house and a few angels, ending with a nude woman in a boat. Towards the front are several clowns, prone male figurines, an apple and a windmill. On both sides of this world, Ben has blended realistic and fantasy figurines, the ordinary and the magical. Rainbows in nature bridge the opposites of fire (as light) and water (as vapor), here bridging the two sides of the sandplay. Two feminine figures have been deliberately undressed while the males remain clothed, reflecting Ben's natural curiosity at this age regarding sexual differences. New objects, a gold-roofed house and a windmill, a house with "wings" moved by air in front center, may symbolize spirit (Figure 10.12). In the same week, Ben came twice more and made four sandplays with new objects and groupings. His final sandplay of this stage in the dry sandtray contrasts a group of dried fruits, pods and nuts (inferring potential growth) on the front left with a group of 12 differently colored horses lying prone in the front-right area (inferring potential action). Between these groups, a small blue creature in a green pumpkin hat marks center. Ben has explored hierarchies of power from the divine, to superheroes, dwarfs and humans, in a world where fantasy and reality co-exist. His ego directed him towards increased independence in preparation for a transition to the patriarchate.

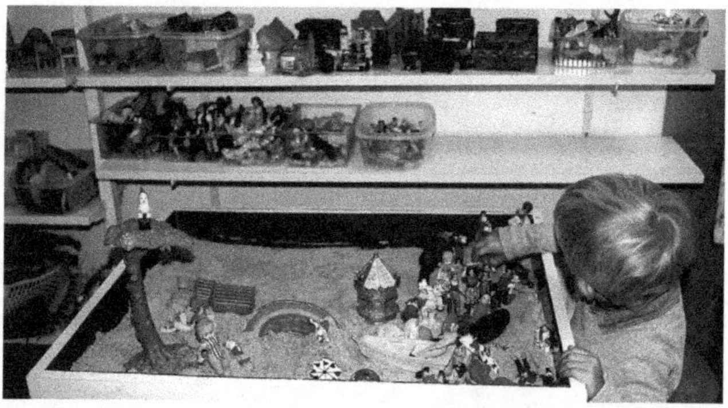

Figure 10.12 *Ben: Age three years seven months, The rainbow connection*

Stage Two: Paving the hero's path (from four years four months to four years six months old)

Four months later, Ben returned and worked intensively for two months, with 11 visits and 14 sandplays, using both sandtrays four times. His images overflowed with figurines and contrasted feminine and masculine, life and death, humans, superpowers and the divine, and tiny Smurfs and other small creatures who look up at stronger forces, perhaps realistically assessing the dangers of leaving the protective matriarchate.

Batman faces his opponents on his way to reach the chief, Sandplay 8

In the first of two sandplays, Batman, leaning on the far-left edge, faces several rows of fierce warriors and chthonic men, and four cacti. They block his path to a Native American chief (Great Father) and two wigwams in the front-right corner. Like Theseus, who conquers six dangerous criminals on his way to his father in Athens, Batman must overcome these dangers and reach the chief in transition to the patriarchate. The matriarchal phase that Ben must leave seems symbolized by a racing-car driver near Batman who faces three Native American women, a wheelbarrow and a white totem in the front left. Opposite, the chief sits near two wigwams, perhaps one for men and one for women. Above the chief, a small blue egg on the sand in the shade of a pink umbrella is protected by two policemen dressed in black, two birds perched high above the egg, other figurines and a second white totem. The egg may imply a time of incubation until Ben is ready to leave the matriarchate (Figure 10.13). Ben's second sandplay in the dry tray is gentle and feminine, with seed pods, two pine trees and a palm, white, yellow and red flowers, a pink butterfly, a shovel and two blue rakes lying near a sand hill in the far left, balancing the aggressive masculine energies of the first (not shown).

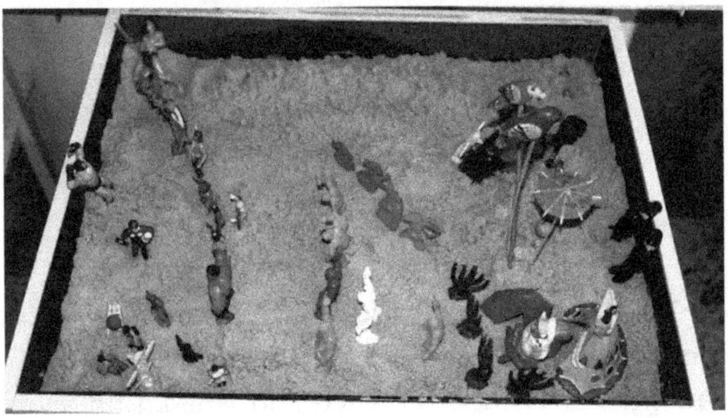

Figure 10.13 *Ben: Four years old, Batman faces his opponents*

The *Ice Age*, Sandplay 10

Ben created two densely packed sandplays inspired by heroic themes, conflictual forces and love between masculine and feminine in an animated film, *Ice Age*. The wet sandtray is divided vertically by a row of angels into left and right sides, implying equal opposites. The dry tray is divided horizontally into far and near areas, perhaps implying unequal power, divine above and mundane below. In the wet sandtray, the frame above the sandtray is emphasized by figurines standing on the right and front edges, sleeping angels, ghouls, superheroes and two dresses that clothed two "Anastasia" figurines. Inside the tray, on either side of the central row of angels, a prominent object is surrounded by different kinds of men or superheroes, and a few pairs of women. A round castle on the far right contains two black policemen and a gold and silver harlequin. Around the castle are a witch, a ghoul and two women, and on the edge above are the Green Hulk and Superman. In the front left, a large red crab is encircled by a cone shell, Pegasus, three men, a tin man and a woman. In the front-left corner, Tarzan hangs precariously outside the tray and, in a gesture of masculine comradery, is helped into the tray by Aladdin, who is supported by two Jasmine figurines. But nearby stands Jafar, a scheming male counterpart of the witch in the far right. In the front-right corner, a chaotic group of masculine figurines has no feminine presence to offer the hero a flaxen thread to emerge into order. A graceful dancer in the far left could represent the flowing feminine movement needed for transition (Figure 10.14).

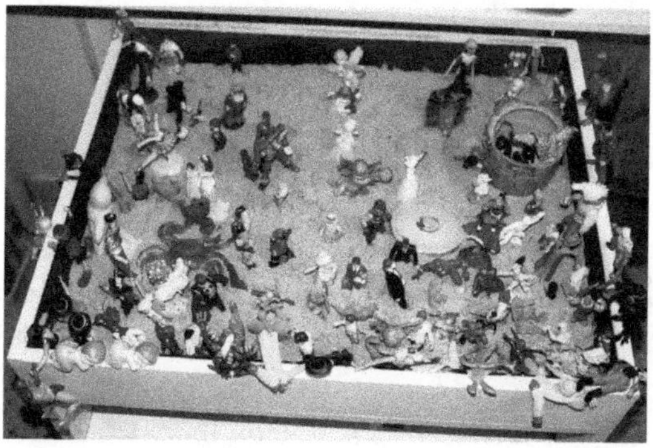

Figure 10.14 *Ben: Age four years four months,* Ice Age

In the dry sandtray, a threatening cow skull, large clam shell and spider conch, framed by dark nuts, dried fruits and natives, loom up in the far area, behind innocent small creatures and small shells positioned along the front area, a dramatic horizontal contrast between above and below. Directly below the skull and clam shell, a smaller white clam shell with a very small shell on it mirror the large skull and clam, and are surrounded by cartoon creatures, a ghost, a spiky white creature, the blue creature with a green hat, a wolf in overalls, a mask, a smiling hamburger and the head of ET. The contrast of dark and light, power and vulnerability, is gentle, but also indicates the danger that the natives in the far right may have to face (Figure 10.15).

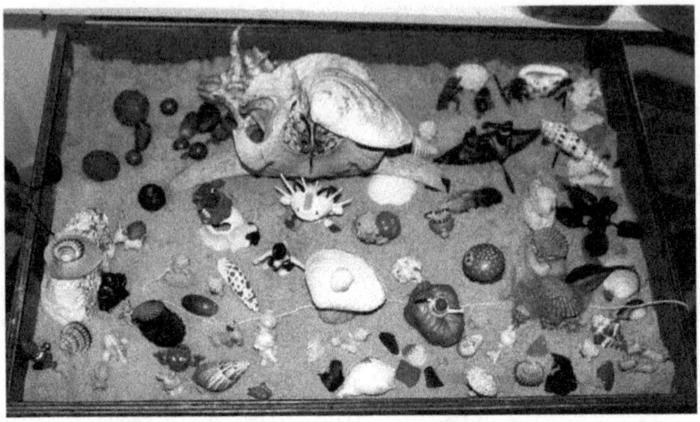

Figure 10.15 *Ben: Age four years four months, Contrasts of dark and light, small and large*

The Big Green Car, masculine energy, feminine approval, excitement, Sandplay 11

One week later, Ben brought a huge shiny green car with him and placed it in the central front area of the sandtray, with many superheroes and several dragons. He balanced the masculine presence with feminine figurines, two Jasmines and many pretty girls around the car, and other feminine figurines on the white cow skull behind the car and nearby, perhaps for their approval and encouragement of potential heroes. An inverted pyramid and a round white igloo behind the skull might signal the death and rebirth that a hero must endure. Above three undressed Anastasia figurines and a gypsy in the far right, Ben has balanced on the sandtray edges a red heart, a sun lying flat with a blue star on it, four tiny Jizo figures and a clock. Two Jizo are on the sand near some tiny mushrooms. A silver pendant hangs outside the tray, near the dresses that Ben removed from the Anastasia figurines, a red pendant on one dress, and two cacti lying prone. His title was "The Big Green Car." We looked at the work together (Figure 10.16).

Vanity, the shadow side of feminine beauty may lurk beneath women's support of heroes. The shadow side of men's heroism is hubris, and denial of danger and death (Homer, 1990, 1991). The presence of many beautiful women, a rainbow, two red ceramic containers, a pumpkin, large red apples and strawberries adds to the symbolism of the archetypal feminine. Their proximity to many heroes recalls the Greek myth of the "Judgment of Paris," a beauty contest between three goddesses, Hera, Aphrodite and Athena, like the three Anastasias. At a wedding feast, Eris, Goddess of Discord, was not invited but she came anyway, and threw her gift, a golden apple inscribed "to the fairest," towards the guests. Paris, a mortal hero was appointed by Zeus to judge who would win. Hera and Athena offered bribes of wealth and power to Paris, but Aphrodite offered him Helen the most beautiful woman in the world for his wife, already married to King Menelaus of Sparta. Paris chose Aphrodite as the most beautiful and carried Helen off to Troy. To retrieve her, the Spartans gathered a heroic army and embarked on the ten-year Trojan War.

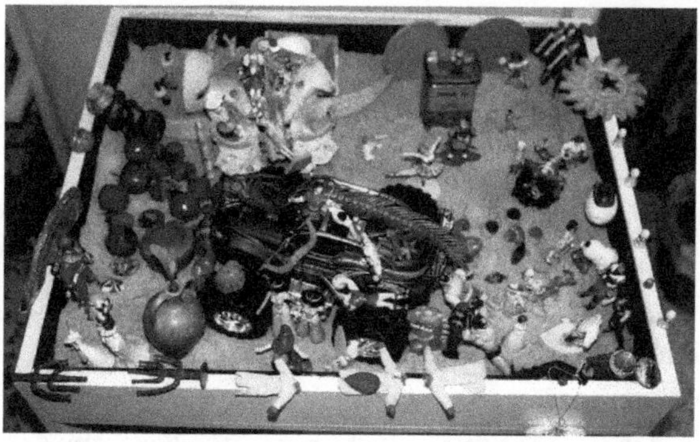

Figure 10.16 *Ben: Age four years five months, The Big Green Car*

Ben's sandplays were often divided into left and right sides, with figurines pointing to specific directions. Jung attributed primary significance to movements, markings or objects connected with either the left or right sides. "The left, the 'sinister' side, is the unconscious side. Therefore, a leftward movement is equivalent to a movement in the direction of the unconscious, whereas a movement to the right is 'correct' and aims at consciousness" (Jung, 1953, para. 166). Jung added:

> The left-hand is inauspicious and awkward; also, it is the side of the heart, from which comes not only love but all the evil thoughts connected with it, the moral contradictions in human nature that are expressed most clearly in our affective life. (Jung, 1954/1966, para. 410)

A man entered a castle and his sword broke, four and a half years old, Sandplay 15

In the left, less conscious area of the dry sandtray are two horizontal rows of figurines. In the front-left row, a large black ceramic whale lies on a mosaic of white and dark pebbles with two tiny metal soldiers behind him, a seal and walrus in front, all facing right, towards consciousness. In the rear second row of archetypal figures, the Eiffel Tower is first, followed by a small African male god, two Cretan snake goddesses on either side of a green Statue of Liberty, a jade Kwan Yin, the Cretan disk with its undeciphered spiral and, in the center, a large golden Buddha. To the right of the Buddha are two lizards, green and red, and two quartz crystals, one white, one pink. In front of the Buddha, a small bear holds a tree trunk. In the center of this group is the hero, a Roman soldier with a broken sword facing the black whale, seal and walrus. Ben titled this sandplay "A man entered a castle and his sword broke." Among the three Roman soldiers with swords on the shelf, Ben chose the one whose sword was actually broken. A sword, symbol of a hero's masculinity, authority, strength and courage, divides body and soul, a first recognition of the opposites, and signifies penetrating insight (Cooper, 1978, p.167). A solar hero fights dragons with his sword and defends the forces of light against the forces of darkness. A broken sword symbolizes the destruction of those qualities which must be reconstructed by personal valor (Cirlot, 1971/1996, p.325). A small boy on the path of heroic masculine independence might feel unready to leave the personal mother, or feel guilt and fear of punishment—a loss of masculinity. The black whale in this sandplay may be the "magical threshold," a transit into a sphere of rebirth symbolized in the universal womb image of the "belly of the whale." Campbell (1949/1973, p.90) states that "the hero, instead of conquering, is swallowed into the unknown and would appear to have died. This motif emphasizes that the passage of the threshold is a form of self-annihilation." The physical body of the hero may be slain and dismembered (p.91).

Ben has chosen three large sea mammals—Whale, Walrus and Seal. All are totemic animals who live in the oceans, symbol for the great unconscious or nature itself. The Whale communicates in song, knows the depths, and migrates annually between the earth's polarities, from feeding in polar areas to breeding in tropical waters, and back. Walrus and Seal give birth on shore. In folk tales and myth, they are shape-shifters, selkies, who take on human form and marry humans, but can return to their original form and to the sea. Their heads, bobbing up and down in the waters, have inspired tales of mermaids and mermen, half-human, half-fish creatures. The males fight savagely but are also playful and protect their pups. A boy might choose them in a sandplay as an alternative to mermaids, who are frequently chosen by girls (Figure 10.17).

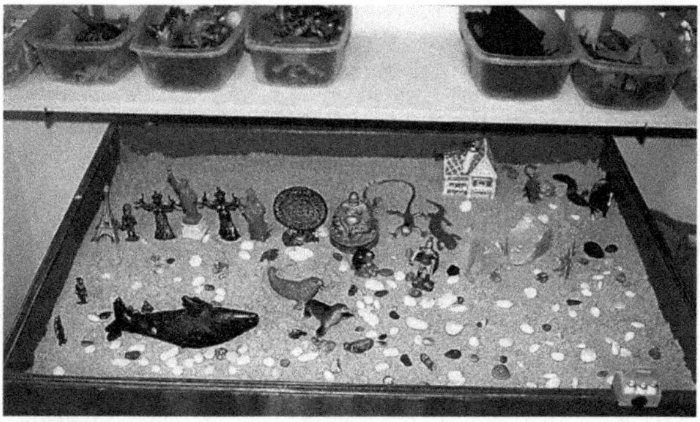

Figure 10.17 *Ben: A man entered a castle and his sword broke*

Three symbols on the sidelines of this sandplay may relate to the mother–son relationship. A case of milk bottles balanced on the front-right edge remind a small boy of his dependence on the mother. The gingerbread house in the far-right corner contains a deceptive witch who tempts Hansel and Gretel to eat many sweets, and then imprisons Hansel, like a seductive mother who will not release her son. While Hansel is being fattened for eating, Gretel, the young feminine, tricks the witch with cunning to light the oven, pushes her in, frees her brother, and, together, brother and sister find their way home (Grimm Brothers, 1981, pp.48–58). The green grasshopper on the roof of the gingerbread house predicts stages of metamorphosis. Its egg, buried and dormant for ten months during fall and winter, hatches in spring into a nymph, and then matures into a grasshopper that can leap and fly. Ben's sandplay the next week was full of movement, with running horses and a few traffic signs, near a yellow chick. Nine months before, in Sandplay 7, the last in Stage One, the horses lay immobile on the sand.

The Golden Ribbon, Walrus and Seal, 4 years, 5 months and 2 weeks old, Sandplay 17

The wet sandtray can be divided into left and right sides, and four groups with content that juxtaposes spiritual, mythological-magical and realistic events that can be seen by the eyes, or by imagination, by the unconscious or by transpersonal powers. Each group is differentiated by the amount and type of its objects. An invisible line from a dark closet with a sleeping angel on it in the far center to a small green dragon on the front-center edge seems to infer left and right sides. A large red house on the left side is visually prominent. A seal and walrus face each other on its roof, two birds hovering above them and three Smurfs nearby on the sand. A golden ribbon encircles them. It begins and ends beyond the left sandtray edge like a spiritual thread binding together all things in existence. Gold, the color of solar light and divine intelligence, and the ribbon's rounded form may symbolize the archetype of the Self (Cirlot, 1971/1996, pp.119, 316). The walrus and seal on the roof can be seen only by the birds or other powers above, giving these sea mammals a spiritual context. On the far right, a human event is formed as a rectangle by rows of objects. A red lantern connects a horizontal row on the far-right edge, with a green dragon, two natives, one in a canoe, and Bart Simpson, and a vertical row with a king and queen facing right towards small children and elves. In a third scene in the front-right corner, Mickey and Minnie Mouse, Donald Duck and a vase topped by a devil mask form a row facing another row of celestial powers in the sand—a blue sun, two moons and two stars. In a fourth encounter in the front center, on a pebble mosaic, Erik and a man with a rifle on his shoulder face two small dragons, one green and one purple, sitting on the front edge. A large green dragon intrudes from the front-left corner edge of the sandtray (Figure 10.18).

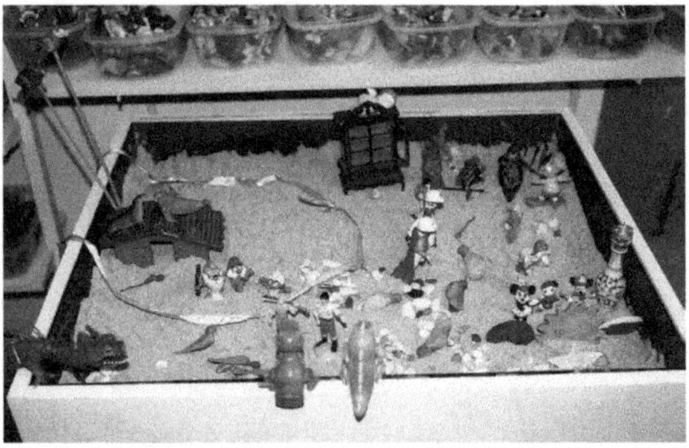

Figure 10.18 *Ben: The golden ribbon*

The bad soldiers want to steal all the fish from the fisherman, four and a half years old, Sandplay 19

Ending Stage Two, in the dry sandtray, objects are grouped from left to right, and from far to near, creating vertical and horizontal axes that intersect and form a cross, symbol of the ability to tolerate the opposites (Weinrib, 1996). A horizontal row of 14 sticks runs across the sand like railroad tracks, from a large mound of white bones and skeletons in the front-left corner to a little red-clothed fisherman on the front-right edge, his fishing line in a white pebble pool below. In the center, two groups straddle the tracks. In front, the three Roman soldiers, two with raised swords, face an innocent-looking "family" composed of Bart Simpson on a red skateboard, his sister Lisa, an elf, a Smurf, Donald Duck and Minnie and Mickey Mouse dressed as firemen. These small creatures, many with red hats, are not equipped to fight soldiers with swords. They stand behind a Bar-Mitzvah boy wearing black and white, reading a Torah portion to celebrate his passage to manhood at age 13. Four red fruits near them point diagonally up towards the right, to outside reality. Red and white, the alchemical albedo and rubedo together, signify the integration of lunar and solar, passive and active, feminine and masculine (Ehlers, 2022, pp.121–122). Bones, skeletons and whiteness can indicate the end of a stage of life and mortality. Resurrection and redness appear in the fisherman's clothes, the Roman soldiers, red hats and red apples. The fish on the fisherman's line, fruit of the unconscious, also enriches life (Steinhardt, 2009). Here the white and red are still separate. Two young males, the Bar-Mitzvah boy and the fisherman are used by Ben for the first time. The fisherman meditates and looks inward, the opposite of the expectations of a Bar-Mitzvah boy, to transition into the masculine world. Ben is four and a half years old. His psyche guides his fishing in the unconscious, in the first half of Neumann's "Magic Warlike" Early Childhood II Play stage in which a boy lessens dependence on the mother, and begins a gradual transition from matriarchate to patriarchate (Figure 10.19).

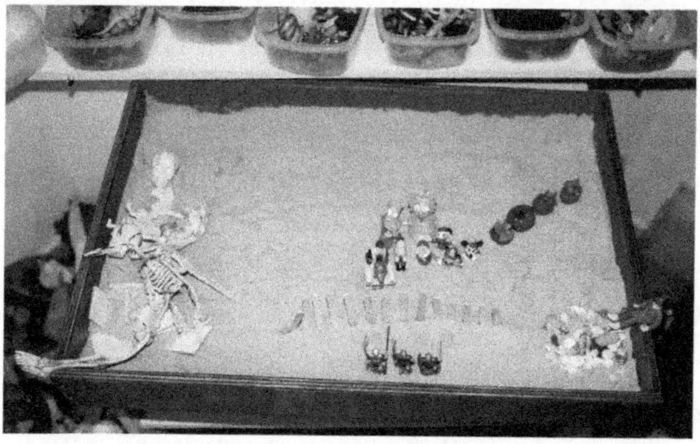

Figure 10.19 *Ben: Age four and a half, The bad soldiers want to steal all the fish from the fisherman*

Stage Three: Transitioning from heroic battle to rational thought (four years six months to four years seven months old)

In a period of six weeks, Ben came six times and made nine sandplays, with themes of opposites of large and small, aggression and passivity. His first and last sandplays of this stage, Sandplays 20 and 25, are discussed with reference to sandplays in between that moved the process forward.

The song of the giants, Sandplay 20

In Sandplay 20, in the wet sandtray, ten huge creatures face the rear—a gorilla, triceratops, winged unicorn, coiled snake, coiled centipede, two turtles, two frogs and a snail. Fourteen tiny creatures—Mickey and Minnie Mouse, Donald Duck, eight Smurfs, Bart and Lisa Simpson, and a robot—look up and observe them, like the young Theseus meeting six dangerous criminals on his road to Athens. Ben called this sandplay "The song of the giants" (Figure 10.20). He continued with themes of conquest in the next four sandplays. Superheroes conquer Ben's green "Killer Truck" and dragons, human Roman soldiers conquer the globe with the approval of four farm women, like the Transformative Mother who supports masculine development. But the Roman soldiers also find themselves in a green forest, opposite the same massive pile of white bones and skeletons of Sandplay 19 (Figure 10.19). The Great Mother presides over life and death and is stronger than any human hero. In one sandplay, Tarzan observes superheroes while hanging from the tall tree which first appeared in Ben's fifth sandplay, at age three years eight months old. He used this tree without mention 13 times more until his final sandplay at age seven, and again in two sandplays done spontaneously at age 12 and 14. The tree's height and wide green canopy suggest a mythological world tree, which in many cultures is considered a world center. Its canopy and trunk support the heavens, its roots touch water and the underworld, and it connects heaven, earth and the underworld. An eagle resides on it above, and a snake below.

Sandplay 25 introduces visible divinities, four Kachinas, Native American nature gods, lined up on the far-right edge, distant observers of the ninja fighters, superheroes, Green Hulk, Batman, Superman, Rocket-man and Hercules in the front row. Ishtar, a blue metal Middle

Eastern fertility goddess stands alone in the front-right center behind Batman, as if in silent approval of the row of heroes who face the "audience" like actors at the end of a play, waiting for applause. A small green dragon heads a vertical row of superheroes up the right edge. Spiky toothpicks in the left rear and downwards close a circle of all the objects (Figure 10.21).

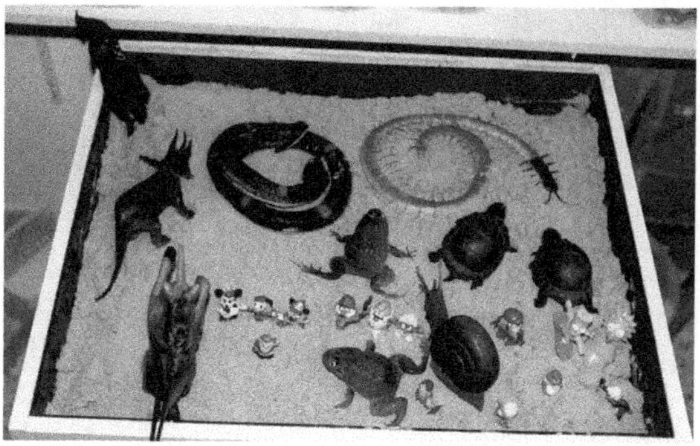

Figure 10.20 *Ben: The song of the giants*

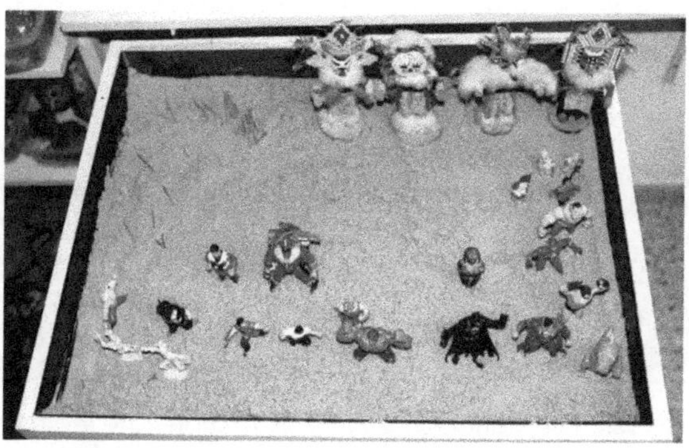

Figure 10.21 *Ben: Age four and a half, Sandplay 25, Kachinas, Ishtar and superheroes*

Stage Four: From Imagined Heroism to Building a Stronger Ego, four years seven months to four years nine months old

In these two months, Ben made 13 dramatic, thoughtful sandplays, with themes of transition from imaginary to realistic appraisal of heroism. Small creatures in a large, powerful world must learn to protect the treasures fished up by the fisherman from the unconscious. Four sandplays are discussed, with reference to the sandplays in between.

The fisherman's line reaches the center, four years eight months old, Sandplay 26

Ben used both sandtrays today. The first in the wet sandtray was dominated by a large red house and two large castles in the far center, with trolls, apples, strawberries, empty benches and 20 tiny animals placed on both sides of the tray (not shown). Then, in the center of the dry tray, Ben built a round pool of white pebbles and fish-shaped brown seed pods. Behind the pool, the seal and the walrus, guardians of the unconscious, together for the third time, face opposite directions, far and near, as if protecting the fish in the center. The fisherman sits on the left edge, but his line with a fish on it extends to the center of the tray, over the pool. He contemplates the pool, the fish and his line, over this round central pool symbol of the Self. Sharp toothpicks in the sand on the right near two tiny creatures may be defense weapons (Figure 10.22).

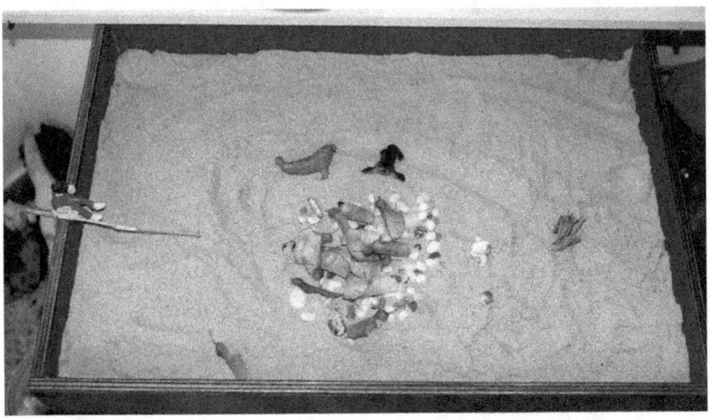

Figure 10.22 *Ben: Sandplay 26, The fisherman's line reaches the center*

Six introspective sandplays followed, juxtaposing large and small objects in rows or pairs. In two sandplays, the great cow skull, again in the far-left area, hovers above 19 houses and cute animals, and in the next sandplay looms over eight large rocks and cute animals. In three more sandplays, a blue pool of water is opened in the front-left corner, once for the fisherman, then for Donald Duck and then for two crocodiles staring at a row of soldiers, never used before.

Superheroes compete on the cow skull, four years nine months old, Sandplay 31

The cow skull stands alone in the center of the wet sandtray, a placement that mirrors the mosaic pool alone in center in Figure 10.22. On the skull, several small masculine figurines compete to knock each other off the skull. Eight pieces of sea glass in a row define a boundary in front of the skull, separating a conscious front area from the skull, perhaps the underworld beyond. In Jewish tradition, stones are left on a grave after a visit (Figure 10.23). Two weeks later, in the center of the dry sandtray, a king and queen hold their wedding, with a metal chair and a Roman soldier near each (not shown). A row of small animals along the front edge witness the wedding, confirming this central event, the coniunctio between the archetypal masculine and feminine.

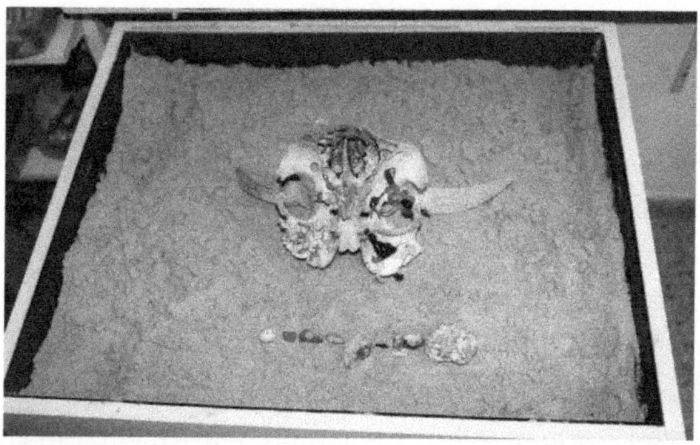

Figure 10.23 *Ben: Sandplay 31, Superheroes compete on the cow skull*

Birthday celebration with 11 boats, Sandplay 33

Three months later, just before his fifth birthday, Ben made a beautiful, joyous and almost abstract sandplay. Eleven boats and a lifesaver fill the entire right side of the wet sandtray. Familiar figurines sit in the boats—elves, Smurfs, soccer players, Roman soldiers, Minnie and Mickey Mouse, Donald Duck, natives and the king, as if celebrating before vacation. Two Playmobil® doctors and an old man with a backpack are new. A sea-glass mosaic paves the front-left area, with 18 large red fruits just above it. Seed pods and pebbles are strewn along the middle area. The sand on the left side is wet but no blue area or depth is seen (Figure 10.24).

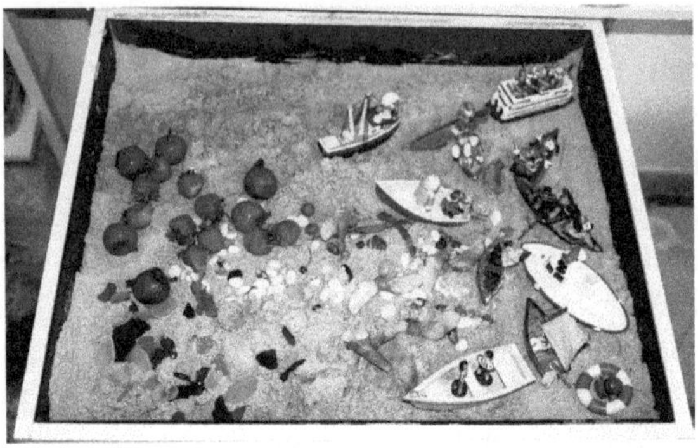

Figure 10.24 *Ben: almost five years old, Birthday celebration with 11 boats*

Stage Five: Order, destruction, collaboration with the spirit of nature, five to six years old

Between Ben's fifth and sixth birthdays, he visited only six times and made nine sandplays, with a seven-month break in between. Three themes predominated—Ben's resonance with the fisherman, a need to witness external destruction of scenes that told stories, and the creation of new abstract aesthetic images. Five sandplays are presented.

Order, destruction and chaos, five years two weeks old, Session 34

Ben made two sandplays in the wet tray, both overflowing with objects, the first very organized, the second chaotic. The tall tree and a container filled with water are present in both. He paid great attention to detail in the first sandplay and divided it into three vertical areas: a row of volcanoes behind a stone wall along the left side; down the center a bridge between a portal, tall tree and castle; and the fisherman fishing from the right edge in a water-filled plastic box inside which are a native family in a canoe, two seals and a walrus, and an alien. From outside the container, a pretty lady peers in. Then Ben removed all the objects except the tall tree and placed a bird on its canopy. He scattered trees on the ground around the tall tree as if uprooted, and threw large shells and a huge mound of skeletons, bones and the cow skull in the far-right corner. In the front-right corner he placed a ceramic bowl of water with a small ceramic canoe and two tiny creatures. On the left, red flowers replace the red volcano, a red ribbon encircles treasure in the front-left area. In the far right, two dragons escape their cage and two large soldiers aim rifles at them. The collapse of Ben's carefully planned first world is witnessed by a king and princess from a high bridge on the left edge, like the aftermath of a tsunami or earthquake (Figure 10.25).

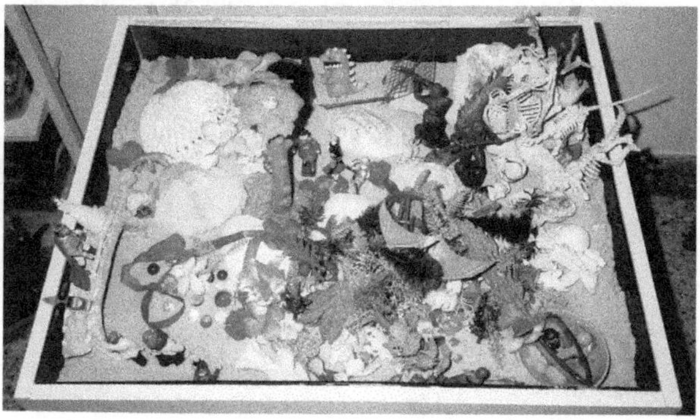

Figure 10.25 *Ben: Age five years two weeks, Sandplay 34, Destruction and chaos*

Three sandplays: Peaceful nature, the Hero, the Fisherman, five years one month old, Session 35

Four days later, Ben made three sandplays, two in the wet tray and one in the dry tray. He first reconstructed the forest that had been destroyed four days before, filled the center with trees and flowers, and hung Tarzan from the tall tree and placed a crate of milk bottles on its top. He rebuilt a cage of dinosaurs and dragons in the far center, and added a group of men nearby. In the far-right corner, a wigwam, a feminine container, replaces the deathly mound of bones. The Native American chief sits nearby. Several men in the front area stand with their backs to the forest. There is no feminine presence. Volcanoes and bonfires in the front-left corner are separated from the forest by two bridges, a stone wall and a portal (not shown). He cleared the tray and gathered sand into a mountain for the first time, built a fence around it and poured water over the top. The tall tree, now on the far right, shelters a large soldier aiming a rifle beyond the tray. On the mountain peak, a strong man in a bright green shirt (the color of the tree top) sits alone on a metal chair facing the far-left edge, an empty cage and two volcanoes that have crushed a large dragon and a pile of bones. The man does not see the visible sparkling treasure on the mountain's front slope, a metal scale with two children, or an alien on a horse, two small soldiers in a wagon and fish-shaped seed pods on the ground. Ben left this scene intact (Figure 10.26).

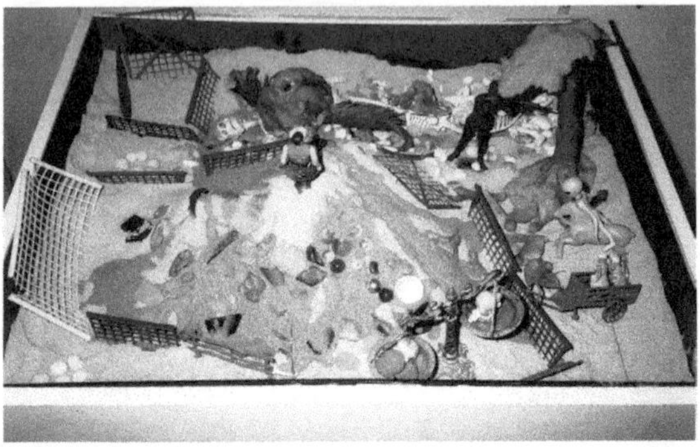

Figure 10.26 *Ben: Age five years three weeks, Sandplay 2 of 3, The man on the mountaintop*

In the dry tray, he constructed a low central mound covered with shells, coral and stones, as if under the sea. A ceramic bowl on the left contains water, crabs, fish and stones. A large plastic container on the right contains water, mud, fish, a lobster, an octopus and crabs. A small compact mound of shells on the front-right edge looks as if it washed up on the shore. Ben asked me to photograph his hand holding the fishing rod over the mound. He is the Fisherman (Figure 10.27).

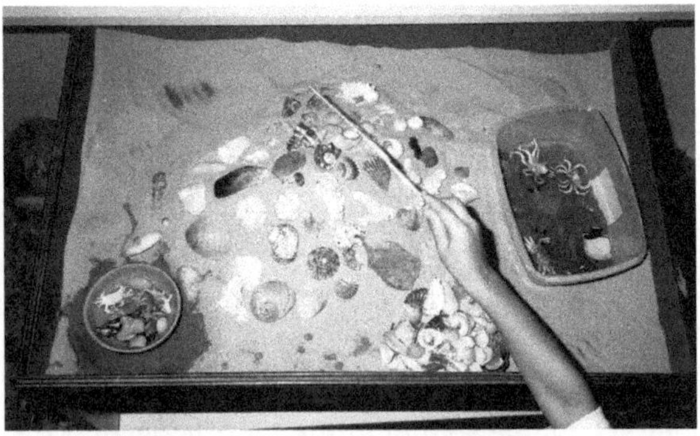

Figure 10.27 *Ben: Age five years three weeks, Sandplay 3 of 3, I am the Fisherman*

This low "submerged" mound balances the first high mountain, and honors the fisherman's patience and Ben's intuitive trust in the unconscious.

In these two sandplays, the height and depth of center are in balance. The strong man's contemplation of crushed dragons is balanced by the inner contemplation of the fisherman in Ben's psyche (Steinhardt, 2009).

Deluge, Sandplay 36, five years two months old

Two months later, Ben flooded two sandplays made a week apart. All his familiar superheroes, dragons, Mickey and Minnie Mouse, Bart and Lisa Simpson, babies, cars, the red house, stones, walls, volcanoes, witches and ghouls, shells, bones and the cow skull were covered with mud. Like a god punishing the world, Ben ended an era, drowning powerful creatures and tiny heroes alike (Figure 10.28). Eight months later, a new order of life in the sandtray emerged. Campbell (1949/1973, p.197) describes the end of battle and the hero's return as the Magic Flight. Supernatural patrons approve the hero's success, but demons will try to prevent him from bringing his trophies back to his world. Before he crosses the threshold of return from the mystic realm, he is still in the underworld. Much destruction can ensue before he enters the land of common day (p.216).

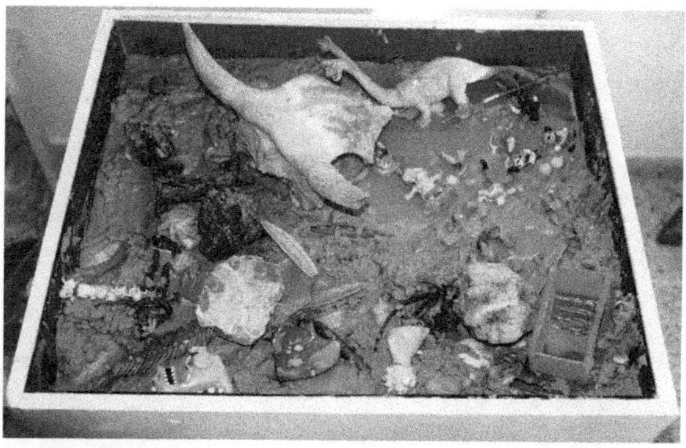

Figure 10.28 *Ben: Age five years two months, Sandplay 36, Deluge*

Shimenawa, Symbolic Transition to the Masculine, Sandplay 39, five years 11 months old

After an eight-month break, Ben returned one month before his sixth birthday and made two ethereal sandplays, two weeks apart, both filled with crystals, stones, trees and flowers. Guided by instinct and psyche, he resolved his ideas in several consecutive sandplays with a common theme. In Sandplay 38, treasure on the left side is separated by a fence from trees and flowers, a few feminine figurines, two closed castles covered above with an abalone shell and a cave in the front-right corner. These large, closed-off representations of the feminine as container might indicate a change in relation to his personal mother. Two weeks later, in session 39, an impersonal objective reality fills the sandplay surface, arranged in areas, each composed of a specific element. In the far left are flowers, white pebbles, shells and a rainbow. Along the right edge is a forest of different trees. In the front-left area, crystals and precious stones define a spiritual area for two Kwan Yin figurines (the Asian Goddess of Compassion), three angels, a black egg, a white egg, a golden basket and the gingerbread house. Almost unseen in the center of the sandtray are symbols of pure fire and light, a Menorah, a blue crystal ornament and a silver star. In the front-right corner, the large plastic container now contains five masculine symbols, two fire-breathing dragons, a black horse, a smaller blue animal and, in their center, a white unicorn. The golden ribbon from Sandplay 17 (Figure 10.18) stretches horizontally over the front of the tray and falls outside the left and right edges. It resembles a non-material boundary in the air above the sandplay, a shimenawa rope that bounds a temple's sacred space in the Shinto religion, representing "the mystery of the boundary between the two worlds—the existent nonexistent line" (Campbell, 1949/1973, p.213). In Japan, the shimenawa marks the miracle of light's return when Amaterasu, the sun goddess, leaves her dark cave. Above temple doors, a straw rope stretches over the threshold of return, as a sign of her resurrection (Figure 10.29).

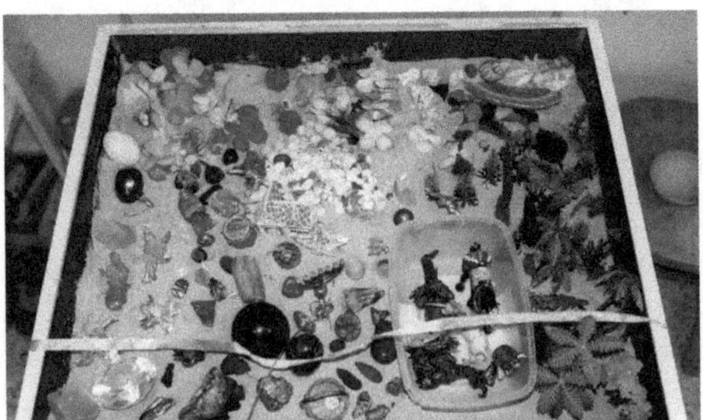

Figure 10.29 *Ben: Age five years 11 months, Sandplay 39, Shimenawa*

Stage Six: Leaving the world of sandplay, six to seven years old, six sandplays

An Enjoyable Country, Sandplay 40, six years two weeks old

The wet sandtray is clearly organized into left and right sides. A central vertical row of archetypal figurines, the King, Queen, Pink Fairy, a Sorcerer and Sorceress face right, towards a Bar-Mitzvah boy, flanked at a distance by two Roman soldiers. Mickey and Minnie Mouse and Donald Duck watch the Bar-Mitzvah ceremony while hanging in the air on two metal plates on scales behind the boy, like spectators in the balcony of a synagogue. A tall woman and a girl in a red dress walk towards the front of the sandtray as if the "feminine" is leaving. The "outer reality" of the Bar-Mitzvah scene on the right is the opposite of a scene on the left of Ben's inner life: two water-filled plastic containers, with sea creatures and four Smurfs in the left container, and four naked children in the right container, guarded from behind by a knight with a sword, from the heroic mythological realm (Figure 10.30).

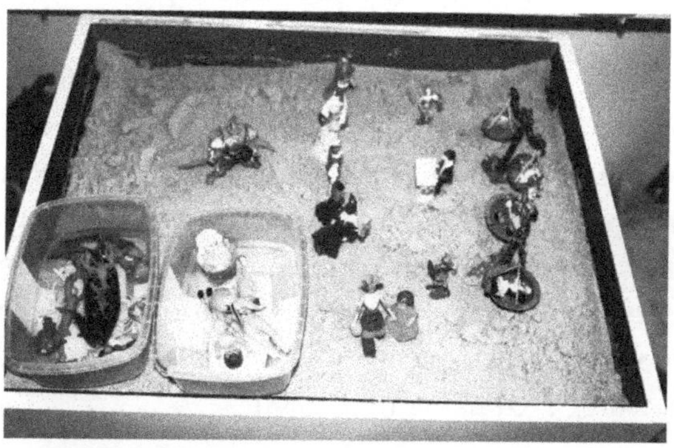

Figure 10.30 *Ben: Age six years two weeks, Sandplay 40, An enjoyable country*

Seven months later, in three sandplays spaced a month apart, Ben revived his old forms and figurines for one last look before leaving. He flooded the first sandplay, leaving a few superheroes, Smurfs, the tall tree and Tarzan standing upright in the mud. In the next, he filled the far and right area of the sandtray with huge frogs, turtles, the large winged horse and a centipede, a glass mosaic in the front area and rows of colored marbles and precious stones. In the third, Roman soldiers and small angels guard the overturned cow skull in the far-right area, the glass mosaic again paves the front left, and Poseidon, God of the

Sea, stands alone with a globe in the far left, the powerful masculine controlling the world.

The last sandplay, Sandplay 44, one week before Ben's seventh birthday

In a final sandplay, the psyche often revisits themes or symbols from the very first sandplay, or from a past turning point. The structure of Ben's last sandplay at age seven was similar to Sandplay 25 (Figure 10.21) at four years seven months old, that concluded Stage Three. The metal masks of his very first sandplay at age two years five months old are again present and have moved from the front-left corner to a distant observation point on the far edge, appropriate to Ben's ego development and growing emotional, spiritual and cognitive abilities. The masks are intersected with corks, containers and a tall feminine-shaped vase closed with a cork. Two Smurfs guard an open passage in the far-right corner, which leads to the world outside the sandtray. The numinous masks above contrast with the conscious "marketplace" world below: a bird cage and golden objects on the right edge, a glass mosaic in the front-left area for the third time, two tiny new creatures on a bench opposite a table with food, milk bottles and, behind them, two blue porcelain vases. A transparent plastic table with a plate on it and an empty chair mark the front center. The front-right corner is filled with a basket of food, musical instruments, a triple spiral and a metal sundial. The center is empty (Figure 10.31). After the formation of the Ego–Self axis, the aware Ego, not the Self, is the initiator and executor of the vital will of the personality (Neumann, 1973/1988).

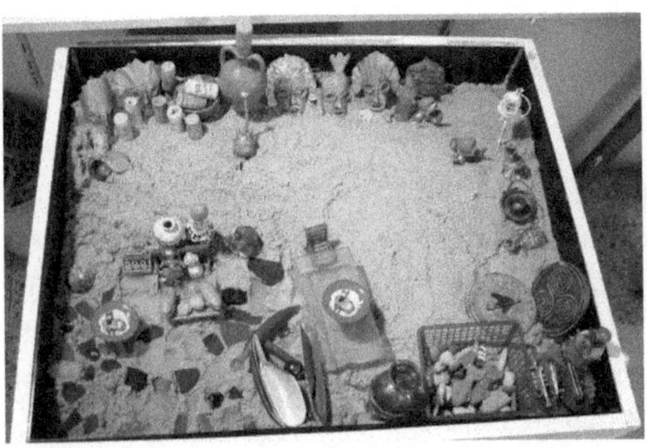

Figure 10.31 *Ben: Almost seven years old, Masks in the round of return*

We shall not cease from exploration
And the end of all our exploring
Will be to arrive where we started
And know the place for the first time.

(T.S. Eliot, 1943)

Ben, an afterward, age 12 and age 14

Ben was 12 years old, excited that he and his family were leaving for a month-long trip abroad. He disappeared into the studio and made a lush, organized jungle scene that fills most of the front of the dry sandtray. Along the far edge, a long strip of blue crepe paper becomes a swirling river where a large shark on the left faces a native in a canoe. Two small fish swim away to the right. The tall tree with a gorilla on it and a large elephant divide the jungle into two triangles, on a diagonal from the front-right corner to the far-left corner. On the right side, trees and flowers conceal tigers, lions and natives. On the left side, a glass mosaic again paves the front area. Several small natives behind four bears and the elephant move towards the far-left corner and the shark. Ben seems to have released his emotional trepidation and excited anticipation in this sandplay before this major journey (Figure 10.32).

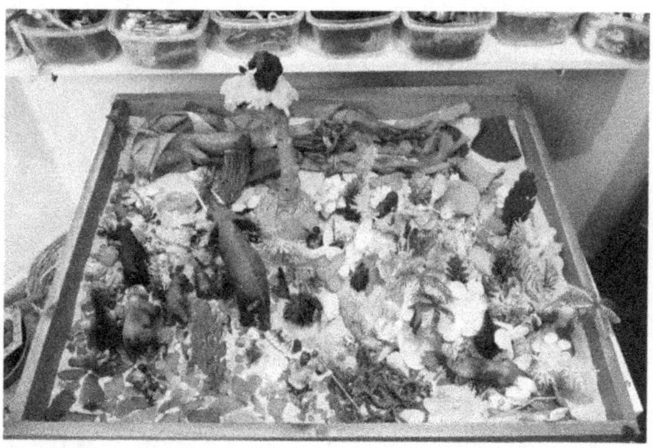

Figure 10.32 *Ben: Age 12, before a family trip abroad, Jungle, river and shark*

Memories of the trip, Ben age 14 years nine months

Three years later, Ben made two more spontaneous sandplays with fences, two weeks apart. A zoo in the dry sandtray has nine enclosures for different animals, and various people observing from outside the cages. This may be a memory of a zoo visited by the family two years before, but could also symbolize Ben's growing ability to observe and compartmentalize his own emotions and instincts from different points of view. The bears have a small cage in the far left, the giraffes in the far right, and a peacock has its own cage. Turtles, lemurs, penguins, birds and gorillas have many visitors. But in the largest cage in the front-left corner, two small elephants stand behind the tall tree, and a large elephant faces the far-right corner. Inside their cage is a tiny human, a professor, perhaps sensing these Great Mothers as symbols (Figure 10.33).

The Statue of Liberty commands the center of a large wavy water area made of blue crepe paper stretching from the far edge to a small dock area in the front of the sandtray. This blue crepe paper, once a dangerous river with a shark is now transformed into a wide, welcoming harbor with a central feminine guardian of freedom. Four boats with men standing in them, two on either side, point towards her. The sand of the entire front dock is covered over by white, brown and blue fences. Six men stand on the flat fences on the left as if on a boardwalk. Around a table laden with food on the right, three women and one black-suited man stand (Figure 10.34). Ben later became interested in music, psychology, literature and theater, and writing stories.

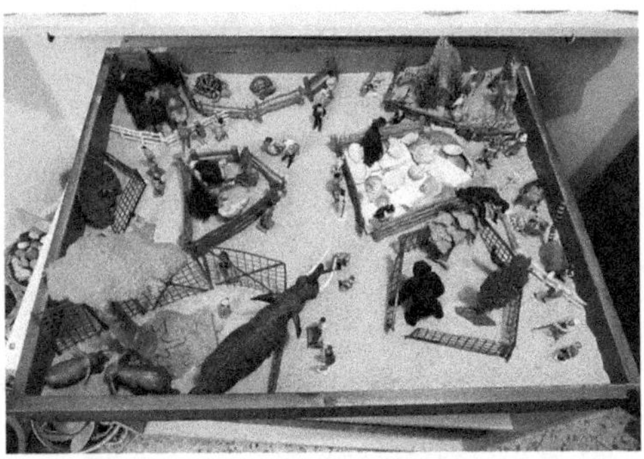

Figure 10.33 *Ben: Age 14 years nine months, Zoo*

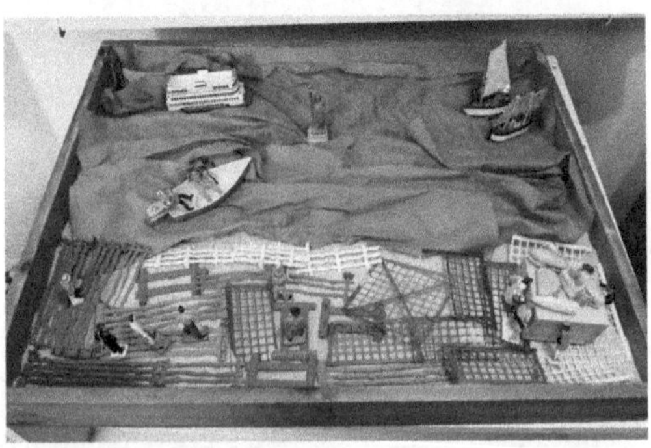

Figure 10.34 *Ben: Age 14 years nine and a half months, The Statue of Liberty*

MAYA, a girl's spontaneous developmental sandplay process from two years ten months to 11 years six months old

Maya played in my studio from the age of two years ten months, to 11 and a half years old, the years that Neumann defines as stages of Early Childhood I and II and Middle Childhood. During these nine years, she often worked alone and called me to look at her work and photograph it when she finished. Around age seven, she began to dictate stories about her sandplays. Altogether she made 39 sandplays and many paintings that expressed verbally untranslatable emotions. As the eldest of three girls, with a sister born when she was one year and three months old, and another sister when she was six years old, her reactions to changes in family structure took form in the sand. When her parents' relationship became difficult, Maya's awareness of their estrangement was expressed in her sandplays. She and her sister received individual art therapy to help them through their parents' divorce, unconnected to any work she did in my studio. Thus, her attachment to sandplay was secure and familiar, and her images authentic. At the time of this writing, Maya had begun work in a helping profession and gave her consent to include her childhood sandplays and their stories in this chapter. I have organized her sandplays into seven stages, based on Neumann's age-appropriate developmental characteristics (1973/1988), the intervals between sandplays and the themes that defined each stage.

Neumann's outline (1973/1988) of stages of archetypal and ego development in children are better adapted to boys rather than to girls, but in his book *Fear of the Feminine* (1994, pp.3–63) he described stages of feminine development, from matriarchal "moon consciousness" to the development of patriarchal consciousness, "as a relative liberation from the unconscious...in which the ego has at its disposal a differentiated system of consciousness" (p.93). Separation from the mother and the matriarchate and transition to the patriarchate may be easier for a boy who is always different from the mother and can more easily identify with the patriarchal society we live in. A girl remains the same as her mother, although she may separate from her.

Jones (in Mitchell and Friedman, 1994) identified differences between boys and girls in the uses of sand, water and objects, and in choice and organization of objects, spatial organization and comprehensive understanding of a scene. In her research of five age groups between one year old and 18 years old, she found that girls used miniatures to portray dyadic and family relationships, and interactions emphasizing cooperation. They built dramatic scenes around which they could tell stories, while boys often enacted their dramas physically with the objects. In "Middle Childhood," girls formed islands and water areas more often than boys.

Maya's relationship to sandplay, and natural stages in her process

Maya's pre-verbal experience of "loss" began with the birth of her first sister and a move to a new apartment. She "lost" the loving neighbor who had cared for her, and she "lost" her mother to her baby sister. Her sandplays before age six express her sense of loss, as well as the normal developmental stages of a young girl who was loved by both her parents and extended family. After age six, her sandplays and stories mirror the birth of her second sister, the deteriorating relationship between her parents and her concern and fear for the family. In her last sandplays, her hope for her parents' reconciliation overshadowed expression of her personal themes. In her sandplays, Maya consistently expressed the feminine tendency towards relationships, from diffuse compositions of objects at age three to a later comprehensive view, scenes of pairing, face-to-face interactions and groupings in various relationships. Her stories evolved from simple tales with positive endings to complex detailed descriptions. She divided her sandplays into left and right sides intuitively, with subdivisions of several scenes on each side. Around age four, she gathered mounds of sand, filled containers and buried things she was afraid of, such as dogs. At age nine, she began to bury white and black eggs, stones and a red diamond to represent the family as "treasure," and sometimes created maps to find them. When her parents' conflict threatened to split the family, her sandplays expressed this in dramatic splits of the sand surface, exposing a gap of the sandtray's blue bottom. After age seven, mounds became islands rising up from the blue depths into consciousness. Her final isolated island at age 11 and a half, in the far left with a king and queen in an alchemical pool was viewed by figurines from previous sandplays placed on the front and right side shores. A small mermaid accompanied her in 16 sandplays, but disappeared when she was ten years old, no longer present to view the disappointing reality of family impermanence.

Maya's family visits, natural developmental sandplay and the changes in family structure are mirrored in seven sandplay stages. There are six sandplays in each of the first six stages, and five in the final stage. In

Stage One, there are long intervals between sandplays, from age two and a half to four years and three months (Neumann's Early Childhood I, Age 1–2 and 3–4). Stage Two was more intense and continued from four years and five months old to four years and nine months. A year later, Stage Three began at age five years 11 months, and continued until six years nine months (Early Childhood II, Age 3–4 and 6–7). Stage Four ("Middle Childhood," Age 6–7 to 11–12), from age seven and a half to eight years 11 months, was characterized by hope that her parents would resolve their differences. The themes of Stage Five, from age nine to nine years ten months, moved between hope and denial. In Stage Six, from nine years 11 months to ten years two months, the split in her parents' relationship was dramatically depicted. Finally, in Stage Seven, from ten years two months, to 11 and a half years old, Maya's sandplays show that she was able to adjust to external reality and to self-preserve.

Stage One: Early Childhood I (two years ten months to four years three months)

Maya was two years and ten months old. She mixed sand and water into mud in a plastic tub on the floor, placed eight round plastic discs and a white igloo in two rows on the mud. She added a cluster of short colored pegs in the front-right corner. Their shapes could represent an intuitive sense of gender opposites, the round discs and igloo representing the feminine, the oblong pegs the masculine (Figure 10.35).

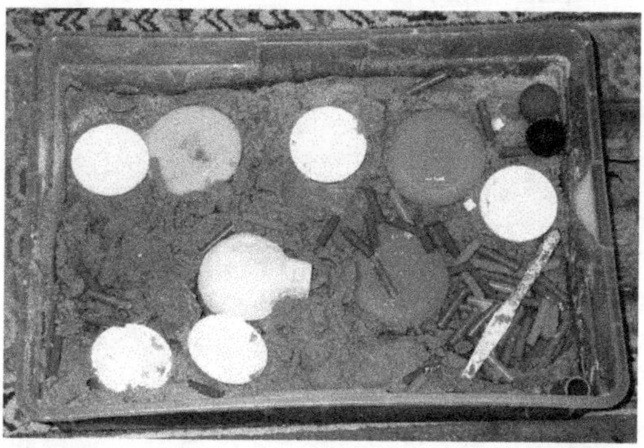

Figure 10.35 *Maya: Age two years ten months, Sandplay 1, Mud, discs and pegs*

Nine months later, at age three years seven months, she divided the space in the dry sandtray horizontally, leaving the rear area empty, with three groupings in the front and an expanded choice of objects. On the front left, a rake has uncovered blue stripes on the sandtray bottom. In front center, five white discs from her first sandplay are each decorated with one oblong peg and a piece of sea glass. A sixth red disc is empty. In the front right is a group of cute animals, elves, a hamburger, wolf, big bird, wooden puppet and orange cat.

Her next sandplay a month later is a dramatic prominent sand mound in the center punctured by the colored pegs, like spikes into a pregnant belly. Two metal chairs and two pink shoes in the right center introduce the theme of pairing. The mound is encircled by feminine symbols of food, furniture, a whale and dolphin on the left, a crib and cow in center, which might represent a sense of being replaced by her younger sister. Masculine symbols cover the far and front-right areas with frogs, turtles, giraffes, horses, crocodiles, worms and a lion racing towards the far right (Figure 10.36).

After another month, the front area of the sandtray becomes a sand sea divided by a solitary blue dolphin in a blue pool on the left, and a group of small, partially buried fish in the front center. The dolphin points to a guitar, fish and mushrooms in the far left, but most importantly to a straw basket with tiny babies and milk bottles elevated on a sand-filled container. Tables, plates, tubs of food and two metal chairs nearby might represent her mother and baby sister. Almost unseen in the far-right corner, a small red-headed mermaid holds a red string tied to a baby's pacifier, near a small red heart-shaped mirror. The mermaid, dolphin and mirror imply reflection, moon consciousness and receptiveness of the conscious psyche to receive messages from the unconscious, and express them in form (Figure 10.37).

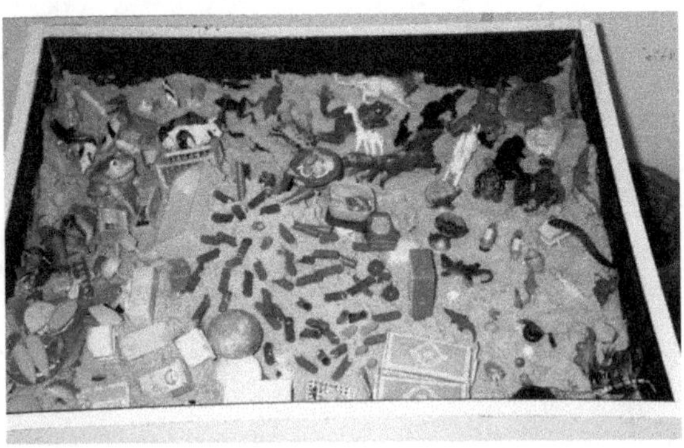

Figure 10.36 *Maya: Age three years eight months, Sandplay 3, Mound, pegs, wild animals, baby crib*

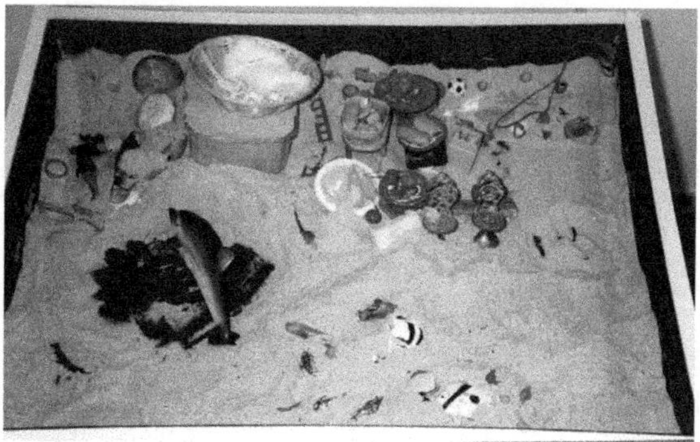

Figure 10.37 *Maya: Age three years nine months, Sandplay 4, Dolphin, mermaid and mirror*

A significant split in Maya's fifth Sandplay contrasts a colorful column of containers, food, gold objects, two pretty girls, babies, tables, chairs and a baby carriage on the left, with empty sand and a sand-filled container on the right that conceals buried dogs and animals that Maya is afraid of. An overturned cow and empty white container lying on a green rake convey a sense of desolation and loss compared to the rich left area, which may reflect love of the new baby and loss of the love that was hers before her sister's birth. The small metallic containers glow like reflective moonlight and are most often used by girls rather than boys (Figure 10.38).

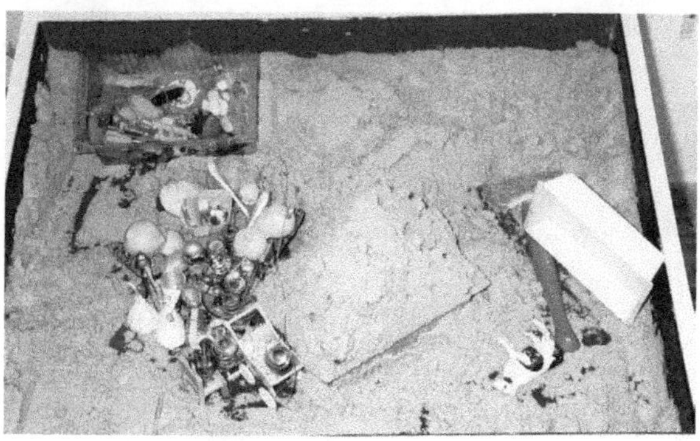

Figure 10.38 *Maya: Sandplay 5, Burying fear*

Stage Two: From age four years five months to four years nine months

Five months later, in Sandplay 7, the Little Mermaid has moved forward. She dives into her own blue pool towards two fish and some stones, surrounded by gold metal objects and a glass gold-roofed house. She might go unnoticed in the clutter of many dark objects on the left edge, many furniture objects and mirrors in the far center, and sleeping father and mother figurines. A group of fairy-tale figurines along the front-right edge face the mermaid (Beast, Snow White, Dorothy, the Pink Fairy, Wicked Witch, Tin Man, Cowardly Lion, Eric, and a lighthouse) and may represent the imaginary companions that children interact with that help develop their own inner voice. Mermaids exist half in water and half out, linking consciousness and the unconscious. She may replace the large dolphin of Sandplay 4, guide to the unconscious, in the same place eight months ago. Maya's frequent use of this mermaid, popular with girls of this age, could symbolize freedom to explore the unconscious sea of the imagination, just at the age of transition to the patriarchal and rational thought. Girls often learn to censor outspoken expressions of emotion, but imagination is uncensored (Figure 10.39).

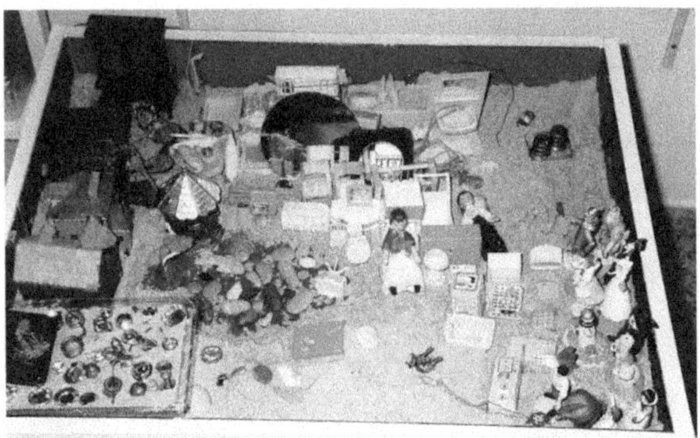

Figure 10.39 *Maya: Age four years five months, Sandplay 7, "Mermaid"*

The Little Mermaid is more visible in Sandplay 8, in her pond surrounded by open space. Large objects again crowd the left edge, leaving the rest of the sandtray empty. A theme of surface visibility and a hidden or unknown aspect underneath is shared by the mermaid, whose lower body can be concealed under water, a partially buried fisherman in the far-right corner and a partially buried cave in the front-right corner. This may suggest interest in the lower body of the masculine and the feminine womb, rather than a theme of descent (Figure 10.40). The numinous presence of two goddesses, a red clay European Venus of Willendorf and a green jade Kwan Yin, Eastern Goddess of Compassion who "hears all prayers," support the mermaid in her pool in Sandplay 9. These archetypal feminine divinities stand in front and behind the mermaid, holding her and Maya physically and spiritually, beyond the personal mother (Neumann, 1983). The pattern of support of a central figurine by two figurines on either side is repeated twice more. In the front-left corner, Dorothy stands between the Tin Man and the Pink Fairy at the entrance of a cave, implying descent into an unconscious earth womb of sleep and dream. Along the left edge, Pinocchio, Jafar, Belle, a bride in a closed castle, three bridges and a cowrie shell, lead upwards to two cages in the far-left corner. One encloses dogs and farm animals. In the second cage behind a fence, Beast stands between two dead tree trunks looking into his magic mirror that reflects anything that he would like to see in the outside world. Beast may represent a young girl's fascination and fear of the masculine, and acceptance when he is transformed into a prince as she makes the transition to the patriarchate (Figure 10.41).

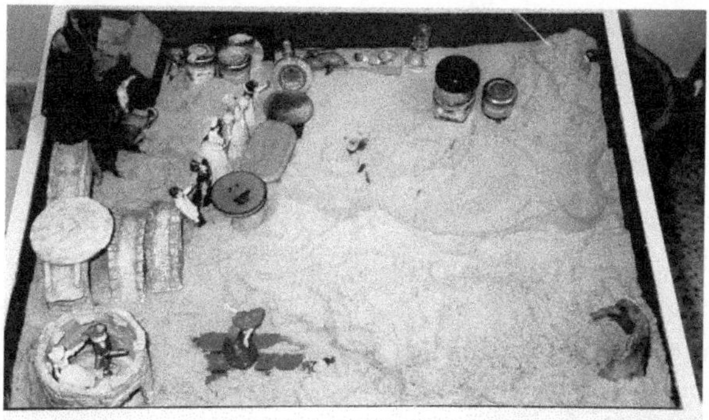

Figure 10.40 *Maya: Sandplay 8, Mermaid, fisherman and cave*

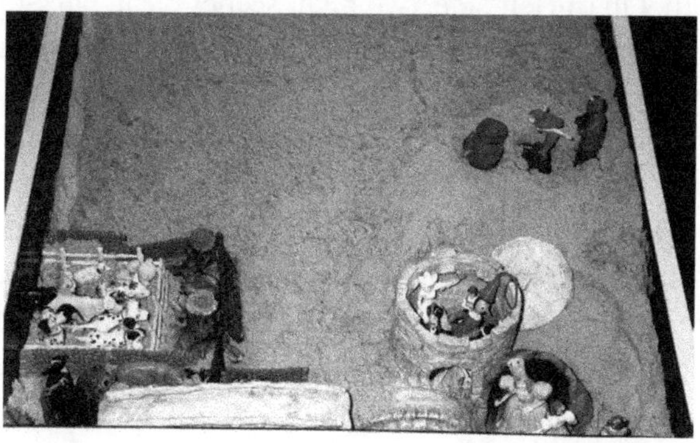

Figure 10.41 *Maya: Sandplay 9, Mermaid between goddesses, Kwan Yin and Venus of Willendorf*

Mermaids

A mermaid is a young sea goddess, beautiful, alluring to men, not yet a siren but connected to Aphrodite, Goddess of Love, born of the sea. Her curves resemble a crescent moon. She often holds a harp to accompany her singing, and a mirror into which she gazes as she combs her long hair. She is said to save lost souls in a sea storm. Mermaids, Tritons and merpeople have the upper bodies of humans and fish tails in their lower extremities. Their tails are always in water, linking them to the sea and access to the deep unconscious, to our ancient origins in water and to our present human birth from a watery womb. Mermaids are said to lure men down to the depths with their song. For centuries, humans have longed to see merpeople. Tales of sightings and reports of their capture seemed to corroborate their existence (Scribner, 2020). The mermaid, being half human and half fish, can move easily between consciousness and the unconscious, which is one goal of therapy. This young mermaid figurine from the 1989 Disney film *The Little Mermaid* can symbolize dreaming, intuition and deeper knowing (Sidesinger, 2016).

Sleep, dream, night and fairy tales

Maya is four years and ten months old, in transition from the matriarchate to the patriarchate. In Sandplay 12, three scenes of sleep, night and dreams can represent the underworld predicted by the cave of Sandplay 9. A large central silver star radiates soft light and points towards a "cave" made of purple cloth taped over the front edge, covering two tepees and several sleeping girls. The mermaid is alone in a well to the right of the cloth. On the left side, two night scenes recall fairy-tale themes. In front, three bears sit at a table with many empty chairs. In the original British folktale of the Three Bears, written by Robert Southey in 1837, the bears were male, very orderly and neat. Their home was invaded by a nasty old woman, who, 20 years later in a second version, became a young girl. In a third version, a sweet but undisciplined girl named Goldilocks enters this male citadel uninvited, unguided and unprepared. She eats the Bears' food and falls asleep in the bed of the smallest Bear. The angry Bears wake her and she jumps out the window and runs away (Steel, 1922). In a scene in the far left, Superman sleeps face down on a large yellow sun, blocking its light, between two overturned trees, like Beast and his mirror standing between two dead trees in Sandplay 9. Behind Superman, a large mermaid is buried in sand under a rainbow, two yellow stars, a moon, a stewardess in pink and a bride with flowers who are both wide awake. The bride with her flowers approaches the dormant Superman and his pillow of masculine sunlight, perhaps rousing Maya's dormant masculine consciousness. Her father is becoming increasingly dominant in her family. In the private world of Night, Maya and her mermaid can dream solutions for the challenging interactions of Day. Neumann states that in transition to the patriarchate a girl can become dominated and servile. But Maya has received archetypal feminine support as she begins to comprehend masculine values (Figure 10.42).

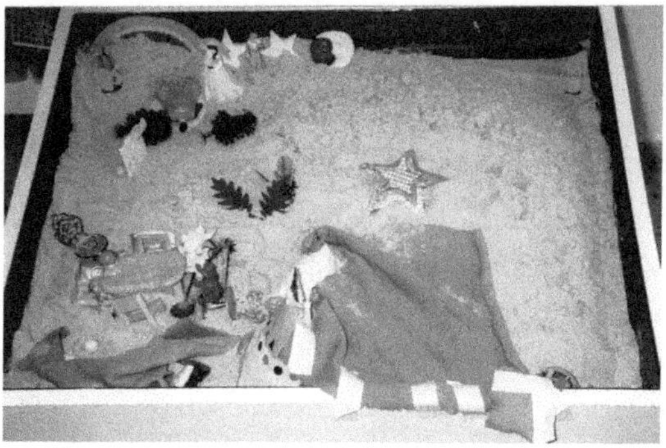

Figure 10.42 *Maya: Age four years ten months, Sandplay 12, Sleep, dream, night and fairy tales*

Stage Three: Transition from Matriarchy to Patriarchy

Two days before the birth of her second sister, Maya was almost six years old. On the left side of Sandplay 13, four pairs of feminine figurines, including Belle in her yellow dress, seem to wait in anticipation amid bedroom and bathroom furniture, a television and jewelry that no one looks at. The pink and blue fairies nearby seem more alert. On the right side is a hospital scene. A doctor faces a patient on a bed surrounded by medical equipment. Above the hospital are the mermaid and a baby in a crib. A group of farm animals invade the far-right corner towards the hospital. A girl sits near a sand-filled wheelbarrow, like Maya playing her thoughts in the sand. Belle in her blue dress reads a book in the front-right area, encircled by animals, a king, samurai and two Japanese women. Her book, like Beast's mirror, takes her to distant places (not shown).

Birth of a second sister

Sandplay 14, done two months after her sister's birth, seems ambivalent, or confused, in an unfamiliar family structure. Belle in her yellow gown is the center of a cross, formed by a horizontal double row of precious stones and a vertical row consisting of women, food, babies and an igloo. Above her are two pretty girls, a baby on a bench and a table of food. Below her is the igloo and near the front-center edge, a crib full of babies. The babies, food and Belle form a vertical boundary between the left and right sides. Four scenes on the left side are social but ambivalent. A group of four women sitting on separate chairs face each other. On a white cloth on the sand, Jasmine sits near lots of food while two Japanese women and a samurai stand above her. On a second white cloth in front are an empty table and four chairs. Nearby, behind the crib of babies, a black horse (masculine energy), a spinning wheel (associated with feminine fate) and a second igloo that joins the first, like two cold breasts, may anticipate the end of her naïve feminine childhood. On the right side, access to the openings of four "containers" is blocked as if imaginative depth and dream is no longer an option. A cave opening is filled with dark blue marbles, chains tie a castle shut, a black round stone blocks a well, and a yellow flower-shaped ribbon blocks a second well. There are two humans on the right side, a tiny baby on a bench opposite a plate of food and a Native American chief facing the horse. Yellow, the color of Belle's gown, the "flower" blocking the well's depth and Superman's sun pillow, is a central ray in the rainbow and can lean towards warm or cool, warm emotions or cool thought, intuition or spirit (Figure 10.43).

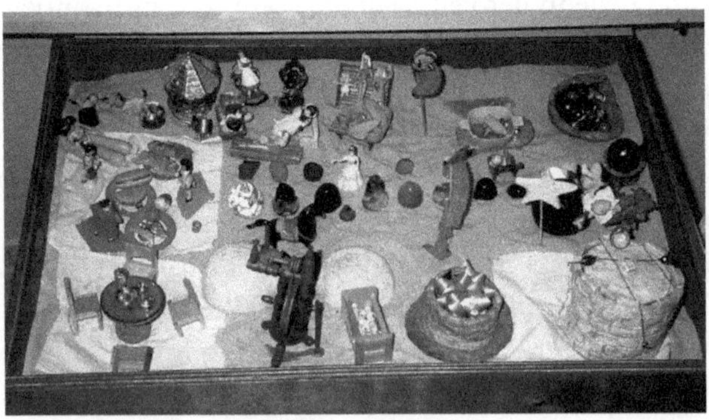

Figure 10.43 *Maya: Age six, Sandplay 14, A new family structure*

The ascent of Aladdin and the development of consciousness in the feminine

Aladdin, symbol of masculine power, dominates Maya's fifteenth sandplay. She is six and a half years old. He fishes from a high bridge over a chasm of blue water filled with fish, sea creatures and ducks. Two Jasmine figurines stand on either side of the bridge like lions, guarding a king's throne. To the left, the spinning wheel points to the stone castle with a white dove on its roof. In front of the bridge, a high white soccer net separates the water from a group walking left. Hercules, Belle in her yellow dress and Mulan approach two smaller bridges, a gingerbread house and the blue fairy prone on the sand. In front, two stars, red and blue, are joined by a purple feather. Purple, as the opposite of yellow, is the color of inspiration and magic, blending the red blood of life and the blue of thought and contemplation. A purple cloth canopy covered dreaming little girls in Sandplay 12. All the objects on the left side are large and dominant but the fewer, smaller objects on the right side reveal a development of consciousness and intuition in the feminine. A black hour glass in the far right measures time. On the right edge are four discs from Maya's first sandplay, four years ago, filled with sand, a peg and feather in each. They frame two tables. On one stands a large stone owl, and on the other a large stone eagle. Around the owl table are the large black horse, a pretty girl in a chair, a baby in a crib and an empty bench. Seated at the eagle table are three Anastasia figurines. Between the tables are three black and white Dalmatian dogs (Figure 10.44).

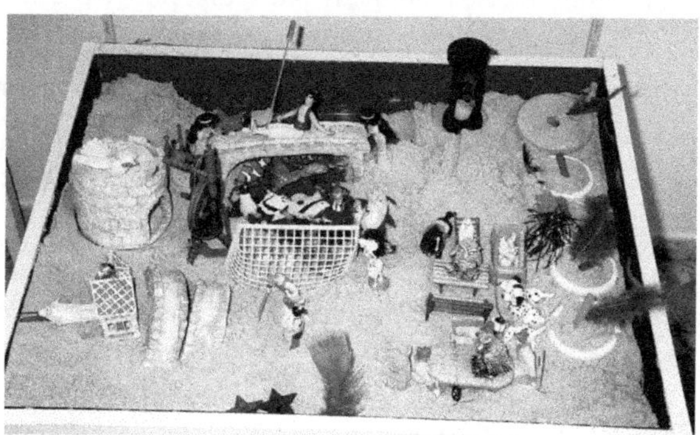

Figure 10.44 *Maya: Age six and a half, Sandplay 15, The ascent of Aladdin*

Maya's choice of objects in these two groups is significant. Neumann (1994, p.17) states that the eagle, horse and dog can symbolize penetration of masculine energy into a young girl's unconscious.

> The eagle is an archetypally masculine symbol of the sun, the heavens and the spirit; the owl, on the other hand, symbolizes night and the archetypal Feminine. Moreover, as a symbol of wisdom of the nocturnal, the owl in itself is not associated with any negative symbolism. (Neumann, 1994, pp.41–45)

The owl is also the symbol of Athena, Greek Goddess of War, handicraft and strategy, the feminine intuition that "sees" in the dark and can comprehend dark unconscious processes. The spinning wheel and owl recall the myth of Arachne, a mortal weaver who challenged the goddess Athena to a spinning contest. Athena's tapestry depicted the perfection of the gods, but Arachne won the contest with a tapestry that depicted the love affairs of the gods. In anger, Athena turned her into a spider, hanging forever on her web while spinning it. In the air, not being grounded, is similar to a girl's transition from the matriarchate, still not connected to the patriarchate.

Maya dictated her first story after making Sandplay 17. Belle, this time in a red dress, emerges from the right side of a large forest and sees Beast, his house and strawberry garden.

> Once there was a beautiful girl named Belle. She went to pick strawberries but a forest blocked her path. She didn't notice the animal that stood near his house and kept looking at himself in a mirror. Belle went to the strawberry fields and picked three strawberries. Suddenly the animal said, "What are you doing with my strawberries?" She replied, "I picked only three strawberries for my father." The Beast said, "But you know this is my field?" Then they went into the animal's house and talked. Belle was very afraid of him. Then she got used to him. And then suddenly he kissed her and turned into a prince. They fell in love and married and lived in great happiness until today.

She then replaced Beast in the sandtray with a figurine of a charming prince.

Stage Four: Rainbows, witches and stones, seven years six months to eight years 11 months

The years from age 6–7 until 11–12, "Middle Childhood," are archetypally termed "The Great Father" stage and the Ego stage is termed Solar Warlike (Neumann, 1994). Neumann describes the Paternal Uroboros as a strong symbol of instincts, different from the maternal instinct and similar to Hades who abducts the young girl Kore-Persephone supported by Gaia, Mother Earth, in defiance of Demeter the Elementary Mother. The mother may need to hold her daughter close, but the girl must break away in order to develop. Her identification with the symbiotic paradise of Mother–Daughter is ending (Neumann, 1994, pp.18, 268). The Paternal Uroboros that activates the Father archetype is a strange new unknown numinous inner force, but a normative and essential stage in a girl's development. Its role is to "penetrate," and although it can awaken great fear, it can also be interesting. Neumann (1994, pp.14–22) stresses the importance for a girl to experience this force that is larger than her, without a sense of rape or inferiority.

At seven and a half years old, Maya created Sandplay 18, a small island on the left side of the sandtray, with a sign on it labeled "Island," separated from the outside sand by a narrow moat filled with fish and dolphins. Maya formed 29 large colorful flowers from round cloths, inserted a colored peg in the center of each and arranged them on the outside sand. Three butterflies land on a few. Running across the center, a horizontal row of human figurines begins with two Jasmine figurines on the island, facing a small ceramic house. A bridge connects the island to the outer sand on the right. On the bridge, Belle, in her yellow dress, gazes down at Eric, who faces the mermaid looking at the water with Mulan behind her. On the right surrounded by flowers, a prince and white princess gaze at each other. Along the front edge, a row of four women—a pretty girl and three Anastasia figurines–gaze towards the island, past a rainbow and large yellow sun. Belle, Mulan and these four women witness the first meeting of Eric, a human man, and the mermaid. But the mermaid directs her gaze at the water, perhaps a wish to return to the original sea, the mother's protective womb, or Maya's wish to be an only child, not feeling replaced by another sister, not having to move to a new developmental stage and not having to witness her parents' conflicts (Figure 10.45).

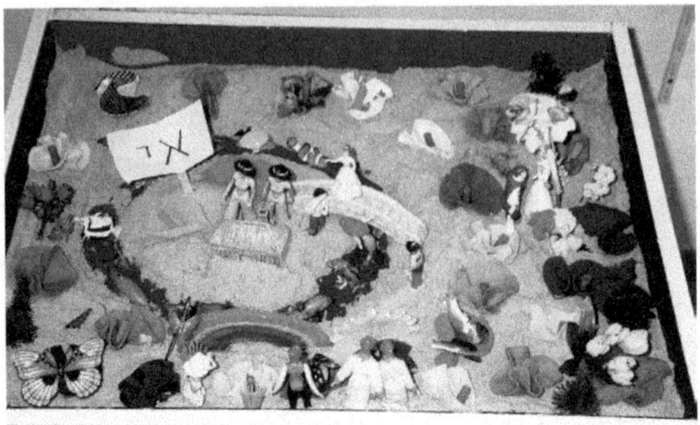

Figure 10.45 *Maya: Age seven and a half, Sandplay 18, The beautiful island*

She dictated a story:

> A few days ago on a most beautiful island there were many, women, healthy and whole, and even a bride and groom under a flowered umbrella. And do you know what? There is water around the island, and do you know who lives in the water? The Little Mermaid, The End.

Nine months later in Sandplay 20, at age eight years two months, the split between Maya's parents is represented by two large yellow suns far apart on the rear edge. They create a symmetrical structure of left and right sides around a central mound enclosed in a ring of sand with three witches who peer towards the mound from the rear. Three red and two blue marbles are evenly spaced in the front of the sand ring. Water appears in three pools—a central small round pool between the suns, and two vertical oblong pools on the left and right sides. Mulan lies prone above the left pool, a crystal, amethyst and black stone on its banks. At the bottom, four dwarfs face her. The mermaid is alone in the empty water on the right, facing four small marbles on the sand below. In front of each long pool are a house and a car. Two of the witches are dressed in black, one with a broom and one with an apple, on either side of a third witch seated on a metal chair who beckons with her finger towards whatever is within the mound. The witches may be invoking an evil spell, making them guilty of the split between the parents. Or they represent the "evil woman" who bewitched Maya's father. They may be inviting Maya to join the dark feminine and work powerful magic to prevent her parents' divorce (Figure 10.46).

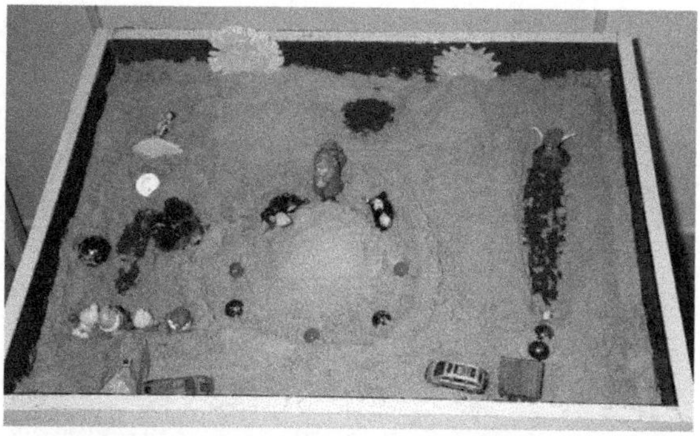

Figure 10.46 *Maya: Age eight years two months, Sandplay 20, Two suns and three witches*

Four months later, Maya made two sandplays in her 21st session. The first dramatically expresses the split between a stormy reality and hopeful fantasy, but in the second sandplay two beautiful white stones are suddenly discovered and, like the Philosopher's Stone, will help Maya to cope with transition to the patriarchate and with the irreconcilable split between her parents.

In the first sandplay, Belle faces the sea in her yellow dress, standing on a long central bridge between two worlds. Behind her on the rear edge, a large sun and a rainbow hide a lightning cloud, a stormy world behind the rainbow. Three couples—a bride and groom not facing each other, one Jasmine separated from Superman lying face down, and a second Jasmine separated from Eric—ominously mirror Maya's parents' separation. A white horizontal fence separates this bleak world from a charming sea in front, full of starfish, dolphins, a seahorse, colorful fish, a small castle and, on the left, the mermaid and prince together on benches above the water near the gold-roofed house, an empty table and four chairs. (Figure 10.47).

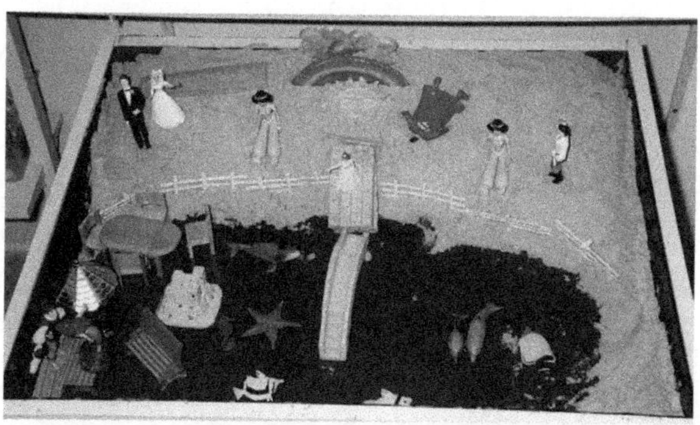

Figure 10.47 *Maya: Age eight and a half, Sandplay 21a, The last rainbow*

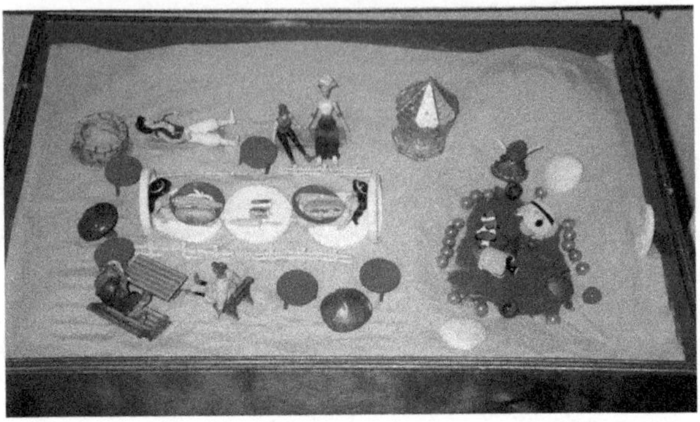

Figure 10.48 *Maya: Age eight and a half, Sandplay 21b, Two white stones*

In her second sandplay, two Jasmine figurines, like Maya and her sister, enjoy a picnic together in a fenced-off area. Outside the fence are several figures: Beast sitting near Anastasia, two women in the center—an unclothed Anastasia that may represent Maya's mother, and a figurine of a tall colorful woman who might represent her father's girlfriend. Nearby, Aladdin lies down alone on a bench. On the right side, the mermaid is also alone in a large pool filled with fish. Two smooth white stones on either side of the pool are the focus of Maya's story (Figure 10.48).

> Once there were two sisters who wanted to have a picnic at the sea. They ate very tasty food. Then they walked and saw starfish and seahorses, and even blue and red pearls in the water. They kept walking and suddenly they saw two beautiful smooth white stones. They took the stones back to the picnic table and continued eating. And then they saw it was dark and went home and said in their hearts: we had a wonderful day at the sea. I'll always remember that day.

Six months later, at almost nine years old, Maya's inner sense of desolation is expressed in Sandplay 22 (not shown). A storm cloud covers the sun in the far center, and in the far right a deserted castle is surrounded by sand. On the left edge, Jasmine and Aladdin face each other near an empty crib, each holding a baby. A bridge leads from a sand island in front to the storm cloud. A second Jasmine in a rowboat on the left, gazes at the Jasmine–Aladdin couple. Maya's story was entitled "The White Egg."

> Aladdin and Jasmine sat on their porch and played with their baby. Suddenly, there was a sand storm. They hid inside a hill opposite them, where they always hid during sand storms. They went inside the hill but the sand filled the opening. They dug and dug but they couldn't reach a place where there was no sand. Suddenly, they saw a white egg, and decided to take it. When the sand storm ended, they took the egg and then the egg stopped glowing and it looked like a rotten egg. And then they put it back and learned their lesson not to take anything from its place.

An egg cannot incubate when it is removed from the warmth of a protective nest. It begins to rot, the life within it dies, as the life of Maya's family died when the family container disintegrated. Yet the first stage of blackening in the alchemical process is putrefaction or rotting, the nigredo. Jung, quoting Maria Prophetissa, writes that the secret lies in knowing about the "Hermetic vessel." The vessel must be

> completely round in imitation of the spherical cosmos, so that the influence of the stars may contribute to the success of the operation. It is a kind of matrix or uterus from which the *filius philosophorum*, the miraculous Stone, is to be born. Hence it is required that the vessel be not only round but egg-shaped. (Jung, 1953, para. 338)

The Philosopher's egg is the vessel within which the Philosopher's Stone is born. This stone has the power to turn base metals into gold or silver and enables transformation.

Stage Five: Middle Childhood

Maya is almost nine and a half years old. The left side of Sandplay 24 is visibly colorful and attractive. An opening of blue water on the rear edge, in the same place as in Sandplay 15, is filled with fish, a starfish and dolphins. But they point upwards as if the water is flowing out of the sandtray. In the front-left quadrant, seven colorful glass stones and marbles are arranged in a square. The colorful surface may divert attention from two quadrants on the right side defined by deep lines cut into the sand, under which Maya has buried two black stones and two black eggs. In the squared furrow in the far-right corner, a flat round sand circle, enclosed by five holes that Maya made with her fingers, conceals and protects the black stones like a hamsa. In the front-right corner, a deep squared blue line encloses a mound that conceals the black eggs. As if buried deep inside a pyramid, these precious stones and eggs will move through the dark underworld, surviving the destruction and present tension in the family (Figure 10.49).

The Little Mermaid (her twelfth appearance) and Eric face each other in Sandplay 25, on either side of a large central mound, she on the left and he on the right. But they are hopelessly separated as the entrances to a possible tunnel under the mound are clogged with sand. They can never meet again. They are also blocked off from the blue waters in the far and near areas, each one standing in a long sandbank reinforced with stone walls that touch the sandtray's edges. In the far sea, six fish swim separately. In the center of the front sea, a whale faces towards the mound between two dolphins swimming in opposite directions. Yet 15 evenly spaced green trees have sprouted on the mound, giving hope for the future. The blocked portals recall Maya's story of a sand storm and rotten egg, blocking her transition to the patriarchate (Figure 10.50).

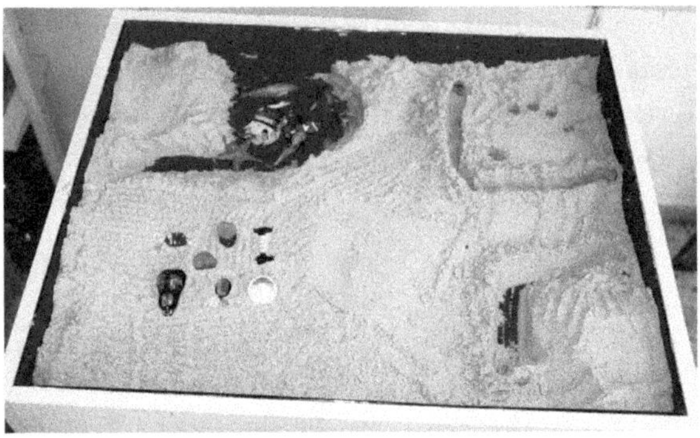

Figure 10.49 *Maya: Age nine and a half, Sandplay 24, Two buried black stones, two buried black eggs*

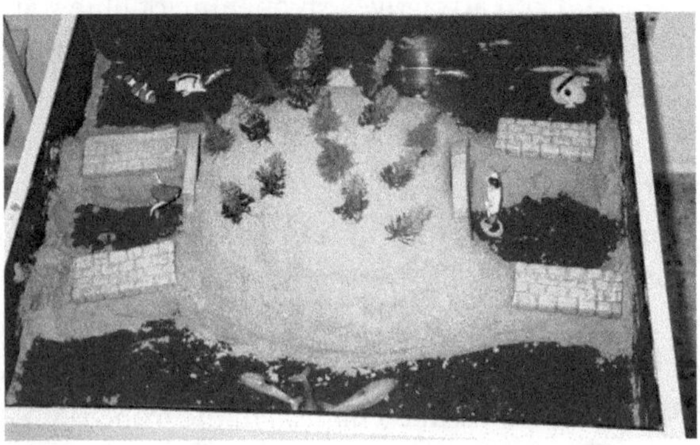

Figure 10.50 *Maya: Sandplay 25, Eric and the Mermaid cannot meet*

Two weeks later, in Sandplay 27, a symmetrical Self-tray illustrates a great drama. Queen Jasmine sits on her throne on a central mound, above a magic stone buried underneath her. A large yellow sun empowers her from behind, but also conceals a storm cloud and two small houses. In front of the mound, three guards and a second Jasmine, the queen's twin sister, guard the queen and the buried stone. In front, a prince arrives at a forest searching for the stone. Scenes in the four corners complete the mandala structure but are not part of Maya's story. In the two far corners, familiar figures sit with food-laden picnic tables, Aladdin, Eric and Belle in her blue dress on the left and the mermaid (her fourteenth appearance) who jumps into a tiny pond observed by a small girl. On the right, Belle in her yellow dress, Anastasia with no dress and Beast sit at their table. Large, deserted houses in the front corners and a second tiny pond and small old house on the right complete the sandplay (Figure 10.51).

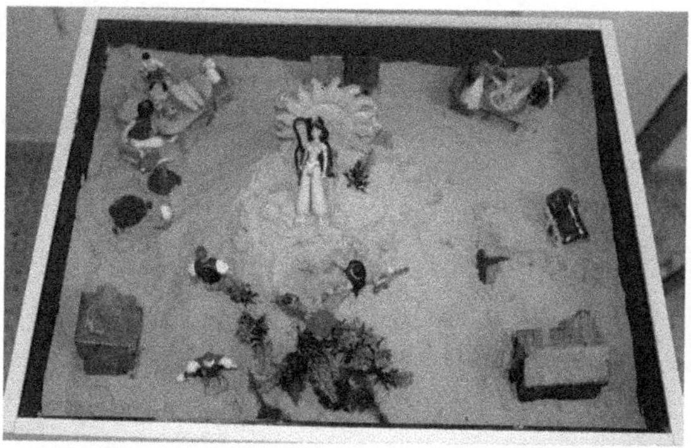

Figure 10.51 *Maya: Age nine years eight months, Sandplay 27, The Queen hides the magic stone*

Once upon a time there was a queen who sat on a mountain. She had three guards and one woman guard who was her twin sister. Everyone loved the queen because she guarded the Enchanted Stone. A little prince came from far away to the forest around her mountain. The guards saw the prince from above. The prince climbed and climbed and cut down all the trees with his sword. He passed the first guard with no problem. He passed the second guard too. But the third guard was very strong and he couldn't pass him. Although he was wounded, he went around the guard and then the queen saw him and immediately went to hide the magic stone. She said to her twin sister, "Sit in my place." The prince arrived and saw the sister

> and thought she was the queen. He said to her, "Can you tell me where the magic stone is?" The queen's sister said, "Yes," but she had prepared a trick. Meanwhile, all the guards returned to their stations. She took him straight down. They walked for half an hour and saw the first guard and they began to duel. The queen's sister went to the queen and said that they would have to help the guards. Of course, the queen was the strongest of them all, and knew Capoeira, and she approached the prince. He saw her, and she saw him. The prince immediately knew that he could not stand against her and that he would have to go. But he went around the trees to the other side of the mountain and began to look for the magic stone. But until today he never found it.

Maya's heroine is no longer compliant. She is a queen who can use cunning or strength to cope with conflict and with the masculine. Maya is painfully aware that her parents are fighting over property, and not fighting to unite the family. I wrote down her story and read it back to her. This provided a sense of order and helped her share her inner reality with me without addressing the external struggle. The magic stone as the central point of a spontaneous mandala suggests that, in Maya's psyche, masculine and feminine are able to unite, although in reality her parents are divided. Jung (2014, para. 636) describes the diamond thunderbolt, the dorje in the center of a mandala, as a symbol of the perfect state of unification of masculine and feminine. "The world of illusions has finally vanished. All energy has gathered together in the initial state."

Stage Six: Six sandplays and spoken stories

Maya's sandplays provide form and stable boundaries for her spontaneous stories with themes of family conflict, hope and longing for a peaceful solution. But their sequence follows the stages of dissolution of the family. Her stories are summarized below together with spoken quotes.

Maya and her sister improvised a story "The Red Diamond" for their joint sandplay. A father, mother and their five-year-old son Miki visit an enchanted pool which was the source of all the treasures in their home. A second family couldn't find their bathing suits and did not come. Other people were in the pool. Miki went in but fell and hit his head on something hard. His father lifted a stone and saw it was a Red Diamond. When he showed it, everyone began to fight for it.

> Miki took the diamond and crawled out of there while the others continued fighting. Then he showed them the diamond and said, "It belongs to the one who found it." At home Miki was happy, his parents were angry. Miki kept the diamond in his room and slept with it each night. He was angry at it because it had hurt his head but he also loved it.

The painful blow to Miki's head from the red diamond is like the pain of crystal-clear consciousness. Magical objects in Maya's stories have shifted from stone to egg, from white to black, and now to a Red Diamond. Jung writes that the diamond's "hardness, transparency, and rubeous hue" makes it an excellent symbol for the Philosopher's Stone (1953, para. 511). The extended families were now part of the feud between the parents.

After Maya's tenth birthday, the parental split manifested clearly in Sandplay 31, "The war that makes love impossible." A large vertical central ocean splits two vertical sandbanks along the left and right sides containing all the sand. A spikey yellow sun leans on the far center edge. In the water near the sun, a large blue dolphin (from Maya's fourth sandplay) and three whales form a group. Elsewhere in the water, two pairs of smaller fish point left, and three metal golden fish point right. Figurines of equal numbers and types are crowded onto each sandbank: picnic tables, horses, several women and a man, huts on the front left, a castle in the far right. Yet the left side seems fragile, less in control, needing stone walls to reinforce it. Snow White, Dorothy, Eric and an unclothed Anastasia sit at a table. Below them are a groom, two unclothed Anastasias, a gypsy, a pretty girl and two white horses, with two small round huts in the front-left corner. The right sandbank needs no supporting walls. Two Jasmines, a princess and Aladdin (perhaps Maya's father) sit casually at their table with two pretty girls and a baby in a crib behind them. In the far-right corner, Belle in her yellow gown peeps out of a stone castle. The strong black horse stands near her. The enmity between the parents and their families is reflected in Maya's story, closing with an unrealistic happy ending (Figure 10.52).

In her story, Princess Ella and Prince Joseph meet by chance near a well in a forest and fall in love. They promise to meet in three days but discover that their countries are going to war. Crying, Ella tells her father, the king, that she loves Joseph and might not see him again because of the war. The king replies that the other country was cruel and not nice, and forbids Ella to meet Joseph near the sea as they had planned. Ella says to the king, "All right," but in her heart she knows she will go to meet him. Meanwhile, Joseph tells his mother the same thing. The queen does not agree. Joseph says, "All right," but knows that he will go to meet Ella. Three days later, Ella and Joseph are prevented from leaving their castles. Each one thinks about the other.

> The war began, and they could see each other with binoculars. They were happy that neither of them had remained alone at the meeting place. Then the queen took away Joseph's binoculars and put him in a shelter so he would not be wounded. Ella's father, the king, did the same thing. Three days later, the war ended, they met secretly and got married. The king and the queen looked for their children and found them getting married. They were very happy about this and told them that they would make a regular wedding for them. And they lived happily ever after.

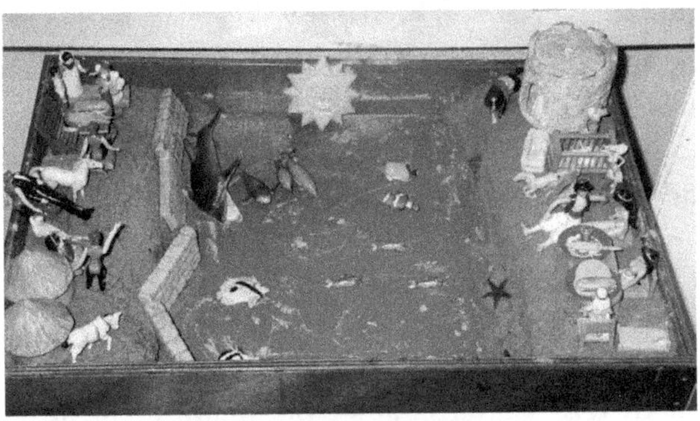

Figure 10.52 *Maya: Age ten, Sandplay 31, The war that makes love impossible*

The next week, in the dry tray, Maya emphasizes respect for the treasures of nature and imagination, not greed for material possessions. In her story, two men seek treasure in an African country, "Congo," ruled by a king with many diamonds and jewels. On the left, Tarzan hangs from a tall tree near a portal to a blue pool surrounded by flowers. In the center, the two men ignore the pool and gaze beyond a forest at a cave in the far-right corner fenced off by strong walls. Peering into the cave are a small king and Anastasia. In Maya's story, aggressive plants, perhaps the Great Mother of the Plants, ensnare the two men and pull them down into an underworld of treasure, where they decide to take nothing (Figure 10.53).

Two people arrived at the jungle on the same day, and a very scary surprise waited for them. A fox and a wolf blocked their way. They cleared the path and reached a lake, and saw many unexpected animals, but the animals were peaceful and they crossed the lake. But some plants grabbed them. It took a while to get free. They walked until they reached a mountain full of thorny trees. Luckily, they had swords and cut their way through. Then some flowers caught their feet and pulled them down into a secret opening in the mountain. They entered and walked through canals and came to a tunnel. Inside were many jewels, but they couldn't take anything. They went back to their countries and told their king that they brought back nothing, but that they had seen animals that no one had ever seen. There were flowers there that grab your legs and don't let go. Why should we steal jewels? The jungle needs to be as it is, beautiful, full of trees, flowers and animals. But the king said, "I don't know what you want, but I want treasure!" But the king's soldiers said to him, "If you try to go, we won't let you pass. Because the jungle has to remain as it is, a mysterious jungle." End.

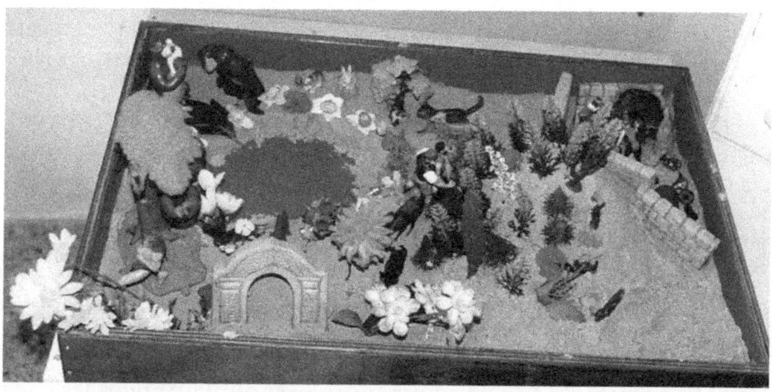

Figure 10.53 *Maya: Sandplay 32, Mother Earth protects her treasures*

Sandplay 34 illustrates a story within a story, of a man holding a "treasure map" near a portal that leads to a flowering jungle on the left side of the sandtray (not shown). Grandfather Yaakov tells his five-year-old grandson that his great-grandfather gave him a treasure map, and that he had looked for it and found the right place. Then he stopped telling the story and said, "It's a surprise, you will know tomorrow."

But the next day Grandfather Yaakov said, "Your great-great-grandfather gave the map to me, and you will get it when you grow up and do with it whatever you want." Years passed and the little boy grew up. He had the

> map in his hand and was curious to know what the treasure was. He reached the jungle and went to a grove of trees and flowers where the treasure was hidden. He dug and dug, but instead of treasure he found a piece of paper, and this was written on it: "Treasure is not the most important thing in the world. The family, brothers, sisters and friends are more important than treasure." And then he said to himself, "The treasure that I now hold in my hands is the most beautiful treasure that I have ever held, because it is wise and full of love." End.

Stage Seven: Final Stage, from ten years two months to 11 years six months

Maya had to stop going to the piano lessons she loved. In her next sandplay, "Music, the Good in People," she enclosed six musical instruments on cloths on the sand and five musicians in a circle around them with stone walls and wooden sticks. In the far-left corner, she added a row of eight dark green trees of the kind found in cemeteries.

In Sandplay 36, the portal that led to a treasure map in a forest is now in water between a large mound on the left surrounded by water and a small mound attached to the far-right corner. Behind the portal, a large round mirror bridges the mounds and invites Maya to focus on herself rather than on those on the mounds. On the large mound, a white princess is the central figure of a group with a Japanese man and woman and two houses on either side. In front of her a white horse faces left towards a large dark house with a wooden hammer stuck in the sand, and a blue crystal ball hanging from it. Involved with themselves, no one faces the gold-roofed glass house, a table and chairs on their right. A row of sticks (from the previous musical sandplay) encircles the bottom of the mound with three small houses, and two rows of seven precious stones just above. On the small corner mound, Aladdin and a yellow dog sit in front of a dark forest, between two small houses. A dark house and a lighthouse are hidden in the trees. Maya's story is unfinished.

> Once there were two islands that were close to each other. On the small one was a forest. The other had a castle where a beautiful girl lived. In the forest lived a handsome boy. One day the girl from the castle went for a walk and by mistake entered the forest and there she met the boy from the forest. They fell in love and the next day the king...

The next week Maya and her sister made Sandplay 37, and then took turns improvising a story about two separate kingdoms who were not friends and not enemies. Two girls, one from each kingdom, meet near a well and become good friends, but the parents of each kingdom forbid them to see each other. The story begins three years later when the girls meet again and keep their friendship secret so they won't be separated again. The sandplay's mandala structure has four corners, each with a separate theme, around a central pool with a fisherman who seems oblivious to the corners packed with figurines and objects that continue along the edges. Stone walls and fences block communication between all the corners. In the far left, walls enclose a queen, her castle, a princess near a well, many houses and a lighthouse. Diagonally opposite in the front-right corner, a king and prince stand face to face among houses, furniture and a castle. In a forest in the far right, a witch near a gingerbread house beckons with her finger at a pretty girl. Diagonally opposite the witch are 20 cars in a parking lot in the front left. Under the cars, a Red Diamond is buried (Figure 10.54). The fisherman has actually heard the girls talking and tells the king and queen. Maya and her sister continue to improvise the story:

> The king and queen say to the girls, "If you want to be friends, you must go to the witch's forest and ask her for a magic potion and drink this together in one gulp." But many cars blocked the road to the forest. So the king and queen gave them a second task: get rid of the cars, and start to dig there and find the Red Diamond. But they found the way into the forest and went to the witch's house. They asked her for the magic potion, but the witch gave them a potion that put them to sleep for two hours. When they awoke, they realized that the witch didn't know how to read. They asked for the poison bottle, drank it and pretended to be dead. When the witch turned her back, they ran out of the forest and went to find the Red Diamond. They asked the drivers to drive their cars out of the area. They dug into the earth, found the Red Diamond, put it in a bottle and went to the king and queen. Their parents couldn't believe it and said, "Okay, you win: you have completed all the tasks, now you can be friends."

Perhaps only the magical Red Diamond can alleviate Maya's pain and growing sense of hopelessness. There was no story for Sandplay 38, which she did alone. A wide diagonal river from the far left to the near-right corner extends beyond the sandtray, creating two triangular sand areas with no bridge. In the far left of the river, large sharks, whales and dolphins block the exit. On the front left of the smaller sand triangle, a king and queen stand at opposite ends separated by 14 different houses, with Eric in the middle. They face the larger sand triangle on the right, on which a large sand pyramid stands. The red diamond is buried beneath it. Above and around the pyramid are three couples, two lightning clouds looming behind and the glass gold-roofed house. This "house" was once a perfume bottle that belonged to my mother. Maya placed it in Sandplay 7 six years ago near the Little Mermaid, both used for the first time. It could carry a deep feminine protective transference, like the two goddesses that supported the mermaid in Sandplay 9, or like Glinda, the Good Witch of the North (in *The Wizard of Oz*) who appeared in several early sandplays and is paired here with a bearded sorcerer. There are two other couples: a strong man in a green shirt opposite a sorceress and the white princess with a strong supportive man (Figure 10.55).

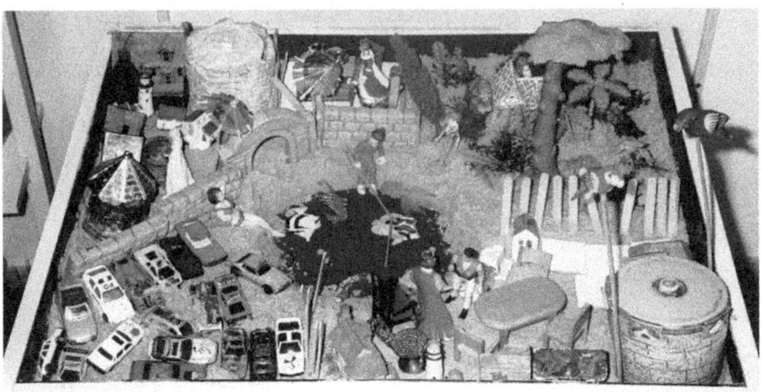

Figure 10.54 *Maya: Sandplay 37, Red Diamond of Friendship; War between the King and Queen*

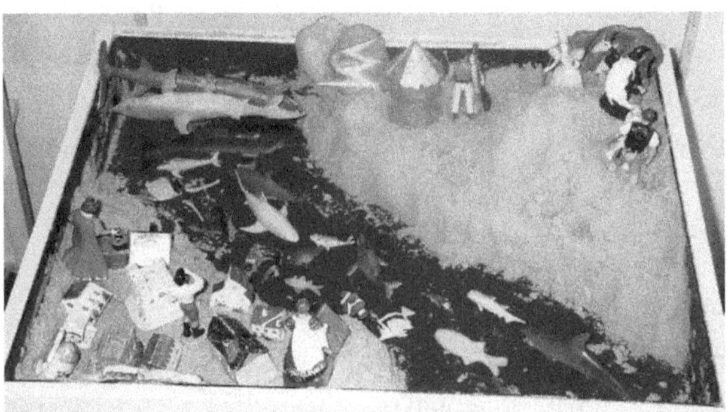

Figure 10.55 *Maya: Age ten and a half, Sandplay 38, The Red Diamond is buried under a sand pyramid*

Maya's final sandplay when she was 11 and a half years old, establishes the growth of a positive masculine and feminine relationship within her psyche. A king and queen face each other standing in a ceramic pool of water, an "alchemical bathtub," on the top of a large round isolated mound in the far left surrounded by a clear blue semi-circle of water. Two bonfires and a guard stand below them, like a memorial to an ideal but dead past. The placement of the mound and the semi-circle of water resemble the structure of a sun, often drawn by children in the upper left corner of a paper. A sun, or this round mound rising up from the sea, surrounded by a large amount of deep blue water, may evoke reflection or purification of violent energies in the waters of past sandplays. The blue water semi-circle also shapes a narrow beach in front that widens into a land area reaching the far-right corner. Ten green trees and four dead tree trunks are spaced out along this area. In the front left, the fisherman and Aladdin sit together. In the center, the two Jasmines and Anastasia face the island near a large picnic lunch. Four large houses on the right edge might represent the parents' separate houses, and the houses of the grandparents on either side. Two lighthouses in the front-right area may indicate that caution is necessary for Maya to deal separately with each parent. A solitary yellow dog under a portal observes the mound, no longer near Aladdin in Sandplay 26 two years ago, when the split became clear. Maya's mother adopted a similar dog after the divorce. Finally, the man in a green shirt, in a wooden boat in the spot where a bridge and a mirror had been, gazes to the left at the island (Figure 10.56).

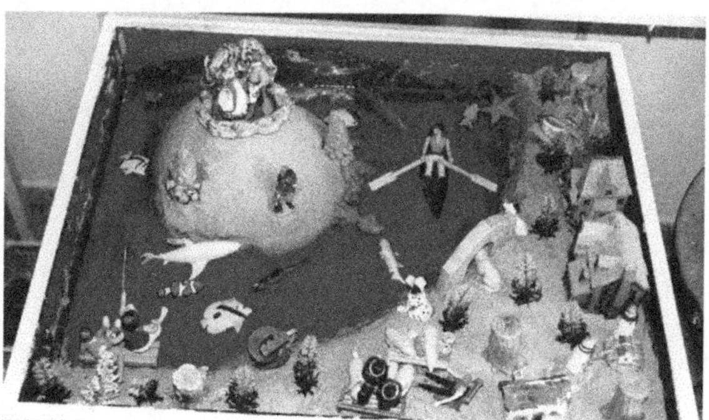

Figure 10.56 *Maya: Age 11 and a half, Final sandplay, The Alchemical King and Queen*

Conclusion

Maya's early exploration of sand, water and objects encouraged her authentic self-expression in sandplay. Her images progressed according to the stages and characteristics of girls, outlined by Neuman and by Jones, as compared to the sandplay of boys. At about four years old, preceding her transition to the patriarchate, a deep connection to the archetypal protective feminine and to the mermaid, was established in her psyche. Fairy godmothers and goddesses supported Maya as she coped with the impermanence of her parents' marriage, through her distress and hope for reconciliation, which dominated her sandplays before she was able to focus on herself. A sequence of alchemical eggs and precious stones supported her process of individuation, and helped overcome "servitude" to the father image to the detriment of the feminine. In her final sandplay, a new male authority in a green shirt rows a boat and looks at the king and queen in their pool on an isolated mountain top. He may be the inner prince who liberates her from her controlling father, such as Eros was to Psyche at first. The green of his shirt suggests growth upwards still attached to a beneficial earth goddess. She and her prince are ready to undergo additional developmental stages until they find a mature relationship together.

PART 4

SANDPLAY AND MYTHOLOGY

11

Sandplay and Myth: Bridging Consciousness and the Self

This chapter is dedicated to the memory of Yonat Fischer, dear friend and colleague, inspired teacher of sandplay and Greek mythology, who, on November 26, 2022, departed this world.

Greek mythology

> *The wonder is that the characteristic efficacy to touch and inspire deep creative centers dwells in the smallest nursery fairy tale—as the flavor of the ocean is contained in a droplet or the whole mystery of life within the egg of a flea. For the symbols of mythology are not manufactured; they cannot be ordered, invented or permanently suppressed. They are spontaneous productions of the psyche, and each bears within it, undamaged, the germ power of its source.*
>
> (CAMPBELL, 1949/1973, P.4)

I discovered mythology when I was ten years old, in my parents' bookcase. An abridged version of *Mythology: Timeless Tales of Gods and Heroes* (Hamilton, 1942) introduced me to forceful, jealous and devious shape-shifting gods whose magical powers surpassed those of Superman, Wonder Woman and Batman. They had evolved at the beginning of time and were rarely penalized for their violent or crafty deeds, unlike mortals punished for their arrogance. The godly intergenerational family feuds and schemes among each other were fascinating, yet something—an invisible substance in between the lines—seemed to be missing in the version I read. Forty years later during my sandplay studies, I found what I had searched for in Jungian interpretations of the myths. In the curriculum of the two-year sandplay training program that I founded at a college in Tel Aviv in 2003, I included fairy tales and several Greek myths. Fairy tales were referenced when they corresponded with themes in a sandplay case, but the heroes and heroines of the Greek myths needed their own space. Edinger (1994) summarizes C.G. Jung's view that

> mythology is the self-revelation of the archetypal psyche. Jung conceived of the human psyche as consisting of two interpenetrating levels, the personal and the archetypal (or transpersonal). The personal level derives from the immediate experience of one's own life history. The deeper, archetypal level does not have its source in personal experience, but is an innate psychological structure, present at birth and common to all human beings, just as the physical structure of the body is. This inner structure is composed of the archetypes, universal patterns representing the typical experiences of mankind.

The sandplay training program groups consisted of art therapists, a few psychologists and social workers. Art therapists teach theoretically and experientially. We had 20 wooden sandtrays painted blue inside, sand from a local beach and enough miniatures and natural objects for group use. Four myths were presented each year, illustrated by slides of black-figure paintings of mythical heroes on Greek amphora (570–500 BC). Mythological themes came alive after each presentation through the students' spontaneous work in individual sandtrays.

The first myth of Demeter and her daughter Persephone focused on their relationship, Persephone's abduction to the underworld by her uncle Hades, and Demeter's search for her. The feminine–masculine relationship of Psyche and Eros followed, with Psyche's struggle for individuation. The third myth tells of masculine individuation through Theseus, the hero who kills the Minotaur in its labyrinth, aided by Ariadne, the Minotaur's sister. In the fourth myth, Ariadne, abandoned by Theseus on the island of Naxos, was found by Dionysus, God of Wine and Ecstasy, who fell in love with her and helped her to find healing and joy.

The second-year myths began with Asclepius, God of Healing, followed by the descent of Orpheus into Hades and his loss of Eurydice. Odysseus's long journey home and the triple goddess Hecate, guardian of crossroads, night, magic and boundaries, closed the second year. Edinger (1994) writes:

> From the viewpoint of depth psychology, the gods stand for the archetypes, the basic patterns within the human psyche that exist independent of personal experience. They are the templates on which the individual life is formed. Mythologically, these eternal patterns are thought of as gods, existing in a special place apart from ordinary human experience. The Greeks called that special region Olympus, and thought of it originally as a mountain peak, and later as the whole upper sky.

The great Greek classical myths that describe the creation of the world from Chaos, the births of Titans and gods, and the creation of mankind were at first passed on in oral form by bards. Myths that existed previously during the Paleolithic era until about 10,000 BC, and during the Neolithic era, until about 3200 BC, may have honored a great goddess, a feminine life-giving force evidenced by numerous "goddess" statues and ceramic vessels unearthed in archaeological sites (Spretnak, 1992). Conquerors who invaded middle Bronze Age Greece, from 1200 to 900 BC established a patriarchal culture that imposed a masculine-dominated version of the world, dividing the one great goddess into several goddesses, each with a specific role. About this time, in 800 BC, the Greek poet Homer wrote two epic poems, *The Iliad*, the story of the Trojan War, and *The Odyssey*, the long journey home of Odysseus after the war.

In approximately 730 BC, the Greek poet Hesiod wrote a second epic poem, *The Theogony*, about the origins of creation from Chaos, the successions of Titans and gods, and the war between them won by Zeus, the undisputed ruler of Olympus and the world. The Roman poet Ovid, born in 43 BC, wrote a third epic poem in Latin, *Metamorphosis* or *Transformations*, consisting of a 15-volume history of the world with over 250 myths, from Chaos and Creation until the death and deification of Julius Cesar in Ovid's own time. It was published in Rome in AD 8 and joined the works of Homer and Hesiod as classics that have been read for over 2000 years and translated into many languages. Versions from different eras of history reflect a translator's personality, choices and culture. Often, masculine brutality was softened and the endless rapes endured by women were blurred. A recent translation of the *Metamorphosis* is faithful to Ovid's descriptions of divine violence and rape (McCarter, 2022). *Mythos* (Fry, 2019) is another accurate and entertaining collection of the most well-known myths. In AD 160, Apuleius, born in North Africa and educated in Rome, wrote a novel in Latin also called *Transformations* or *Metamorphosis*, now known as *The Golden Ass*. In it, Apuleius inserted the myth of "Eros and Psyche" as told by an old woman to calm a young girl abducted for ransom on her wedding night by a band of robbers. The entire Latin text including the myth has been translated over the centuries into many versions and languages (Taylor, 1822, pp.66–99).

The symbolic sandplay journey, like a myth, is a story whose themes, stages and events lead to a transformation of character. The unfathomable nature of the collective unconscious is revealed in tales of conflict, relationships and goals of the gods that often resonate with our mortal desires and the paths that our lives take. Unlike mortals, the gods shape-shift and transform themselves frequently to seduce, reward, deceive or punish others, according to their shifting loyalties to each other. Zeus became a golden rain to seduce Danae, an eagle to capture the beautiful Ganymede, a swan to seduce Leda, and a white bull to seduce Europa. Athena, his daughter, angrily transformed the gifted mortal weaver Arachne into a spider when she won a weaving contest against her. She transformed Medusa, a beautiful woman who was raped in Athena's temple by the god Poseidon, into a snake-haired gorgon. Circe transformed the crew of Odysseus into pigs, and later returned them to human form. Daphna, fleeing rape by Apollo, was transformed by her father, a river god, into a laurel tree. Dionysus transformed pirates who kidnapped him into dolphins. As the God of Wine, he enables humans who drink his wine to be transformed by "spirit." Our psyches still struggle with our perceptions of others or with others' perceptions of us. Our relationships, between mothers, fathers, children, families and others, coping with emotional and cognitive development, loyalty, deceit and hubris, and with love requited and unrequited, are all alive in our sandplay journeys and their final transformations. Over the years, there have been many versions of the eight myths summarized below, but the main themes remain relatively unchanged (Graves, 1955/1960).

The myths

Demeter and Persephone

Demeter, Earth Goddess, Goddess of Grain, loved her adolescent daughter Persephone more than anything else. Persephone's father, Zeus, was God of Olympus and Demeter's brother. One day, Demeter left Persephone with some nymphs in a field of flowers and went about her work, nurturing the earth to help things grow. Persephone saw a wonderful flower, and as she bent down, the earth opened, a golden chariot with black horses appeared and her uncle Hades, God of the Underworld, quickly abducted her down to his realm. The earth closed over them, leaving no trace. Demeter, distraught at her daughter's disappearance and furious that no one seemed to know what had happened, stopped eating and searched day and night for her without success. Hecate, the triple goddess, heard Persephone's cries and saw Demeter's grief, and took her to the Sun God, Apollo, who sees everything on earth from above. Apollo said that Persephone was now with Hades, who planned to marry her and make her Queen of the Underworld—a very good match.

Depressed at losing her daughter and angry at the deception of her brothers, Zeus and Hades, Demeter disguised herself as an old woman and found employment in Eleusis, as a nursemaid to Demophon, the young son of King Celeus and Queen Metanira. As a gift to her kind employers, she planned to transform this mortal child into a god by putting him through fire, but she was stopped by Metanira. Demeter then revealed herself as a goddess and demanded that a temple be built for her. But in her sorrow, she neglected earth's fertility: plants died, people starved and no gifts were left as offerings for the gods. Demeter resisted the entreaties of Zeus and other gods, and withheld all nurturance for humans until she could see her daughter again. Finally, Zeus sent his son Hermes, Messenger of the Gods, to Hades, to convince him to let Persephone go. But Hades had enticed Persephone to eat three or four pomegranate seeds, knowing that after eating in the underworld she would have to remain there, further infuriating Demeter. So Zeus sent their mother, Rhea, to talk to her. Happy to see her mother, Demeter agreed that Persephone would stay with Demeter for eight months of the year, and with Hades for four months, a month for each pomegranate seed. Persephone returned in joyful reunion with her mother at Eleusis, accompanied by Hecate in a golden chariot with horses driven by Hermes. Each spring and summer, Demeter is reunited with Persephone. The earth becomes fertile, blossoms and bears fruit. In the winter months, when Persephone withdraws from earthly life and returns to Hades, Demeter also withdraws from her life, and again nothing grows.

This myth presents the reasons behind seasonal change, so important for an agricultural society. But it also presents the relationship between two women, a loving mother and a daughter who has no reason to leave her. Zeus, Persephone's father, and other close relatives seemed to know that Persephone would not voluntarily separate from her mother, although it was time, and colluded to abduct Persephone to Hades' underworld. Gaia-Earth, mother of Rhea who is mother of the gods (Zeus, Hades, Demeter and others) and grandmother of Demeter, prepared the Narcissus flower that snared Persephone. The event itself—Hades in his horse-drawn chariot emerging from the earth and snatching his sister's daughter down to the underworld—seems "not to have been witnessed" by nymphs in the field, or other indifferent goddesses. Hades, the lonely and depressed Lord of Death, enticed Persephone with some pomegranate seeds that would keep her in Hades. In her youth, Persephone represents potential life. As a couple, she and Hades form a cycle between the opposites of life and death. The myth portrays the patriarchy as controlling, sending Persephone from a dominant mother to a dominating husband, who feeds her red pomegranate seeds, a symbol of menstrual blood and of loss of virginity from a fruit with many seeds symbolizing fertility.

But Demeter was victorious when Zeus finally gave in to her demands to retrieve her daughter. This victory, and the three stages of the matriarchal—Maiden, Mother and the Crone Hecate—were celebrated yearly as the Eleusinian Mysteries, at the Temple of Eleusis in a ten-day reenactment of all the stages of the myth: Persephone's abduction by Hades, Demeter's search and Hecate's help to find her daughter, and the joy at her return. Demeter renewed for her worshippers the secrets of agriculture in each stage of the ritual, which explained the seasons for planting, growing and reaping, and Demeter's sadness in winter when Persephone descends to Hades. The celebration was held near the autumnal equinox, to ensure the success of each agricultural year. Afterwards, the gods and goddesses were honored with gifts so they would provide rain, rich crops, health and wealth. Persephone's journey and transformation joins the opposites of masculine and feminine, helpless and powerful, innocent and devious, underworld and upper world, and gods and mortals (Graves, 1955/1960, pp.89–96).

Psyche and Eros (Amor, or Cupid)

H.E. Butler (1910) translated the tale of "Amor and Psyche" in *The Metamorphoses* or *Golden Ass* by Apuleius from the original Latin. Erich Neumann, in his commentary, preferred the Greek name Eros for the god of love, to convey a deeper relationship of the opposites of "Eros and Psyche," Psyche meaning "soul" or "butterfly" in Greek.

The myth begins: "In a certain city there once lived a king and queen. They had three daughters very fair to view..." All were charming but the youngest was so wonderfully fair that men were struck dumb with admiration of her beauty and made pilgrimages just to view her, neglecting the temples of Aphrodite, Goddess of Love. Aphrodite, enraged that the "unlawful loveliness" of a mortal girl had replaced her, ordered her son Eros to cause Psyche to fall in love with most vile creature possible. Eros mischievously used his arrows to cause the gods to fall in love with whomever he chose, but he himself had never felt love except for his mother. Psyche's two older sisters had married, but she remained alone, worshipped but not wooed. Her parents consulted the oracle (the god Apollo), who prophesized that Psyche would wed a monster. The king and queen accepted this terrible prophecy, wrapped Psyche in shrouds, marched her with a crowd of people to the appointed crag on a mountain top and left her there, awaiting her fate. But Eros had seen Psyche's beauty, and instead of a monster, he sent Zephyr, the West Wind, to gently transport Psyche to a beautiful valley with a castle of great beauty and riches. Psyche was received by invisible servants, heard voices and ate wonderful food, but no person was seen. At night, Eros came to her bed and a dark, passionate night relationship began. Each morning, he left before Psyche awoke. But Psyche never saw her husband and became lonely, longed for her sisters and wished to tell her family that she was safe. Eros warned her that her sisters would harm their happiness, but Psyche implored him, and he agreed. Zephyr carried the sisters from the crag to the palace, where Psyche showered them with rich gifts. Later at home, they plotted jealously to make Psyche believe that her husband was the monster. Again, Eros warned Psyche of their evil intent and also informed her that she was pregnant with their child, which should be enough to bring her joy. But Psyche cried, and Eros permitted the sisters to visit. The sisters convinced Psyche that her husband was a venomous snake and their child a monster. They encouraged her to light an oil lamp to see her husband while he slept, and prepare a razor to kill him. At night, after Eros fell asleep, Psyche lit her lamp and beheld a beautiful divine youth. In excitement, she pricked her finger with one of his arrows, fell in love and stooped to kiss him. A drop of hot oil from the lamp fell on Eros's shoulder, waking and wounding him. Furious that he had been disobeyed, Eros flew off to his mother, Aphrodite, to care for his wound.

Psyche found herself suddenly alone in an ordinary landscape with no castle. Tormented by her loss, she tried to drown herself in a river, but the river returned her to the bank. She then saw Pan embracing Echo. Pan advised Psyche to win Eros back by tender submission, like Echo, having a sweet voice, but one that is heard only when reflecting others. Psyche did not answer but continued her journey to her sister's town, and for the first time, she used guile. She told her sister that Eros no longer wanted her, but instead would marry her sister. Overjoyed, the sister went to the cliff expecting Zephyr to carry her to Eros's palace. She threw herself into the wind, but fell and drowned. The second sister perished in the same way. Psyche had now quietly rebelled. At the temples of Hera and Demeter, she sought help to return to Eros, but both goddesses refused. They knew that Aphrodite had sent Hermes to find Psyche, but they chastised Aphrodite for denying her son his passion for Psyche. Aphrodite sought revenge for being shamed by a mortal woman and took the role of a "pitiless wicked stepmother."

Weary and pregnant, Psyche gave herself up to Aphrodite, expecting to die, but instead, Aphrodite beat her and threw grains of corn, barley, millet, poppy seed, lentils and chickpeas into a jumbled heap. She bade Psyche to sort the grains into individual piles until her return that evening. Psyche was overwhelmed, but a horde of tiny ants swiftly separated the heap into individual grains and then left. Aphrodite returned and could not believe that Psyche had separated the grains alone. The next morning, she pointed Psyche to a grove near a river where a herd of golden-fleeced sun rams grazed, and told her to quickly bring back some of their wool. Psyche thought to cast herself from a cliff above the river, but a green reed gently murmured that in the morning sun the rams absorbed heat and became destructive, but later while they slept she could gather the wool clinging to leaves and twigs. She brought the wool to Aphrodite who frowned and suspected that Psyche had received guidance. For the third task, she handed Psyche a small crystal jar and asked her to fill it with icy water from the summit of a high mountain peak, where a black stream flooded the swamps below, flowing into the rivers Styx and Cocytus. Near the peak, the waters, guarded by fierce dragons, warned Psyche not to approach. Suddenly, an eagle, sent by Zeus, seized the urn in its beak and passed through to the waters and filled it. Psyche joyfully returned the full urn to Aphrodite, who accused her of being a sorceress and gave her a fourth impossible task.

Psyche was to take a small casket to Persephone in Hades, to fill with a small portion of her beauty and bring this back to Aphrodite. Psyche immediately went to a high tower to throw herself off. If she was doomed to enter the underworld, she would do it with honor, and this way she would not return. But the tower spoke and directed her to a place called Taenarus, where a path would lead her to the underworld. But first she had to prepare two cakes of barley and mead, carry two coins in her mouth, then walk in silence and ignore the pleas for help from those she encountered on the way—traps devised by Aphrodite to stop her. And in Hades, she must eat only a crust of bread, sit on the floor at Persephone's feet and never open the casket. Psyche descended the path from Taenarus, ignored an old donkey driver, gave one coin to Charon the ferryman to cross the river, paid no heed to the floating dead or weaving women begging for help, gave a cake to Cerberus, the three-headed dog who guards the gates, and entered the house of Persephone. She refused food, ate only a crust of bread, sat on the floor and delivered the casket to Persephone with Aphrodite's message. Immediately, the casket was filled and sealed. Psyche took it and left, gave the second cake to Cerberus, gave the ferryman the second coin and walked quickly towards daylight. But as she approached the conscious light of day, she wanted to beautify herself for Eros with some of the divine beauty concealed within the casket, and she opened it. A cloud of sleep poured over her and she fell, motionless on the path. Eros, meanwhile, had suffered from his wound but more from desire for Psyche. Now that his wound had healed, he slipped away and flew swiftly to her. He wiped the sleep off her, returned it to the casket and woke her, telling her to quickly return to Aphrodite and complete her task. He then flew to Zeus who granted his marriage to Psyche. Hermes assembled all the gods so that all could agree that it was time for Eros to settle down in wedlock to Psyche for all eternity. He consoled Aphrodite that this would be a lawful marriage. Zeus summoned Psyche to heaven and offered her a goblet of Ambrosia, making her immortal. All the gods celebrated their wedding, and soon a daughter was born to them, whose name was Pleasure.

Neumann's commentary on the myth of Eros and Psyche (1973)

"Eros and Psyche, the Psychic Development of the Feminine" relates to myth as the representation of crucial archetypal life experiences—in this case, a young bride married to a monster, a marriage of death of the maiden (Neumann, 1973, p.64). Psyche, a mortal woman born from the earth impregnated by "a drop of heaven's dew," eventually won the contest with Aphrodite, a goddess born from the sea, and became immortal, symbolizing the drop of divinity in each of us. Psyche's journey began with passive acceptance of her marriage to a monster, but instead she was swallowed symbolically in paradise, imprisoned in unconscious darkness while enjoying love. She passively obeyed her jealous sisters to "throw light" on the "monster," perhaps unconsciously resenting being dominated by an unknown husband. Light was the turning point for her. She emerged from darkness and consciously fell in love with a visible Eros, becoming his equal. But Eros based his love on feminine submission. He resisted change to his archetypal status, banished Psyche from paradise and flew angrily home to his mother. Both Psyche and Eros lost their lover and both suffered the pain of loss. But Psyche's loyalty to her divine lover, despite her propensity to suicide, led to transformation and illumination of them both (p.138).

Aphrodite's four impossible tasks forced Psyche into action and despair. But with each of the first three tasks, helpful forces of nature appeared. Instinctual ants connected to earth taught sorting. The small voice of a river reed taught her conscious planning, timing and patience needed to obtain the ram's golden fleece and avoid their deadly aggression. An eagle, Zeus's bird of the air, a masculine aspect of wisdom and spirit, enabled Psyche's journey to continue. She completed her final, most difficult task alone, following instructions from a tower that spoke with a human voice. The tower was a man-made structure, built stone by stone on a foundation. It warned her that desperate people would beg her for help on the way, but these were dangers that Aphrodite put in her path that she must avoid, placing her own interests first. She learned to prepare herself for other dangers, soaking cakes in mead for Cerberus to make him drowsy, and coins to pay Charon who carried her across the river, not eating foods offered by Persephone except for a crust of brown bread which represents the numinosity of the ordinary, sitting only on the floor. She had to remember her goal to return safely and reunite with Eros, and not open the casket of beauty containing Persephone's face cream for Aphrodite.

In Hades, Psyche followed the advice given her. She left the underworld with the beauty cream in a sealed box and almost reached daylight. But in her desire to be beautiful for Eros, she disobeyed and opened the box of divine beauty, releasing the sleep of death. She fell unconscious to the ground. Symbolically, this act represents the death of her old passive attitude. Her "failure," just at the moment of her success, activated Eros who flew to her, incubating a rebirth. Eros was now a committed man who asked Zeus to legalize his marriage to Psyche. The gods approved, and Psyche was transported to Olympus. After their wedding, Eros left his mother, who accepted Psyche, and Psyche gave birth to a daughter, Pleasure, who connects earth–moon consciousness with the solar realm. This consciousness, rooted in the senses but linked to illumination, heals and joins two opposite kinds of consciousness, a Holy Union, Hierosgamos. Jung writes: "Although the opposites flee from one another, they nevertheless strive for balance, since a state of conflict is too inimical of life to be endured indefinitely" (Jung, 1971, para. 307).

Theseus, the Hero and his journey

King Aegeus of Athens had no male heir and consulted the oracle of Delphi. Her words were "Do not loosen the bulging mouth of the wineskin until you have reached the height of Athens, lest you die of grief." Aegeus, not understanding the meaning, went to visit King Pittheus of Troezen who was known as an interpreter of prophesies. Pittheus understood, got Aegeus drunk that night and gave him his daughter Aethra to bed. That same night, Aethra received a dream from the goddess Athena, instructing her to leave the sleeping Aegeus and wade to an island close to shore. There she would pour a libation to attract Poseidon, God of the Sea. Poseidon came and possessed her there. When Aethra became pregnant, Aegeus, afraid of his enemies and wanting to protect the child, warned Aethra and Pittheus to keep secret that he was the father. Aegeus left his sword and sandals under a great rock for his son to retrieve when he was 16 years old and returned to Athens. Theseus was born nine months later, a child with double paternity, with one immortal and one mortal father. When he was old enough, Aethra took Theseus to the rock and revealed his true parentage. He lifted the rock easily, took the sword and sandals and left for Athens with these tokens to meet Aegeus (Graves, 1955/1960, pp.323–344).

Two routes led to Athens. By sea, Theseus would be protected by Poseidon, while the land path around the Saronic Gulf was dangerous. Along the way, there were six entrances to the underworld guarded by six chthonic monsters that beset travelers and killed them. Theseus was young, brave and ambitious, and chose the land route. At Epidaurus, sacred to Apollo and to the healer Asclepius, he met Periphetes, who waylaid travelers and beat them to death with a heavy metal club. Theseus asked to examine the club, then beat Periphetes to death with it, taking the club for his own. Further on, he met Sinis, the "pine bender." Sinis would bend a pine tree to the ground and ask a traveler to help him hold it. When the traveler seized the tree, Sinis released his grip and the traveler would be flung to his death. Theseus tricked Sinis the same way, into being thrown by his own tree. He then slept with Sinis's daughter Perigune, and fathered a son, Melanippus. In Crommyon, the local inhabitants were terrorized by an enormous man-eating pig bred by an old crone named Phaea. He was an offspring of Typhon, the hundred-headed dragon, a monstrous serpentine giant. Theseus killed both the pig and Phaea, and freed the area from them. Theseus's fourth encounter was with Sciron, an old robber who sat on a narrow high rock pass where he forced passersby to wash his feet. When they complied, he kicked them off the cliff into the sea where a great turtle devoured them. Theseus tricked him as well and threw him into the sea. He continued on to Eleusis and met Cercyon, a vicious wrestler who crushed each traveler to death. Theseus overcame him by applying conscious skill rather than brute force, thereby inventing the principles of wrestling. In Eleusis, a robber named Procrustes captured travelers and laid them out on his bed. If the traveler's feet were too long for his bed, he chopped them off. He placed shorter travelers on another bed and stretched them to fit. Theseus forced him to fit his own body to the bed and killed him. "Procrustes's bed" symbolizes an inflexible preconceived attitude that disregards the reality confronted, and brutally forces it to conform to one's preconceptions.

King Aegeus had given refuge to Medea, a priestess with magical powers who fled Corinth after killing her four children in revenge at her husband, Jason, who left her. Medea planned that her son with Aegeus would inherit the throne of Athens. Theseus arrived in Athens unaware of his father's marriage and unaware that Aegeus had caused the death of Androgeus, the only son of King Minos of Crete, by sending him to battle in Marathon. King Minos demanded retribution. Every nine years, Aegeus would send seven maidens and seven young men to Crete to be devoured by the Minotaur, a half-human, half-bull creature who lived in a labyrinth built by the architect Daedalus, in Knossos, Crete. King Minos was the eldest of three sons of Zeus, Lord of Olympus, and the Phoenician Princess Europa, whom Zeus saw picking flowers in a meadow. Zeus transformed himself into a beautiful, gentle white Bull. Europa mounted him, but the Bull ran away with her, and many sea gods and nymphs appeared. Europa realized that the Bull must also be a god. Zeus revealed himself and his love for her, promised her no harm and assured her that their sons would be famous. Europa later married Asterion, King of Crete, who adopted her sons. After his death, Minos took the throne aided by the god Poseidon, and banished his brothers. As a sign of their relationship, Poseidon sent Minos a beautiful white bull that emerged from the sea and asked that he sacrifice the bull. But Minos took the bull for himself and sacrificed an ordinary bull instead. Angry and insulted, Poseidon punished him, with help from Aphrodite, who caused Minos's wife Pasiphae to fall passionately in love with the white bull. At Pasiphae's request, Daedalus constructed a hollow wooden cow that Pasiphae could enter and couple with the bull. She gave birth to their son, the Minotaur, a monster with a bull's head and a human body. Pasiphae nursed him until he grew into a ferocious beast who devoured humans for sustenance. The Delphic oracle advised Minos to ask Daedalus to construct a labyrinth beneath the palace at Knossos, for the Minotaur.

Theseus arrived in Athens just when a third group of young men and women were to be sent to Crete to feed the Minotaur. Medea recognized Theseus. To prevent him from displacing her son as ruler, she told Aegeus that Theseus was a spy and offered him a poisoned drink. But Aegeus recognized the sword he had left for his son years before, dashed the poisoned cup from Theseus's hands and declared him heir to the throne. Theseus volunteered to kill the Minotaur and joined the youths being sent to Crete. He promised his father that if he returned alive from Crete, he would hoist white sails on his boat. If the boat returned with black sails, this would mean that Theseus had been killed.

In Crete, Theseus and the 14 Athenian youths debarked from his ship and were paraded through the town. Minos's daughter Ariadne instantly fell in love with Theseus. Theseus prevented King Minos from raping one of the Greek maidens, and an altercation began between them. To prove his relationship to Poseidon, Theseus retrieved a ring that Minos threw into the sea. He announced that he would kill the Minotaur, but Minos assumed that even so he would never find his way out of the labyrinth. Ariadne, the Minotaur's half-sister, offered to help Theseus if he would marry her and take her with him to Athens. He promised, and she handed him a ball of flaxen thread given to her by Daedalus, architect of the labyrinth. Theseus would simply tie the thread at the entrance of the labyrinth and follow the path of the ball as it rolled along inside. He later could retrace his steps and exit the labyrinth. Theseus found the Minotaur asleep in the center of the labyrinth, killed it with his bare hands and followed the thread back to the entrance. He, Ariadne and the Athenian youths ran to their ship and sailed towards Athens. At the island of Naxos, they stopped to celebrate.

In the morning, Ariadne lay asleep on the beach. She awoke alone. Theseus and the others had sailed from Naxos without her. Some say that Theseus had achieved his purpose, was tired of Ariadne and abandoned her. Others say that the god Dionysus came to Theseus in a dream and told him to leave Ariadne as he wanted her. Theseus, the hero, broke his promise to Ariadne, the helpful feminine, and both would now travel separate paths. That morning, Dionysus returned from adventures in far parts of the world and landed on Naxos. He saw the beautiful Ariadne alone on the beach and immediately fell in love. Their marriage opened a new joyous approach to life for her and helped her to heal (Graves, 1955/1960, pp.103–106). As Theseus and his ship approached Athens, he forgot to raise white sails to indicate that he was victorious. King Aegeus saw a ship with black sails. He believed that his son was dead, jumped into the sea and drowned. Theseus was crowned King of Athens and created a model of government that became a prototype for Greek and Roman culture. He fathered a son, Hippolytus, with the Amazon Hippolyte, who was devoted to the virgin goddess Artemis and rejected love. This angered Aphrodite, Goddess of Love. When Theseus married Phaedra, sister of Ariadne, she caused Phaedra to fall in love with her stepson, Hippolytus. When he refused her, she falsely accused him of rape and killed herself. Theseus believed her lie, banished Hippolytus and prayed to Poseidon for revenge. Poseidon sent a charging bull out of the sea just as Hippolytus drove his horse-drawn chariot along the shore. The frightened horses reared up, Hippolytus fell from the chariot and was killed. Too late, Artemis revealed the truth to Theseus, but the boy was already dead. Theseus's reign signified the rising power of Greek civilization, the end of Cretan domination of the Mediterranean and the transition from a matriarchal to a patriarchal civilization. The later Greek male-dominated culture incorporated the Minoan Pantheon into their culture and changed their myths. Minoan culture declined and disappeared by 1100 BC.

Minoan civilization, Greek civilization and the bull

The bull was a major symbol in myth and in the visual arts throughout the Minoan era (3500–1100 BC). Archaeologist Sir Arthur Evans began excavations at Knossos in 1900, and coined the term "Minoan" after the legendary King Minos. Crete was first settled around 9000 BC by people from Asia Minor. Their knowledge of irrigation, agriculture, animal husbandry and fishing ensured their independence and provided a variety of food products for trade. They also traded their fine pottery, weapons, tools and jewelry at Minoan colonies in the Mediterranean. In Knossos, a high central building was connected to over 1000 interlocking rooms, similar to the labyrinth of the myth, with spacious living quarters, plumbing, storerooms, workshops and spaces for food processing. Large painted murals depicted men hunting, women dancing, ships, dolphins and sea creatures, and a bull-riding sport with acrobats somersaulting off the back of a bull, while grasping its horns. In 1903, two sculpted statuettes of bare-breasted goddesses were discovered at Knossos, each holding a snake in each hand, one with a cat on her head (dated at 1600 BC).

Ariadne may have been a Great Mother goddess who ruled the Minoan Pantheon without a male consort. On frescoes, the goddess is shown among flowers and sacred animals. The meticulous attention to detail, design and color of clothing, hairstyles, jewelry and symbols, such as the labrys, the double-headed ax, a tree, pillar and serpents, indicate that by 3500 BC the people of Crete had built the first advanced civilization in Europe. By 1700 BC, several city-states with large central palaces existed at Knossos, Phaistos and other places. As the Greeks took over, the one great goddess was divided into many different goddesses, each one representing a single trait (Bolen, 1984). Ariadne's power was reduced, but her association with the labyrinth and the ball of flaxen thread continues to represent the helpful anima aiding the masculine ego to find a path through the unconscious. The thread leads to the womb-center of being and, like an umbilical cord, enables return from death into a rebirth of consciousness in the world. Flax is a product of human ingenuity: learning to cultivate the plant, cull and prepare its fibers, spin them into thread and weave them together into a whole totality. The ball of flax is round, like the Self, with a center and periphery. It rolls along as Theseus follows within the labyrinth towards his destiny, mastering the primordial masculine energy of the half-bull monster at the center of the unconscious, and then led by the umbilical cord of flax outwards, to rebirth, ego-directed consciousness and his own refined masculinity.

Ariadne, Mistress of the Labyrinth

Graves (1955/1960, p.106) theorized that Ariadne, meaning "utterly pure," was a great goddess, "the first divine personage of Greek mythology to be immediately recognized in Crete." As "Mistress of the Labyrinth," she presided over a winding dance-ground and a prison for the Minotaur at its center. Ariadne's father, King Minos, was a son of Zeus, ruler of Olympus, and her mother, Queen Pasiphae, was a daughter of Helios the sun god, who drove the chariot of the sun daily across the sky, pulled by four horses. But as a woman, Ariadne's royal lineage did not empower her to decide her own future. Her father appointed her as caretaker of the labyrinth, attending to sacrifices made there to Poseidon or Athena, and to her half-brother the Minotaur, waiting for the youths that fed him every nine years. With Theseus, she could escape Crete. She gave him the flaxen thread that led him to the Minotaur in the labyrinth and back out. He promised to marry her. They left Crete and stopped on the island of Naxos. Ariadne awoke in the morning, alone and abandoned. Some say that, in a dream, Dionysus threatened Theseus to forsake Ariadne, and in his grief he forgot to lower the black sail, causing his father's death. Others say that he simply left her. Fortunately, Dionysus discovered Ariadne, made her his wife and raised her among the immortals. He placed the crown which he gave her at their marriage among the stars as the constellation Corona Borealis (Bulfinch, 1979, p.199). The couple had 12 children.

Ariadne's symbol of thread, fate, weaving and spiders

The Three Fates are the fatherless daughters of Night, who decide on human destiny in the form of thread. Clotho spins the thread of one's existence, Lachesis measures its length, and Atropos cuts it. A thread woven into a single cloth determined the limits of one's life. The spider, who so precisely weaves its web in a single night from silk secreted from glands near its abdomen, is known as a creator in the Native American lore of Grandmother Spider or Spider Woman, and may be thanked for her medicine in keeping other pests away. The spider's web is its home and a place to lay its eggs and trap prey, and as such is a symbol of entrapment. Spinning and weaving, the spindle and distaff, seem to have been invented in the Mediterranean sometime between AD 500 and 1000, and were documented in art around AD 1200. Athena, daughter of Zeus, was patroness of spinning yarn, weaving cloth and of war, all based on strategic planning.

Dionysus, God of Wine, Ecstasy and Love

Zeus took the form of an eagle and flew over his temple. He saw Semele, a priestess at his altar. She had just slaughtered a bull to him and was bathing herself clean in the river. They began a secret affair that was discovered by Hera, wife of Zeus, when Semele was six months pregnant. Hera visited Semele disguised as an old crone and gained her confidence. Semele admitted that her lover was a god, but Hera implied that he might be lying and encouraged Semele to ask him to reveal himself, knowing that exposure to Zeus's thunderbolt would burn her to death. Zeus tried to persuade Semele not to ask this, but she persisted. He hurled his thunderbolt, killing Semele in the fire.

Gaia, Mother Earth, took pity on the unborn child and ordered ivy vines to cover the pillars of the house, protecting the fetus from the flames. Zeus cut open his thigh, placed the fetal Dionysus inside and sewed up the flesh. Three months later, he opened his thigh, and Dionysus was born, his name meaning "twice born." Some say that he was born with horns, around which Zeus wrapped a crown of snakes. Zeus sent him to Ino, Semele's sister, to rear. But Hera discovered this, and Zeus changed Dionysus into a baby goat and sent him to be raised by nymphs in a cave on Mount Nyas. He grew up surrounded by women, often disguised as a girl so Hera would not find him. In the forests, he discovered wild grapes, learned to make wine and began to teach this to others.

In another version of the birth of Dionysus, Hera made the Titans dismember the newborn infant and eat his body parts, except for the heart, from which Zeus reconstituted Dionysus. He threw a thunderbolt at the Titans to punish them and turned them to dust that contained sparks of their energy and parts of Dionysus that they had eaten. The dust was then used to form humans, who now contained both Titan specks and specks of Dionysian energy.

Hera pursued Dionysus relentlessly, drove him mad and caused him to wander from place to place. The Titaness Rhea, his grandmother, healed his madness and aimless wandering. As an adult, Dionysus was described as a beautiful man, sitting on a leopard, his staff wound with ivy. He traveled the world with bands of women called Maenads, who set up places of worship and wild orgies, and instilled the culture of fermenting grapes and wine making.

Drinking alcohol can transform the personality, in moderation to ecstasy, in excess to suffering, violence and madness. Dionysus represents the polarities of inner transformation of the human spirit through wine, believed to contain the "spirit" of the grain from which it is brewed. Transformation can enhance true creativity, which often comes upon us unpredictably. It can symbolize renewal of life, sudden insight, truth and the understanding that brings change. Dionysus presided over ecstatic celebrations in forests beyond the bounds of civilized order and appeared suddenly in new places, causing excitement, joy and terror. While traveling in the Aegean Sea, a band of pirates captured him to sell as a slave for ransom. He covered their ship with creeping vines and wild beasts, and transformed himself into a lion and the terrified pirates into dolphins as they leaped overboard. He then landed on Naxos and discovered Ariadne, whom he married for love rather than for masculine domination and rape, characteristic of other male gods. A temple for Dionysus was built on Naxos. Some say that Perseus, also a son of Zeus, turned Ariadne to stone with the snake-wreathed head of Medusa. Dionysus descended to Hades and retrieved Ariadne and his mother, Semele, and they joined the gods on Olympus.

Asclepius, Healer, God of Medicine

Asclepius's name means "to cut open." His father, Apollo, God of the Sun, healing, truth, prophecy, and music, cut him from the womb of his dying mother Coronis, in the world's first cesarean section. Apollo fell in love with the mortal princess Coronis. When she became pregnant, Apollo returned to Delphi, leaving a white raven to watch over her. In his absence, Coronis fell in love with a mortal. The white raven notified Apollo of her infidelity which so infuriated him that he turned all ravens black. He asked his twin sister, Artemis, Moon Goddess and Goddess of the Hunt, to shoot Coronis with her arrow. A funeral pyre was prepared, and just before the flames consumed her, Apollo rescued his unborn son from Coronis's womb.

Asclepius was raised by the Centaur Chiron, himself a wounded healer, who taught him the art of medicine. It is said that Asclepius also received secret healing knowledge from a snake that licked his ears clean and taught him wisdom, healing and resurrection. Asclepius was once summoned to heal the sick son of King Minos of Crete. He was locked in a room with the boy when a snake slithered under the door. Asclepius killed it, but then a second snake entered with a leaf and placed it on the first snake, who returned to life. Asclepius took the leaf and healed Minos' son with it. Since then, the snake has been associated with Asclepius and healing.

Asclepius's skill was so great that he could evade death and bring others back to life, such as Hippolytus, son of Theseus. Zeus, fearful of overpopulation of humans and that Asclepius could render all men immortal, warned him never to revive the dead without his approval. But Hades worried that dead spirits would no longer come to the underworld. So Zeus slew Asclepius with a thunderbolt. In revenge, Apollo slew the Cyclopes who made the thunderbolt. Zeus punished Apollo by ordering him to serve as a goatherd for a year to King Admetus of Thessaly. Apollo helped Admetus, causing his cows to have twin births, and winning Alcestis for his wife. After a year, Apollo returned to Mount Olympus, and Zeus revived the Cyclopes that made his thunderbolts. To appease his son Apollo, Zeus placed the body of Asclepius among the stars as the constellation Ophiuchus, the Serpent Holder, and made him a god. It was then said that a healer who cured someone who was fated to die challenged divine decree. He would forfeit his own life, dying in place of the cured patient, just as Zeus killed Asclepius after he brought Hippolytus back to life.

Asclepius is also the grandson of Leto and Zeus, parents of Apollo the Sun God and his twin sister, Artemis the Moon Goddess. Leto, daughter of the Titans Croesus and Phoebe, suffered greatly during her pregnancy as Hera, Zeus's jealous wife, cursed her to not find any solid ground on Earth on which to give birth. Zeus secretly created the floating island of Delos for Leto, where she gave birth easily to Artemis. But Hera prevented the Goddess of Childbirth, Eileithyia, from helping Leto with the painful birth of Apollo which lasted for nine days and nights. Artemis then helped deliver her twin brother under a palm tree in the presence of all the gods and goddesses except Hera. This confirmed Apollo's and Artemis's right to be Olympian gods. Hera continued to harass Leto, Apollo and Artemis, and they wandered for years. They were very thirsty when they arrived in Lycia, but peasants stirred up mud in the well so the water was undrinkable. In anger, Leto turned the peasants into frogs. Eventually, Zeus received Apollo and Artemis on Olympus to live as gods but Leto settled in Thebes. There she endured the insults of Queen Niobe who claimed superiority to Leto as she had given birth to seven male and seven female children, not two. In anger, Apollo and Artemis killed all of Niobe's children. Zeus turned Niobe into a pillar of stone to end her grief. It is said that people who passed by could see the stone weep tears.

In Greek sculpture, Asclepius is shown standing, wearing a long cloak open at the chest, holding his staff with one serpent coiled around it. The Rod of Asclepius is today the physician's symbol, a healing scepter entwined with one non-venomous snake. A similar staff, the caduceus, sometimes used as a medical emblem, is winged and has two intertwined snakes wrapped around it. This is the magic wand of Hermes, Messenger of the Gods and the patron of trade. The two snakes that are intertwined around Hermes's caduceus might refer to a myth in which Athena took two vials of blood from Medusa. Blood from the right side had great healing power and could raise the dead, but the blood from the left side was instantly fatal. Athena gave these vials to Asclepius. The "blood opposites" may refer to the snakes on Hermes's caduceus, mirroring unconscious opposites that can be helpful or harmful, depending on the context of their use.

Asclepius was first worshipped as a god in the fifth century BC. In the Greek world, his temples were very popular, with the most important on the island of Kos and at Epidaurus. His cult spread from Greece to Rome in 293 BC, and by the third century AD, 500 temples dedicated to Asclepius were located from Europe to Egypt and as far as Persia. The Asclepieion at Epidaurus held 180 rooms, with a large theater and a tholos, a round underground shrine where snakes were kept. A temple received pilgrims who were chronically ill or dying, and women in labor. After arrival at the site, a pilgrim would pay homage to the gods, perform a prayer or a sacrifice assisted by physicians or priests, give monetary gifts or sleep at the temple. Following this was a stage of "Katharsis" or purification, a series of baths and purging, such as a clean diet for several days and attending a drama in the theater to purge emotions. The patient would then offer money or a prayer, followed by "incubation" or dream therapy. The patient would sleep in the temple, and perhaps during the night a god or Asclepius himself would visit the dreamer. It was believed that Asclepius could cure the sick in dreams or give directions for the appropriate treatment of an illness. If he did not "visit" the patient, while he dreamed, the dream could be discussed in the morning with a dream-interpreter who prescribed treatment.

Hippocrates, father of the "Hippocratic Oath," was born in Kos in 460 BC and claimed to be descended from Asclepius. He observed and recorded descriptions of disease and realized that illness results from natural causes rather than from superstition. In Epidaurus, engraved on marble in 350 BC, are names, case histories and surgical procedures of many patients who were treated and cured at the temple, some while "asleep," possibly induced by opium. In AD 325, when the Emperor Constantine converted to Christianity, the temples became Christian centers. The Temple of Kos was destroyed in an earthquake in AD 544, but Hygieia, the daughter of Asclepius, remained a symbol of health into the Christian era.

Chiron the Centaur, mentor to Asclepius: two "wounded healers"

Chiron the Centaur was born half horse and half human. His parents, the Titan Cronus and the nymph Philyra, were interrupted during their tryst by Rhea, wife of Cronus. To deceive her, Cronus changed himself into a horse. Philyra was ashamed to have given birth to a Centaur and abandoned him. Zeus turned her into a Linden tree and Chiron was reared by Apollo and his sister Artemis, who taught him the arts of music and medicine. He was peaceful and intelligent, and tutored many Greek heroes, such as Achilles, who played the lyre, and Asclepius, whom he raised and trained as a healer. In Greek art, Chiron was portrayed as a man dressed in clothes that covered his human front legs, while behind he was attached to the body and hind legs of a horse. Other centaurs were wild creatures born from a cloud formed by Zeus to resemble his wife Hera, to deceive King Ixion who tried to seduce her. They had the upper body of a man and entire lower body of a horse. Chiron was accidentally wounded in the knee by a poisoned arrow dipped in Hydra-venom, which caused such unending pain that he gave up his immortality. He was the first "wounded healer," curing others despite his own suffering. Zeus placed him among the stars as the constellation Sagittarius or Centaurus.

Orpheus and Eurydice, descent into the underworld

The gods are eternal, but humans descend to Hades only once, in death. Just a few have returned to life on earth. Psyche was sent by Aphrodite to the underworld to fill a small casket with Persephone's beauty cream. She succeeded, but at the last minute, she opened the casket and was covered by the sleep of death. Luckily, Eros saved her and raised her to Olympus.

Dionysus descended to Hades to retrieve his wife, Ariadne, and his mother, Semele, whom he had never seen, and raised them both to Olympus. Odysseus, seeking advice from the dead seer Tiresias, stood at the entrance of the underworld, spoke to Tiresias, his dead mother and others, and left in time. In the following myth, Eurydice and Orpheus are two young mortal lovers who lived briefly, were given a second chance at life, but were reclaimed by the underworld.

Calliope, the eldest of the Nine Muses, goddesses of the arts, married King Oeagrus and gave birth to Orpheus, although some say that Apollo was his father. Calliope loved song, dance and epic poetry. Her son Orpheus showed such poetic skill and grace that Apollo adopted him and taught him to play the lyre. His beautiful music enchanted wild beasts, trees and rocks who moved with the sound of his music (Graves, 1955/1960, pp.111–113). He accompanied Jason and the Argonauts in their quest to obtain the magical healing golden fleece and saved the crew of the *Argo* from disaster with his music, which surpassed the bewitching song of the Sirens. Orpheus fell in love with beautiful Eurydice and married her, but Hymen the God of Marriage prophesied that their happiness would not last. Soon after, Eurydice wandered in the forest with nymphs, when Aristaeus, a shepherd with erotic intentions, began to chase her. As she fled, she trod on a snake, was bitten and died instantly. In his grief, Orpheus sang and played his lyre with such feeling that humans and gods alike were touched. He descended to Hades to find Eurydice. His music charmed Charon, the ferryman, and Cerberus, the three-headed dog guarding the gate to the underworld, and soothed the tortures of the damned. Hades and his wife Persephone were so touched that Hades allowed Orpheus to restore Eurydice to life, on condition that he would not look behind him until he was out in the light of day. Orpheus began walking towards the upper world, but could not hear Eurydice's footsteps behind him. She was still a shade and would become a woman only when she returned to the light. But Orpheus, as he approached the exit, turned to see if Eurydice was really there, and spirits pulled her shadow back to the dead, never to return. Inconsolable at the second loss of his wife, Orpheus wandered, singing a song of mourning, asking to be reunited with Eurydice in death. The Maenads, wild women who served Dionysus, attacked him madly and tore him to pieces. His head fell and floated down the River Hebrus, still singing, and came to rest on the island of Lesbos, where a shrine for it was built as an eternal prophetic oracle. The Muses tearfully collected his limbs and interred them at the foot of Mount Olympus "where the nightingales now sing sweeter than anywhere else in the world" (Graves, 1955/1960, p.112). It is also said that Zeus struck Orpheus dead with lightning, to stop him from revealing knowledge of life after death and the secrets of the underworld to humans. The Orphic mysteries claimed that a life of truth and restraint would be rewarded by salvation in the underworld. Gold tablets were placed in tombs with instructions for finding the way in the underworld after death, to avoid drinking the waters of the well of Lethe that cause forgetfulness, and to drink from the well of Mnemosyne that promotes memory.

The Nine Muses were goddesses of the arts, literature and science, each with a particular artistic domain. They were created from the union of Zeus, god of Olympus, and Mnemosyne, Titan goddess of memory, to celebrate the victory of the gods in their war with the Titans. Zeus wished to calm the horrors of the war with their beautiful voices, dance and the arts. Calliope, the oldest Muse, mother of Orpheus, inspires poetry, music and writing, and inspired Homer to write *The Iliad* and *The Odyssey*. Apollo taught the Muses music and art, and wandered with them on Mount Helicon (Parnasus) where they lived. They also entertained the gods on Mount Olympus.

The epic hero Odysseus

The Greek hero Odysseus fought in the ten-year Trojan War, to retrieve Helen, wife of Menelaus of Sparta who had been kidnapped by Paris of Troy. Odysseus's great-grandfather was the god Hermes, patron of thieves. His grandfather Autolycus, son of Hermes, was a skilled cattle thief. Laertes, son of Autolycus, was father of Odysseus. Odysseus conceived a plan to end the Trojan War, whose final phase was described by the Greek poet Homer in *The Iliad* in the eighth century BC. Homer later wrote *The Odyssey* about the perilous ten-year journey of Odysseus to return home, finally washed up alone on the shores of Ithaca. Paris, son of Priam of Troy, won Helen, already married to King Menelaus of Sparta, when he judged a beauty contest between three goddesses, Hera, Athena and Aphrodite. Hera tried to bribe him with wealth, Athena offered victory, but Aphrodite offered Helen, the most beautiful woman in the world as his wife. Helen was hatched from a swan's egg, the daughter of Zeus and Leda, whom he had seduced in the form of a swan. Aphrodite caused Helen to fall in love with Paris, leave her husband and children, and go with him to Troy (Graves, 1955/1960, pp.631–738). The war began when an army of Greek heroes was sent to retrieve her. After ten years of failure, Odysseus devised a plan to overcome Troy. During the night, the Greek fleet sailed from Troy, leaving behind a gigantic wooden horse on wheels outside the city gates. At dawn, the

Trojans found the horse, believed that the Greeks had left in defeat, leaving the horse as a gift for the gods to grant them a safe voyage home. They wheeled the wooden horse into their city and celebrated the end of the war. But the Greek army was positioned just a few miles away, and hidden inside the horse were Odysseus and his men. They came out of the horse at night, slaughtered the guards and opened the city gates. The Greek army entered the city, killed and plundered, and captured Helen, who was taken back to Sparta (Mavromataki, 1997, pp.244–253).

Odysseus, his crew and 12 ships set sail for Ithaca and sighted land after a few days. With the hubris of conquerors, they went ashore intending to plunder the local Ciconians, who fled to the mountains. They looted the city, ate, drank wine and fell asleep on the shore. Before dawn, the Ciconians returned and killed many of the crew. Odysseus and his remaining men fled to their ships and set sail, carried by the winds to the land of the lotus-eaters where a narcotic lotus plant grew. Some of the men ate the lotus, became addicted and had to be forcibly carried back to the ship and bound to the masts to stop them from jumping into the sea and swimming ashore. After more weeks at sea, Odysseus and his crew landed on an island that was home to the gigantic Cyclopes, rough creatures with a single round eye, who raised sheep and ate wild plants that grew because of the rain sent by Zeus. On the island, Odysseus and his men found a large cave belonging to the Cyclops Polyphemus, son of the Sea God Poseidon. Inside the cave, they found many sheep and slaughtered and roasted a few. Polyphemus returned and closed the cave entrance with a massive rock. With his one eye, he saw the men and asked who they were. Odysseus replied that they were sailors who had come ashore looking for food. Polyphemus was angry that they had eaten his sheep, refused to let them go and ate two men every day.

But while Polyphemus was away, Odysseus and his remaining crew prepared a pointy wooden pole and burned the tip. When the Cyclops returned, Odysseus offered him wine. When he fell asleep, the men took the burning poker from the fireplace and thrust it into Polyphemus's eye, blinding him. He awoke, howling in pain and rage, and demanded to know who had done this. Odysseus shouted out that his name was "Nobody." Other Cyclopes heard the cries and came running to his cave and asked what was wrong. Polyphemus replied that "Nobody" had blinded him, so they laughed and left. At night, Odysseus and his men strapped themselves to the bellies of the sheep. In the morning, Polyphemus moved the rock, let his flocks out to graze with the men carried outside under them. They loosened the ropes and ran to their ships, but Odysseus shouted out to Polyphemus his true name, Odysseus of Ithaca. Enraged, Polyphemus threw massive rocks towards his voice and prayed to his father Poseidon, for vengeance. Consequently, Poseidon created storms wherever Odysseus sailed so that he would never reach Ithaca. His ships arrived at Aeolia, the home of Aeolus, God of the Winds, who gave Odysseus a bag containing the four winds. He instructed him to release them one by one, as each wind would help him sail safely home. Odysseus went to sleep with the bag near him, but two of his men thought that it contained wine and untied it as they neared Ithaca. All the winds roared out at once and drove the ships back to Aeolia. Aeolus refused to assist him again.

Odysseus and his ships again set sail. After seven days, they reached Telepylos, home of the Laestrygonians, a race of giant cannibals. The entrance to their harbor was a narrow passage surrounded by high cliffs. At night, 11 ships sailed into the harbor but Odysseus anchored his ship in the waters outside. Two sailors landed and were taken by a girl to her father's castle. There, a gigantic woman called to her giant husband who snatched up one man and ate him alive. The other ran to the harbor, followed by many giants who hurled rocks at the ships, speared the men and ate them. Odysseus and his ship had anchored outside the island and escaped.

They sailed to the island of Aeaea, home of Circe, a powerful enchantress and sorceress. A few men went to explore the island and were met by wolves and lions who walked on their hind legs like human beings. Circe knew that Odysseus and his men had arrived and received the crew nicely. They entered her palace and were invited to dine. But the feast was drugged, and as they ate, she transformed them with her staff into pigs. One man escaped and reported this to Odysseus who grabbed his sword to rescue them. On his way to the palace, he was met by his great-grandfather, the god Hermes, who plucked from the ground a plant called Moly, with a black root and white flower that only a god can dig up. This plant prevented Circe's magic that changed humans into beasts. Hermes told Odysseus that when Circe realized that her spells did not transform him, he should draw his sword as if to kill her. Then Circe would ask him to be her lover. As predicted, he agreed, on condition that she turn his crew from pigs back to men and restore all the other animals to human form. His stay with Circe was pleasant, and she bore him three sons, but he yearned to leave for Ithaca. Circe counseled him that to avoid Poseidon's wrath, he would first have to sail to the underworld to consult Tiresias, the dead blind seer in Tartarus, a place that no live man had ever entered.

Odysseus and his men sailed to the ocean stream and into the Grove of Persephone, wrapped in mist and fog. Odysseus, with two helpers who carried sheep to be sacrificed, walked on the downward path, and at the point described by Circe, Odysseus dug a pit and poured libations into it for the dead—honey and milk, wine, water and barley. He prayed and sacrificed the sheep to Tiresias, cut their throats over the pit so the dark blood poured down. Many souls swarmed in with an "eerie clamor." Odysseus asked his comrades to quickly flay the sheep, burn them and pray to Persephone and Hades while he prevented the spirits from coming close. But he did speak to a comrade who had died by accident near Circe's palace, and promised to return and bury him. The soul of his mother, Anticlea, approached. He did not know she had died, and with tears pushed her away until Tiresias could drink the blood. Tiresias drank the blood greedily and spoke. He warned Odysseus that Poseidon would make his journey perilous, that in Sicily he would have to prevent his crew from stealing the cattle of the sun god Hyperion, and in Ithaca he would have to kill the men who had taken over his property. But then he would have to travel with an oar on his shoulder until he reached people who had never seen the sea and did not know what the oar was. There he would sacrifice a ram, bull and boar to Poseidon and enjoy old age. But death would come to him from the sea. Odysseus thanked Tiresias. He allowed his mother to drink. She was distressed to see him there, but he explained his purpose. She spoke of his aged father's grief and yearning for Odysseus, and her own grief and heartache for him that brought her life to an end. She did not tell him that suitors had taken over his home, but said that he must quickly leave, and she slipped away. Other famous ghosts came near and told their stories (Homer, 1946/1991, pp.159–178).

Odysseus and his men sailed back to Circe, who warned that new dangers awaited. The first were the winged Sirens with bird's feet and enchanting voices that would lure his men off the ship to their island where they would be killed, unless they blocked their ears with beeswax. The ship approached the Sirens' island, the men blocked their ears, but Odysseus wanted to hear their song which was said to give to whoever heard it foreknowledge of all that happened on earth. He asked his men to tie him tightly to the ship's mast, heard their song and begged to be released. But his men could not hear him and they sailed past in safety. Danger arose again when their ship had to pass between two cliffs guarded by two terrible monsters. Scylla had been a beautiful woman, but was changed into a six-headed dog-like monster with 12 feet who ate sailors off the decks of passing ships. Charybdis was cursed by Zeus with an unquenchable thirst for the sea, and three times a day she created a huge whirlpool that sucked ships into it. Odysseus bypassed Charybdis and sailed close to Scylla, who caught six sailors and ate one in each mouth. Odysseus and his ship had to leave them behind and sailed on towards Sicily. Odysseus forbade his men to steal the cattle of the sun god Helios, but while he slept, a few men landed and slaughtered and roasted a few cows. In the morning, Odysseus was furious at the slaughter. But Helios complained to Zeus, who sank the ship with a thunderbolt and everyone drowned. Odysseus clutched the floating mast as it drifted back into Charybdis's whirlpool, then clung to a tree until it resurfaced and paddled on it with his hands for nine days.

The lovely nymph Calypso lived in Ogygia in a large, sheltered cavern near the beach. She welcomed Odysseus as he stumbled up and offered him immortality if he stayed with her. Seven years later, Calypso would still not release him until Zeus ordered her to let him go. She gave him tools to build a raft and food and clothes for the journey. But on the sea, Poseidon sent a huge wave that almost drowned him. He managed to rise to the surface, shed his heavy clothes and regain the raft. Then the sea goddess Ino appeared beside him and gave him her veil to wrap around his chest, which would save him if he swam again in the sea. Poseidon sent another wave that shattered the raft, and then descended to his undersea palace. As Odysseus swam, the goddess Athena sent a wind to flatten the waves in his path. Two days later, he was cast ashore naked on the island of the Phaeacians and fell asleep on the sand. In the morning, he awoke to the shouts of some girls playing ball. Nausicaa, daughter of King Alcinous and Queen Arete, saw him and had him taken to the palace where he was received kindly. A bard at the court entertained them with "tales of Odysseus and the Trojan War." With tearful eyes, Odysseus revealed his identity and told them the stories of his adventures. The Phaeacians gave him gifts and a ship with an escort who brought him to Ithaca, and left him sleeping on the sand in a cove.

Athena appeared and greatly assisted Odysseus to reclaim his property and meet his wife Penelope, who had been plagued for ten years by over a hundred suitors asking for her hand. She had delayed them by weaving a burial shroud for Laertes, Odysseus's father, and said she would marry when it was complete. But at night she unraveled what she wove in the daytime and the shroud was never finished. Athena transformed Odysseus into an old beggar and sent him to the shack of Eumaeus, his old swineherd. She then told Telemachus, his son, to visit the shack and transformed Odysseus to his normal form. Father and son were reunited and planned to fight the suitors. Odysseus went to his palace disguised as a beggar. His old dog Argus recognized him, but Odysseus ignored him to preserve his disguise, and Argus died of sorrow.

Penelope didn't recognize him, but he told her that her husband was alive, and a hero of the Trojan War. Penelope then set the suitors an impossible task. She would marry the one who could string Odysseus's bow and shoot an arrow through 12 ax-handles joined together. None of the suitors had the strength to do this. They ridiculed Odysseus as he strung the bow, but with one shot he succeeded and then proceeded to massacre some of the suitors who had desecrated his home. Penelope was unable to believe that this beggar was her husband, and tested him. In Odysseus's presence she ordered the servants to remove the bed from her chamber to the hall outside, but Odysseus said this was impossible as he had made the bed from a living oak and it could not be moved. Penelope knew that this was her husband and embraced Odysseus. He told her about his adventures and that Tiresias had prophesied that he would have to journey inland to a place far from the sea, and make a sacrifice to Poseidon. He then massacred the rest of the suitors and killed several treacherous maids. He visited his old father, gently revealing that he had returned. The fathers of the dead suitors wished to avenge their son's deaths, but the goddess Athena ended the conflict and established peace.

Here ended Homer's *Odyssey*, but unfinished strands of his story continued in a lost poem, the *Telegony*, written by Eugammon in the sixth century BC. As Tiresias prophesied, Odysseus traveled inland with a ship's oar and reached a land far from the sea, where people thought the oar was a winnowing fan. He made a sacrifice to Poseidon and married a local princess. It is also said that he ruled Ithaca until Telegonus, his son with Circe, came to find him but then accidentally killed him with a poisoned arrow. Odysseus was buried on Aeaea, Telegonus married Penelope, Telemachus then married Circe, who made everyone immortal.

Hecate, Triple Goddess of the Crossroads, Witchcraft and the Household

Hecate was once a widely revered, beautiful and powerful goddess, honored by Zeus above all others and a welcome guest in Hades. It is said that Hecate, a fourth-generation Titan, helped Zeus become the undisputed ruler of the Universe in the war between Titans and gods. Zeus then stripped the Titans of most of their powers, except for Hecate, who was privileged to transcend the boundaries between sky, earth, the seas and the underworld. Zeus shared with Hecate the power of giving humanity anything she wished, or withholding it if she pleased. The number three, a dynamic number which leads towards change, was associated with Hecate. She was often portrayed with three human heads, or with three animal heads, a snake, horse and boar, or as three women standing closely back to back. She represents the three stages of a woman's life—maiden, mother and crone.

Hecate saw in all directions at once, and into the past, present and future. She noticed detail and took great interest in things that others might think irrelevant. She was guardian of places of transition, roads, crossroads, city walls, borders, doorways and realms outside or beyond the world of the living. Food was left at crossroads where three roads converged, or a pole was hung with three masks to honor her and request her guidance in choosing the right direction. Three-faced masks hung at the entrance of homes prevented evil spirits from entering the household. Dogs always accompanied her, and the howling of a dog heralded her approach. Meat for her dogs might be left at a crossroads, but dogs were also sacrificed to her. Like Hecate, dogs are guardians of the threshold, doors and portals. The three-headed dog Cerberus guarded the entrance of the underworld, the boundary between life and death, and prevented the living from entering Hades and the dead from leaving. Hecate, as Queen of the Night, was associated with witchcraft. She visited cemeteries during the dark phase of the moon with her entourage of ghosts, social outcasts and slaves, and always carried two torches on her journeys. She was described as luminous, a "moon goddess," invisible or glimpsed as a flickering light. As goddess of in-between realms, she mediated between Olympians and Titans and between mortals and divinities. She aided whomever she chose without regard to status, protecting women who made a trip alone at night or individuals who passed through dangerous liminal spaces. If she received a soldier's or sportsman's prayers favorably, she gave victory and prizes. With Poseidon, she gave sailors a good catch, but could take it away. With Hermes, she could increase or decrease a shepherd's herds of sheep and goats.

Hecate's great-grandmother Gaia, Earth Titaness, was Mother of All Life who arose from Chaos, birthed her husband Uranus the Sky God, and with him had 12 Titan children: six brothers, Oceanus, Coeus, Crius, Hyperion, Iapetus and Cronus, and six sisters, Thea, Rhea, Themis, Mnemosyne, Phoebe and Tethys. Rhea and Cronus gave birth to the gods Zeus, Hera, Demeter, Hades, Poseidon and Hestia. Hecate's grandmother Phoebe, oracle and moon goddess, had two daughters, Asteria and Leto. Leto was a devoted mother to Apollo and Artemis, but it is said that Asteria abandoned her only daughter, Hecate. Like Artemis, Hecate remained independent and unmarried, loved dogs and protected women during childbirth. She could ease the pains of a woman's labor and protect or restore the health and growth of a child and anything newly born. Hecate also protected the old and dying and prepared them for a smooth, painless passage into the next life. She might stay with them in the otherworld to help prepare the return to earth in their next life. Thus, she understood the process of death and dying as well as that of birth and new life. She knew medicinal herbs and poisonous plants. Her sacred tree was the centuries-old evergreen yew that regenerates itself when its branches touch ground and sprout new trees. The yew is used to make bows but contains poison. Its boughs were burned on funeral pyres. Hecate is also associated with the cypress tree, symbolic of death and the underworld.

Hecate was worshipped daily as guardian of the Athenian household and its entrances. She could bestow prosperity, bless a family and avert harmful spirits, but could also cause spirits to turn against the family. Each evening, leftovers from supper, the "Deipnon," were placed in the darkness outside the door as an offering to Hecate and her hounds, although the homeless poor whom she blessed might actually eat them. But once in each lunar month on the night of the New Moon, after sunset when no moon is seen, a three-day "Diepnon" began to honor her and the restless dead who traveled with her. A meal of raw eggs, leeks, garlic, onions and fish was placed at a shrine outside each house or at a crossroads. In these liminal spaces, two worlds could meet, "neither here nor there," outside the boundaries of a settlement where spirits could be contacted. Once the meal was offered, people would not look outside, as spirits do not like to be seen and might "long for vengeance."

On the next day, the Noumenia, the first day of the lunar month when the first sliver of moon is visible, amends were made for any wrongdoing of a family member so that Hecate would not withhold favor from them. The family members "transferred" their sins onto a dog who was then sacrificed and its entrails read by the house patron. If the atonement had been accepted, the new month could begin without sin against Hecate or the gods.

The third day of the Diepnon, the Agathos Diamon, was a day of good spirits, purification of the household and reflection on the end of a month and beginning of a new one. Incense was burned and the smoke was moved through the house. All leftovers, ashes, food that had fallen to the floor and waste now belonged to Hecate and were placed at a crossroads and never used again.

Hecate, guardian of liminal spaces, and the sandplay therapist

Hecate's qualities and roles often resonate with the role and presence of the sandplay therapist, guardian of the "free and protected" sandplay setting and the sandtray. In this liminal space, a sandplay image comes into being. The sandplay therapist feels comfortable with those "on the edge of society," those who are different and less fortunate. Hecate takes charge of extraordinary events at a three-way crossroads. What are the three roads that meet in the sandtray and manifest in a client's sandplay? The sandtray is the meeting point of the outer sandplay setting, the therapist's experience of the setting and the patient's experience of his or her inner world. A new world comes into existence in the sandtray at that moment.

Hecate journeys with her entourage, lighting the dark roads of the unconscious with her two torches, opening portals and passages with her key. The therapist's understanding is both a light and a key, perceiving with compassion inner conflicts that others will ignore or deem unimportant, and protecting that which will be born. Hecate's "luminosity" or flickering light is the flicker of insight as it metamorphoses into a positive form or a definable object. Like Hecate, the sandplay therapist's acceptance of the underworld of the unconscious stabilizes the sandplay patient's acceptance of the reality of the psyche. Like Hecate, the therapist pays attention silently to the image from afar, perceives its details and finds interest in what is not obvious, and indirectly reveals what she sees through silent co-transference and joint observation from "above" the completed sandplay. Like Hecate, the therapist may see many directions simultaneously, with a silent presence that supports the client in choosing the right direction in an undisturbed open space that can slowly be filled with meaning. Yet, if Hecate is not honored, she can dispense justice equally. Here, it is not the therapist who needs to be honored, but the psyche and the Self, who can cause illness and dis-ease when demands for honoring the body, soul and spirit are ignored.

Honoring Hecate in a sandplay workshop

At a sandplay conference in Israel, the author led a workshop for about 20 people, honoring the presence of Hecate in sandplay therapy as a force that can embrace change and new beginnings, lead us to see things and ourselves differently, and find greater understanding of ourselves and others. Like Hecate's three-part "Diepnon," there are three stages to the workshop.

The setting and procedure

A black cloth covers a table in the center of the room. One sandtray is placed on it, surrounded with branches of fresh purifying herbs—rosemary, sage, basil and Syrian hyssop. Three other tables covered with ordinary tablecloths are placed at a distance, spaced like a triangle around the center. Miniatures representing Hecate's powers and deeds in her many realms of knowledge are placed on them. The door entrance, windows, the sandtray, tables and objects and the people who enter the room are all purified by brushing them with branches of rosemary.

Various objects are placed on the three tables to represent boundaries, good fortune, the number three, certain animals, fire and light, night and darkness, magic, birth and death, herbal plants, prophecy, the poor, offerings and music, fruits, flowers, trees and spices. A wide range of objects might include walls, portals, keys, doorways, gates, houses, coins, Cerberus, a three-headed snake, a three-headed lion, a three-faced mask, three monkeys, dogs, horses, owls, shepherds, sheep, sailboats, fisherman, athletes, bonfire, lightning clouds, volcanoes, suns, moons in different phases, candles, matches, a cave, demons, witches, a magician, wands, crystals, ghosts, beggars, gravestones, a world tree, an old wise woman, a crystal ball, a women giving birth, babies, young children, young women, mothers, beggars, ghosts, skeletons, wine, musical instruments, spices, flowers, sage, garlic, evergreen branches and rosemary.

The three-day "Diepnon" first honored Hecate with an offering to her, then a sacrifice asking for pardon of misdeeds, ending with a cleansing purification and new beginnings. The workshop follows this structure, but begins with a short lecture with slides to introduce Hecate and her realms of influence. Then people are invited to look at the miniatures in the three locations, noticing but not taking, and return to their seats.

Stage One: Participants choose one miniature or a herb, as an offering to Hecate, or to helpful spirits, and place it in the sandtray. *Stage Two:* Participants choose one object as an atonement for bad deeds, to purify the household, and place this object in the sandtray. Each person can move his or her own objects if needed but not touch anyone else's. *Stage Three:* Participants again choose one object that represents good spirits coming in for the new month and place it in the sandtray. We look at the sandtray; we can move only our own objects as needed. There is no photography. We return to our seats. With eyes closed, each person focuses on the breath and meditates on the three objects that were chosen and placed, and what significance they might have. After a time of breathing and meditation, a hot, dark, thick energy in the room is palpable.

We open our eyes and sit quietly. When ready, each participant can approach the sandtray, acknowledge his or her three objects, and take them back, thank them silently and return them to the table from which they came, releasing them from the role they were given. The sand in the empty tray is marked with tracks of whatever was there, and emits a powerful energy. This tray and its marks are our final group work. The windows are opened to let the excess energy out. We sit silently, without talking, and end with everyone just saying their name, in a round. I thank everyone for being here. We pack up the miniatures in their boxes, cover the tray and leave.

The Greek goddess Hecate reminds us of the importance of accepting change and transitions, helping us to release the past, especially those things that are hindering our growth. She is there for support and to give light, when we must let go of what is familiar, safe and secure, and travel to the scary places of the soul. New beginnings, whether spiritual or mundane, aren't always easy. But Hecate loans us her farsightedness to see what lies forgotten or hidden, and helps to make a choice and find the path. She may shine her torch to guide you while you are in dream or meditation. Her name may mean "The Distant One," but Hecate is always close at hand in times of need, helping us to release the old, familiar ways and find our way through new beginnings.

12

Conclusion: Listening to the Unconscious

In a field in a country far from my home, Jumping Mouse unexpectedly dropped into my consciousness, together with the realization that I would write a new book. Sudden communications from the unconscious are always a surprise, especially when they occur in liminal time and space. They insist that I acknowledge their messages, as if the boundaries of my present realities are in need of a new creative horizon. Jumping Mouse's "wandering" towards individuation suggested that I could relate the sandplay journey to a larger scope of inner and outer journeys that people make in reality, during wandering, quests and pilgrimages, to power spots where they experience transitions to states of intense focus, awareness and clarity. I had noticed that the sandplay therapists that I supervise kept detailed records of their clients' histories and the progression of objects chosen as symbols, with diagrams of their placement. But less noticed was sandplay's abstract language of structure, color, the color blue as the sandtray's interior, number, use of sand and water, and the possible meanings of space, location and transitions within the sandtray and in the process. I asked that my supervisees arrange all the sandplays of a client in short rows of three, from left to right, so we could view them in a complete sequence. Then we could more clearly identify stages and turning points by observing repetition of forms, objects, their relationships, changes and transitions until final resolution. The internal dynamic of a complete sandplay process becomes visible when we take time to re-observe the interactions, repetitions and transitions over several sandplays arranged in a chronological sequence.

Time is a container for our inner thoughts as they move towards conscious awareness. Time that is not measured is essential in a creative process. As a child, I had time to observe plants and living creatures in a wild field a small distance outside the door of my house. Indoors, my unconscious was imprinted with repetitions of movement, contours and colors, tone of voice, silence, grace or abruptness of the people around me, etched in memory and later externalized in drawings, paper images. Time and timing and patience are essential factors in working with clients who create images in art therapy and in sandplay, sometimes extending beyond the therapeutic hour. Events, or bits and pieces of events, buried in the archives of the unconscious take their time to become part of visual expression, coalescing into successive images over time. The painting critique of art school, "When in doubt, leave it out," shifts to "When in doubt, try it out; let things evolve in their own time." Time and impermanence join together as images transition and change, in a sandplay and in life. In a sandplay process, the psyche presents its themes ambiguously at first. Symbols may disappear and are repeated in rhythms; structures change and repeat themselves with small changes. When the ego is stronger, resilience, intention and precision become possible. The non-essential is discarded, choices become emotionally accurate, clarity of intent can coincide with a visit from the numinous. Authentic expression in a sandplay image "feels right." Its own primal truth may remain undeciphered rationally for years, until it is time. Trust in the unconscious brings forth images that dialogue between suffering and unconscious archetypal sources of healing from beyond ordinary life experience. The aesthetic beauty of a new imaginative reality helps to rise above pain and strengthens control over actual life reality.

The golden thread: death and rebirth of a six-year-old boy in sandplay

Prenatal traumas, pre-verbal or conscious traumas are encased deep in memory and stored in certain areas of the body as if they were ongoing. In the "free and protected space," their release into the sandtray can be forceful, while their origins remain initially unrecognized. Royi, a six-year-old hyperactive boy cursed constantly, was violently jealous of his two younger siblings and failed to understand why his mother needed more children. He also lived in fear of death, of being stabbed in the brain. In a recurring dream, he ate a poisoned apple and a hand reached up from a grave to pull him in. In the first nine months of art and sandplay therapy, we worked on his external adjustment to school and friends and how to spend his allowance. He wrote his many curses on slips of paper and put them in a transparent plastic box. His first sandplay after nine months in therapy represented his recurrent fear of death. He dictated a story of a world of giant monsters, skeletons and dinosaurs who procreated, died and returned to life.

> Once there were a few skeletons who gave birth to two frightening creatures. Why did they do this? Because the skeleton, the bat and dinosaur copulated and a colored snake was born and a giant worm. And then they gave birth to dinosaurs, bats and crocodiles. And then there was an earthquake and some of the animals died and some didn't. And then the dinosaurs died and only skeletons remained. And then the dinosaur skeletons arose and lived. And they gave birth to mice and they gave birth to blood-ants, and then to the two biggest dinosaurs. The snake and the worm ate the ants and vomited up their skeletons. And the skeletons grew and grew and became half skeletons, half dinosaurs, half bats and half mice. And then all of them together gave birth to people. And then some of the dinosaurs remained and there was an earthquake. And they died, and humans remained, and they gave birth to new children. And that's how the story ended.

Royi listened quietly and intently as I read his stories back to him, together with other stories such as the Greek myth of Theseus. In one session, he painted his hands with gold paint and asked me to photograph them. As he left the studio, on an impulse I drew an imaginary golden thread in the air, like Theseus's flaxen thread that he unrolled as he walked the labyrinth, killing the Minotaur at its center and exiting safely. I tied one end of the invisible thread to the doorknob of the studio and the other to Royi's hand. The imaginary string would remain tied to the studio door and to his hand as he walked with his mother to their car and drove home. He would return the following week, following the string. His next sandplay introduced themes of strength-giving magical stones, entrapment in a womb-like water world, giving birth and leaving the water world, which may have symbolized his own birth, about which I had not been given information. In his story, the hero was accompanied by another person, perhaps transference to me, a feeling that in his quest for reaching the source of his fears he was not alone.

> Two people went to search for two precious stones that would give them strength and they got trapped in a world of water. A shark swallowed them and one of the people had a bow and arrow. He shot the shark and they got out. The shark became alive again and gave birth to the stones, he vomited them up. Then two fish connected the two stones and that

> gave them strength. And then the two fish gave birth to all kinds of creatures and crabs. And then they connected two other stones and the people got strength. And when they did this, there were many stones. And then they went out of the water world, and all kinds of people were created and whales and everything. And so ends the story.

In a following session, Royi sculpted a "Giant Monster" in clay, and described "her" or "him."

> She lives in the mountains and she is very big, and she is frightening and she is hairy and she is bad. And she leaves tracks and she likes to do bad things. And she wants to cross in the middle of the road on purpose. She passes many lands and she feels good. And she has long fingernails, a red nose, and she wants to do bad things to dwarfs. He is also fat and sometimes he is not dangerous. And he has no tail. And he has no friends. And he has no family.

In a second session with clay, he sculpted his dream of dying and made a sign to mark his grave.

At a meeting with his parents, his mother described her pregnancy and Royi's birth. When she was five months pregnant, amniocentesis, a prenatal test to identify genetic disorders or birth defects in the fetus, was performed. A needle inserted into the uterus to remove some amniotic fluid had injured the head of the fetus. The birth process was difficult. Royi had stopped breathing and was resuscitated. These traumas might explain the incomprehensible fear that had negotiated its way into symbolic form in his dreams, sandplays and claywork. His psyche guided him to create images that we both could see, that expressed visually the attack on him within the womb and his death and resurrection, which had actually occurred. These facts remained untold to him, but as a healing process, together with his parents, we re-enacted a joyous and successful "rebirth" for Royi in the studio. He hid under his mother's skirt, lying close to her stomach, and with father assisting, Royi was "born." He emerged into the space between his mother's legs, healthy and peaceful, received into life with great love.

Royi's story for his fifth sandplay, "The Indian Hero in the Land of Death,"[1] merges his medical history and a mythological hero's arduous

1 The term "Indian hero" has been retained to reflect the language used by the child at the time. For more information about appropriate terms of reference and address for Native peoples, visit: https://americanindian.si.edu/nk360/faq/did-you-know.

ordeal in the underworld, his helpers in the battle to beat death, time as healer (an hourglass) and finally the return home.

> All the dead came, and one Indian hero came too, and on a sign was written: "The Land of Death, whoever enters, it is forbidden to enter, will die there as he passes, he will release the dead but he will die. The dead can return to life only until midnight." The hero went in and kept meeting skeletons and he was terribly afraid. He saw a mummy and ran behind it and broke the hourglass. And then everyone began to wake and they almost ate him. Dinosaur Rex came and swallowed him and good dinosaurs hit Rex on his tail and saved the hero. The hero had magic and he turned the good dinosaur so that he would never die. And then the mummy wanted to catch him and the hourglass killed the mummy, and then the mummy's brother came and the hourglass broke him and he couldn't do anything. And then their father, the biggest skeleton in the world, came and wanted to kill the hero. And then all the dinosaurs fought, and the good ones won, and everyone died except the good dinosaur and the hero. And the two of them went home, and the hero made a place in his garden for the dinosaur to lay his eggs, and he had many children and all of them could never die, and they lived in happiness and prosperity until today.

Two months later, Royi and his parents did a sandplay together with a rainbow in the center. In his last sandplay, he constructed an island with a peak on the left side, with a few scattered bones on it, surrounded by a moat. Two bridges connected it to the right side, where two large human skeletons and two dinosaur skeletons and a skull were scattered around the space. This final "Isle of the Dead" was no longer active in his theater of memory.

Some thoughts

- The client's psyche is the most knowledgeable guide to the creation of each current image, with the foresight to work at a pace suited to each client towards expression of trauma and gradual negotiation of the passage into healing and the return to mundane life.
- The sandtrays and objects become alive in the client's psyche, activated by being touched, chosen and placed with intent.

- The psyche is joined by other archetypal invisible entities that have also become activated.
- Stones, red diamonds and white or black eggs in a sandplay can represent magical powers of healing, protection and transformation.
- Invitations from the unconscious are received in dreams and embodied in sandplays.
- The sandtray holds the tension between a disordered life and the unpredictable inner journey towards healing and order.
- We are in danger of being written out of our own history when others consider our content as not suited to be told, or less valuable, for any reason.
- The image penetrates the heart, even more so when it is beautiful.
- There are as many different styles to making a sandplay as there are patients.
- Thanks to all the theorists, researchers, therapists, artists, wanderers and others, in the list of references in this book. Their work has been helpful in this journey of exploration through the multitude of levels and connections, identifying some pre-conditions and influences on the creation of sandplay images and their maker's quests towards individuation.

References

Abram, D. (1996) *The Spell of the Sensuous: Perception and Language in a More-than-Human World*. New York, NY: Vintage Books.

Abramovich, L. (2015) "Between sand and blue in the closed psychiatric ward: Sandplay therapy with adolescents in a state of psychosis." *Journal of Sandplay Therapy 24*, 1, 133–149.

Aix-en-Provence, ville de Cezanne (n.d.) Atelier de Cezanne. www.cezanne-en-provence.com/en/the-cezanne-sites/atelier-de-cezanne

Albers, J. (1975) *Interaction of Color*. London: Yale University Press.

Ammann, R. (1991) *Healing and Transformation in Sandplay: Creative Processes Become Visible*. LaSalle, IL: Open Court.

Ammann, R. (1994) "The sandtray as a garden of the soul." *Journal of Sandplay Therapy 4*, 1, 46–65.

Ammann, P. (1972) "Sandplay—Dora Kalff." YouTube. www.youtube.com/watch?v=aWd40dMH70c

Apuleius (1822) *The Metamorphosis: or, Golden Ass of Apuleius*, translated from the original Latin by Thomas Taylor. London: Robert Triphook and Thomas Rudd. https://ia801307.us.archive.org/23/items/TheGoldenAss_201509/TheGoldenAsspenguinClassics-Apuleius.pdf

Bachelard, G. (1994) *The Poetics of Space: The Classic Look at How We Experience Intimate Places*. Boston, MA: Beacon Press.

Bachelard, G. (1999) *Water and Dreams: An Essay on the Imagination of Matter*. Dallas, TX: The Dallas Institute of Humanities and Culture.

Bahn, P. and Lorblanchet, M. (2017) *The First Artists: In Search of the World's Oldest Art*. London: Thames and Hudson.

Berman, A. and Hopper, E. (2005) *Edward Hopper's New York*. Portland, OR: Pomegranate.

Bockemuhl, M. (2000) *Rembrandt*. Cologne, Germany: Taschen.

Bolen, J.S. (1984) *Goddesses in Every Woman: Powerful Archetypes in Women's Lives*. San Francisco, CA: Harper and Row.

Bradway, K. (1991, reprinted 2022) "Transference and countertransference in sandplay therapy." *Journal of Sandplay Therapy 31*, 2, 95–101.

Bradway, K., Signell, K.A., Spare, G.H., Stewart, C.T., Stewart, L.H. and Thompson, C. (eds) (1981) *Sandplay Studies: Origins, Theory and Practice*. San Francisco, CA: C.G. Jung Institute.

Bradway, K. and McCoard, B. (1997) *Sandplay: Silent Workshop of the Psyche*. London: Routledge.

Bulfinch, T. (1979) *Myths of Greece and Rome*. London: Penguin Books.

Butler, H.E. (trans.) (1910) "Amor and Psyche." *The Metamorphosis: or, Golden Ass of Apuleius of Madaura*. Oxford: Clarendon Press.

Cage, J. (1961) *Silence: Lectures and Writings*. Middletown, CT: Wesleyan University Press.

Callaway, E. (2014) "Homo erectus made world's oldest doodle 500,000 years ago." *Nature*. https://doi.org/10.1038/nature.2014.16477

Campbell, J. (1949/1973) *The Hero with a Thousand Faces.* Princeton, NJ: Princeton University Press.

Calvo, P. and Lawrence, N. (2022) *Planta Sapiens: Unmasking Plant Intelligence.* London: Little Brown Book Group.

Carey, H. Jr. (2015) "The Navajo Four Sacred Colors." Navajo People. https://navajopeople.org/blog/the-navajo-four-sacred-colors

Cirlot, J.E. (1971/1996) *A Dictionary of Symbols.* London: Routledge.

Cooper, J.C. (1978) *An Illustrated Encyclopaedia of Traditional Symbols.* London: Thames and Hudson.

Connelly, D. (1994) *Traditional Acupuncture: The Law of the Five Elements.* Columbia, MD: Traditional Acupuncture Institute.

Cowart, J. and Schneider, P. (1992) *Matisse in Morocco: The Paintings and Drawings, 1912–13.* New York, NY: Harry N. Abrams.

Davis, M. (1992) *Play and Symbolism in Lowenfeld and Winnicott.* London: The Dr Margaret Lowenfeld Trust.

Davis, M. and Wallbridge, D. (1989) *Boundary and Space: An Introduction to the Work of D.W. Winnicott.* London: Karnac Books.

Deloria, V. Jr. (2006) *The World We Used to Live In: Remembering the Powers of the Medicine Men.* Golden, CO: Fulcrum Publishing.

Devereux, P. (1990) *Places of Power: Secret Energies at Ancient Sites: A Guide to Observed or Measured Phenomena.* Blandford Press.

Eastwood, P.S. (2002) *Nine Windows to Wholeness: Exploring Numbers in Sandplay Therapy.* Honolulu, HI: Sanity Press.

Edinger, E.F. (1972) *Ego and Archetype: Individuation and the Religious Function of the Psyche.* Boston, MA, and London: Shambhala Publications.

Edinger, E.F. (1994) *The Eternal Drama: The Inner Meaning of Greek Mythology.* Boston, MA: Shambhala Publications.

Ehlers, L. (2022) *Alchemy and Individuation: The Colors of Transformation.* Oberlin, OH: Analytical Psychology Press.

Eliot, T.S. (1943) *Four Quartets.* New York, NY: Harcourt, Brace and Company.

Freedle, L.R. (2019) "Making connections: Sandplay therapy and the neurosequential model of therapeutics." *Journal of Sandplay Therapy 28*, 1, 91–109.

Freedle, L., McGee, M.B., Blechman, S., Souza Jr., J. and Zandbergern, D.L. (2021) "'The lava ate my school':The use of group sandplay to reduce anxiety and post-traumatic stress in displaced elementary school students." *Journal of Sandplay Therapy 30*, 2, 128–147.

Fry, S. (2019) *Mythos: The Greek Myths Retold.* London: Chronicle Books.

Gallegos, E.S. (1987) *The Personal Totem Pole: Animal Imagery, the Chakras and Psychotherapy.* Velarde, NM: Moon Bear Press.

Goldsworthy, A. (1990) *A Collaboration with Nature.* New York, NY: Harry N. Abrams.

Gormley, A. and Gayford, M. (2020) *Shaping the World: Sculpture from Prehistory to Now.* London: Thames and Hudson.

Graves, R. (1955/1960) *The Greek Myths.* London: Penguin Books.

Gray, M. (2007) "The Power of Place, Pilgrimage and the lure of sacred sites." *Interalia Magazine.* www.interaliamag.org/articles/martin-gray-the-power-of-place-sacred-sites-and-the-presence-of-the-miraculous

Grimm Brothers (1981) *The Complete Brothers Grimm Fairy Tales.* New York, NY: Chatham River Press.

Hamilton, E. (1942) *Mythology: Timeless Tales of Gods and Heroes.* New York, NY: Little, Brown and Company.

Harner, M. (1990) *The Way of the Shaman.* San Francisco, CA: HarperOne.

Hegeman, G. (1992) "The sandplay collection." *Journal of Sandplay Therapy 1*, 2.

Hillman, J. (1990) *The Essential James Hillman: A Blue Fire.* London: Routledge.

Homer (1990) *The Iliad*, translated by R. Fagles. New York, NY: Viking Penguin.

Homer (1946/1991) *The Odyssey*, translated by E.V. Rieu (1946). Revised D.C.H. Rieu (1991). London: Penguin Books.

Ingerman, S. (2008) *Shamanic Journeying.* Boulder, CO: Sounds True.

Jackson, B. (2008) "Mapping the Cycle of Sandplay Process." In R.R. Mitchell and H.S. Friedman (eds) *Supervision in Sandplay*. London: Routledge.

Jackson-Bashinsky, B. (1994) "Off on a tangent." *Journal of Sandplay Therapy 4*, 2, 48–67.

Jones, L.E. (1986) "The development of structure in the world of expression: A cognitive-developmental analysis of children's 'sand worlds.'" Doctoral dissertation, Pacific Graduate School of Psychology, Menlo Park, CA. Dissertation Abstracts International. University Microfilms No. 8303178.

Jung, C.G. (1953) "Individual Dream Symbolism in Relation to Alchemy." *Psychology and Alchemy. Collected Works Volume 12*. London: Routledge & Kegan Paul.

Jung, C.G. (1954/1966) *The Practice of Psychotherapy: Essays on the Psychology of the Transference and Other Subjects. Collected Works Volume 16*. London: Routledge & Kegan Paul.

Jung, C.G. (1960) *Structure and Dynamics of the Psyche. Collected Works Volume 8*. New York, NY: Bollingen Foundation.

Jung, C.G. (1971) *The Collected Works of C.G. Jung: Volume 14: Mysterium Coniunctionis*, translated by R.F.C. Hull, edited by G. Adler and H. Read. Bollingen Series XX. Princeton, NJ: Princeton University Press.

Jung, C.G. (1973, reprinted 1992) *Jung Letters, Volume 1, 1906–1950*, edited by G. Adler and A. Jaffe, translated from the German by R.F.C. Hull. London and New York: Routledge.

Jung, C.G. (1997) *Visions: Notes of the Seminar Given in 1930–1934 by C.G. Jung, Volume 1*, edited by C. Douglas. Bollingen Series XCIX. Princeton, NJ: Princeton University Press.

Jung, C.G. (2002) *The Earth Has a Soul: The Nature Writings of C.G. Jung*, edited by M. Sabini. Berkeley, CA: North Atlantic Books.

Jung, C.G. (2014) *Collected Works of C.G. Jung, Volume 9 (Part 1): Archetypes and the Collective Unconscious*. Princeton, NJ: Princeton University Press.

Junge. M.B. (2010) *The Modern History of Art Therapy in the United States*. Springfield, IL: Charles C Thomas.

Kalff, D.M. (1980) *Sandplay*. Boston, MA: Sigo Press.

Kalff, D.M. (2020) *Sandplay, A Psychotherapeutic Approach to the Psyche*, translated by B.L. Matthews. Oberlin, OH: Analytical Psychology Press.

Kandinsky, W. (1914, republished 1977) *Concerning the Spiritual in Art*. New York, NY: Dover Publications.

Kimmerer, R.W. (2013) *Braiding Sweetgrass: Indigenous Wisdom, Scientific Knowledge and the Teachings of Plants*. Minneapolis, MN: Milkweed Editions.

Lahad, M. (1997) "The Story as a Guide to Metaphoric Processes." In S. Jennings (ed.) *Dramatherapy Theory and Practice, Volume 3*. London: Routledge.

Lang, A. (1898/2017) *The Fisherman and the Genie, an Arabian Nights Tale*, illustrated by H.J. Ford. Warwickshire, UK: Pook Press.

Lowenfeld, M. (1979) *The World Technique*. London and Boston, MA: Institute of Child Psychology/Allen & Unwin.

Lowenfeld, M. (1935/1991) *Play in Childhood*. New York, NY: Cambridge University Press. Originally published by Mac Keith Press.

Lowenfeld, M. (1993) *Understanding Children's Sandplay: Lowenfeld's World Technique*. London: Dr Margaret Lowenfeld Trust.

Mavromataki, M. (1997) *Greek Mythology and Religion*. Athens: Haitalis Editions.

McCarter, S. (trans.) (2022) *Metamorphosis, by Ovid*. London: Penguin Random House.

Mitchell, R. and Friedman, H. (1994) *Sandplay: Past, Present and Future*. London: Routledge.

Mitchell, R. and Friedman, H. (2007) *Supervision of Sandplay Therapy*. London: Routledge.

Montecchi, F. (2004) "Transference, counter-transference, resistance: From relationship to representation." *Journal of Sandplay Therapy 8*, 2, 55–70.

Muniz, V. (2010) *Waste Land*, directed by Lucy Walker. US: Arthouse Films.

Neumann, E. (1971) *Amor and Psyche: The Psychic Development of the Feminine*. Princeton, NJ: Princeton University Press.

Neumann, E. (1973, reprinted 1988) *The Child, Structure and Dynamics of the Nascent Personality*. London: Maresfield Library/H. Karnac.

Neumann, E. (1983) *The Great Mother: An Analysis of the Archetype*. Princeton, NJ: Princeton University Press.

Neumann, E. (1994) *Fear of the Feminine*. Princeton, NJ: Princeton University Press.
Newman, H. (2018) *Earth Grids: The Secret Patterns of Gaia's Sacred Sites*. Glastonbury, UK: Wooden Books.
Oda, T. (1997) "Aggression and containment in sandplay." *Journal of Sandplay Therapy 6*, 2, 51–69.
Oldenburg, C. and Oldenburg, A.G. (1992) *Claes Oldenburg: September 18–October 17, 1992*. New York: Pace Gallery.
The Oxford Dictionary of Current English (1992) New York: Oxford University Press.
Perry, B.D. (2006) "Applying Principles of Neurodevelopment to Clinical Work with Maltreated and Traumatized Children." In N.B. Webb (ed.) *Working with Traumatized Youth in Child Welfare*. New York, NY: Guilford Press.
Richards, M.C. (1989) *Centering in Pottery, Poetry and the Person*. Middletown, CT: Wesleyan University Press.
Ronnberg, A. and Martin, K. (eds) (2010) *The Book of Symbols: Reflections on Archetypal Images*. Cologne, Germany: Taschen.
Ryce-Menuhin, J. (1992) *Jungian Sandplay: The Wonderful Therapy*. London: Routledge.
Sandner, D. (1979/1991) *Navajo Symbols of Healing: A Jungian Exploration of Ritual, Image and Medicine*. Rochester, VT: Healing Arts Press.
Sandplay Therapists of America (n.d.) "About the Journal of Sandplay Therapy (JST)." www.sandplay.org/journal/about-the-journal
Schutz, K. (2012) *Vermeer: The Complete Works*. Cologne, Germany: Taschen.
Schutze, S. (2021) *Caravaggio: The Complete Works*. Cologne, Germany: Taschen.
Scribner, V. (2020) *Merpeople: A Human History*. London: Reaktion Books.
Seuphor, M. (1956) *Piet Mondrian: Life and Work*. New York, NY: H.N. Abrams.
Shahn, B. (1957, reprinted 1972) *The Shape of Content*. Cambridge, MA: Harvard University Press.
Shamdasani, S. (2015) "Jung's practice of the image." *Journal of Sandplay Therapy 24*, 1, 6–21.
Sheldrake, M. (2020) *Entangled Life: How Fungi Make Our Worlds, Change Our Minds and Shape Our Futures*. New York, NY: Random House.
Sidesinger, T. (2016) "Reflections on mediating the analytic process as imaged in the mermaid." *ARAS Connections* special issue. https://aras.org/sites/default/files/docs/00093Sidesinger.pdf
Smithson, R. (1972) "The spiral jetty." Holt/Smithson Foundation. https://holtsmithsonfoundation.org/spiral-jetty-1
Spretnak, C. (1992) *Lost Goddesses of Early Greece: A Collection of Pre-Hellenic Myths*. Boston, MA: Beacon Press.
Steel, F.A. (1922) "The Story of the Three Bears." *English Fairy Tales*. Global Grey. www.globalgreyebooks.com/english-fairy-tales-flora-annie-steel-ebook.html
Steinhardt, L. (1997) "Beyond blue: The implications of blue as the color of the inner surface of the sandtray in sandplay." *The Arts in Psychotherapy 24*, 5, 455–469.
Steinhardt, L. (2000) *Foundation and Form in Jungian Sandplay*. London: Jessica Kingsley Publishers.
Steinhardt, L. (2007) "The Art Therapist as Sandplay Supervisor." In R.R. Mitchell and H. S. Friedman (eds) *Supervision in Sandplay*. London: Routledge.
Steinhardt, L. (2009) "Following the fisherman image in sandplay therapy." *Journal of Sandplay Therapy 18*, 1, 7–16.
Steinhardt, L. (2013) *On Becoming a Jungian Sandplay Therapist: The Healing Spirit of Sandplay in Nature and in Therapy*. London: Jessica Kingsley Publishers.
Steinhardt, L. (2016) "Casting an invisible net into an invisible unconscious ocean, catching a reflection of the psyche on an invisible map." *Journal of Sandplay Therapy 5*, 2, 179–189.
Steinhardt, L. (2018) "A Symbolic Pilgrimage to the Sea." In D.N. Sherwood and B.C. Jackson (eds) *Into the Heart of Sandplay*. Oberlin, OH: Analytical Psychology Press.
Steinhardt, L. (2020) "Jasmin, thirteen sandplays: From divination to archetype." *Journal of Sandplay Therapy 29*, 1, 71–90.
Steinhardt, L. (2023) "The color blue: Its physiological and psychological impact as the inner surface of the sand tray in Jungian sandplay." *Journal of Sandplay Therapy 32*, 2, 37–57.

Talamini, M. (2010) "The body unveils what the mind holds: The case of Diana." *Journal of Sandplay Therapy 19*, 2, 41–59.

Taylor, T. (trans.) (1822) *The Metamorphosis, or Golden Ass, and Philosophical Works of Apuleius*. London: Robert Triphook.

The Arabian Nights (1910/2017), illustrated by C. Emerson and L. D'emo. Warwickshire, UK: Pook Press.

The Canadian Encyclopedia (2017) "Totem Pole." www.thecanadianencyclopedia.ca/en/article/totem-pole

Turrell, J. (2023). *James Turrell: A Retrospective*. Los Angeles, CA: Los Angeles County Museum of Art.

Violatti, C. (2021) "The Meaning of European Upper Paleolithic Rock Art." World History Encyclopedia. www.ancient.eu/article/787/the-meaning-of-european-upper-paleolithic-rock-art

Von Franz, M.L. (1997) *Archetypal Patterns in Fairy Tales*. Toronto: Inner City Books.

Wagoner, D. (1972) "Lost." In *Riverbed*. Bloomington, IN: Indiana University Press.

Warhol, A. and Figura, S. (2022) *Andy Warhol: Campbells Soup Cans: MoMA One on One Series*. New York, NY: The Museum of Modern Art.

Weber, B. (2013) "Neil Welliver." In *See It Loud: Seven Post-War American Painters*. Exhibition catalog. New York, NY: The National Academy Museum.

Webster's Collegiate Thesaurus (1976) Springfield, MA: Merriam-Webster.

Weinrib, E. (1983) *Images of the Self*. Boston, MA: Sigo Press.

Weinrib, E. (1996) "The shadow and the cross." *Journal of Sandplay Therapy 5*, 2, 23–29.

Welliver, N. (1999) *New Paintings*. New York, NY: Tibor de Nagy Gallery.

Wells, H.G. (1911/2016) *Floor Games and Little Wars*. Springfield, IL: Monroe Street Press.

Wheelwright, J. and Schmidt, L. (1991) *The Long Shore: A Psychological Experience of the Wilderness*. California: Sierra Club Books.

Willis, R. (2013) "The magic of sand." *1843 Magazine*. www.1843magazine.com/content/features/anonymous/sand

Winnicott, D.W. (1971) *Playing and Reality*. London: Tavistock Publications.

Winter, R. (1999) "Sandplay and ego development." *Journal of Sandplay Therapy 8*, 1, 91–103.

Winter, R. (2002) "September 11th, the day and the experience." *Journal of Sandplay Therapy 11*, 1, 17–22.

Winton, A.G. (2016) "The Bauhaus, 1919–1933." The Met, Heilbrunn Timeline of Art History. www.metmuseum.org/toah/hd/bauh/hd_bauh.htm

Subject Index

Author Index